ALLE ZEIT WACH 1842

P. Schmiedek K. Einhäupl C.M. Kirsch (Eds.)

Stimulated Cerebral Blood Flow

Experimental Findings and Clinical Significance

With 97 Figures and 48 Tables

Springer-Verlag
Berlin Heidelberg New York London Paris Tokyo
Hong Kong Barcelona Budapest

Prof. Dr. Peter Schmiedek
Neurochirurgische Klinik
Klinikum Großhadern
Marchioninistraße 15
8000 München 70

Prof. Dr. Karl Einhäupl
Neurologische Klinik
Klinikum Großhadern
Marchioninistraße 15
8000 München 70

Priv.-Doz. Dr. Carl-Martin Kirsch
Radiologische Klinik
Klinikum Großhadern
Marchioninistraße 15
8000 Münchn 70

ISBN-13:978-3-642-77104-0
eISBN-13:978-3-642-77102-6
DOI:10.1007/978-3-642-77102-6

Softcover reprint of the hardcover 1st edition 1992

Product Liability: The publisher can give no guarantee for information about drug dosage and application thereof in this book. In every individual case the respective user must check its accuracy by consulting other pharmaceutical literature.
The use of registered names, trademarks, etc. in this publication does not imply, even in the absence of a specific statement, that such names are exempt from the relevant protective laws and regulations and therefore free for general use.

The logo on the cover was designed for the meeting and represents the lateral aspect of the brain at rest (bottom) and during stimulation (top).

Typesetting: Fotosatz Reiter, Berchtesgaden
2125/3335-543210 – Printed on acid-free paper

List of Authors and Participants

Altehoefer, C., Department of Nuclear Medicine, Technical University of Aachen, Aachen, Germany
Back, T., Max-Planck-Institute of Neurogical Research, University of Cologne, Cologne, Germany
Baethmann, A., Institute for Surgical Research Ludwig-Maximilians-University, Munich, Germany
Bares, R., Department of Nuclear Medicine, Technical University of Aachen, Aachen, Germany
Batjer, H., Department of Neurological Surgery, University of Texas, Dallas, U.S.A
Bauer, C., Institute for Surgical Research, Ludwig-Maximilians-University, Munich, Germany
Boerschel, M., Department of Neurology, Ludwig-Maximilians-University, Munich, Germany
Bishop, CCR., Department of Surgery, St. Thomas Hospital, London, UK
Bouvard, G., Department of Nuclear Medicine, CHU Côte de Nacre, Caen, France
Brandt, TH., Department of Neurology, Ludwig-Maximilians-University, Munich, Germany
Buell, U., Department of Nuclear Medicine, Technical University of Aachen, Aachen, Germany
Carter, Ph., Department of Neurosurgery, University of Arizona, Tucson, U.S.A.
Celsis, P., Department of Neurology, CHU Purpan, Toulouse, France
Chambers, I., Department of Neurosurgery, Newcastle General Hospital, Newcastle Upon Tyne, UK
Chollet, F., Department Neurology, CHU Purpan, Toulouse, France
Coull, F., Wessex Neurological Center, Southampton General Hospital, Southampton, UK
Dahl, A., Department of Neurology, The National Hospital, University of Oslo, Oslo, Norway
Derlon, JM., Department of Neurosurgery, CHU Côte de Nacre, Caen, France
Dickman, CA., Department of Nuclear Medicine, University of Arizona, Tucson, U.S.A.
Diener, HC., Neurologische Universitätsklinik, Essen, Germany
Dietz, H., Department of Neurosurgery, Hannover Medical School, Hannover, Germany
Dirnagl, U., Department of Neurology, Ludwig-Maximilians-University, Munich, Germany

Droste, DW., Department of Neurosurgery, Technical University of Aachen, Aachen, Germany
Einhäupl, K., Department of Neurology, Ludwig-Maximilians-University, Munich, Germany
Fink, GR., Max-Planck-Institute of Neurological Research, University of Cologne, Cologne, Germany
Fitch, W., Wellcome Surgical Institute, University of Glasgow, Scotland
Friberg, L., Department of Clinical Physiology and Nuclear Medicine, Glostrup Hospital, Glostrup, Denmark
Fürst, H., Department of Surgery, Ludwig-Maximilians-University, Munich, Germany
Gaab, MR., Department of Neurosurgery, Hannover Medical School, Hannover, Germany
Graham, RD., Wellcome Surgical Institute, University of Glasgow, Scotland
Grond, M., Max-Planck-Institute of Neurological Research, University of Cologne, Cologne, Germany
Gratzl, O., Department of Neurosurgery, University of Basel, Basel, Switzerland
Haase, J., Department of Neurosurgery, Årlborg, Denmark
Haberl, R., Department of Neurology, Ludwig-Maximilians-University, Munich, Germany
Hacke, W., Department of Neurology, University of Heidelberg, Heidelberg, Germany
Harders, AG., Department of Neurosurgery, Technical University of Aachen, Aachen, Germany
Harms, A., Department of Neurology, Humboldt-University, Berlin, Germany
Haubitz, B., Department of Neuroradiology, Hannover Medical School, Hannover, Germany
Heissler, HE., Department of Neurosurgery, Hannover Medical School, Hannover, Germany
Heiss, WD., Max-Planck-Institute of Neurological Research, University of Cologne, Cologne, Germany
Holl, K., Department of Neurosurgery, Hannover Medical School, Hannover, Germany
Houtteville, JP., Department of Neurosurgery, CHU Côte de Nacre, Caen, France
Iadecola, C., Department of Neurology, University of Minnesota, Minneapolis, U.S.A.
Isensee, K., Department of Nuclear Medicine, Technical University of Aachen, Aachen, Germany
Kane, PJ., Department of Neurosurgery, Newcastle General Hospital, Newcastle Upon Tyne, UK
Kaiser, HJ., Department of Nuclear Medicine, Technical University of Aachen, Aachen, Germany
Kempski, O., Institute for Neurosurgical Pathophysiology, University of Mainz, Mainz, Germany
Kim, P., Department of Neurosurgery, University of Tokyo, Tokyo, Japan
Kirsch, CM., Department of Radiology/Nuclear Medicine, Ludwig-Maximilians-University, Munich, Germany
Kleiser, B., Department of Neurology, University of Ulm, Ulm, Germany

Kuschinsky, W., Department of Physiology, University of Heidelberg, Heidelberg, Germany
Kummer, v. R., Department of Neurology, University of Heidelberg, Heidelberg, Germany
Labhorde, G., Department of Neurosurgery, Technical University of Aachen, Aachen, Germany
Lechevalier, B., Department of Nuclear Medicine, CHU Côte de Nacre, Caen, France
Leinsinger, G., Department of Radiology/Nuclear Medicine, Ludwig-Maximilians-University, Munich, Germany
Lienau, N., Lederle Company, Wolfratshausen, Germany
Lissner, J., Department of Radiology, Ludwig-Maximilians-University, Munich, Germany
Lovick, AHJ., Department of Neurosurgery, Southampton General Hospital, Southampton, UK
Marguth, F., Department of Neurosurgery, Ludwig-Maximilians-University, Munich, Germany
Mendelow, AD., Department of Neurosurgery, Newcastle General Hospital, Newcastle Upon Tyne, UK
Morin, P., Department of Neurology, CHU Côte de Nacre, Caen, France
Müller, HR., Department of Neurology, University of Basel, Basel, Switzerland
Müller-Brand, J., Department of Nuclear Medicine, University of Basel, Basel, Switzerland
Nelson, RJ., Department of Neurosurgery, Frenchay Hospital, Bristol, UK
Nemati, MN., Department of Neurosurgery, Hannover Medical School, Hannover, Germany
Nyberg-Hansen, R., Department of Neurology, The National Hospital, University of Oslo, Oslo, Norway
Paulson, OB., Department of Neurology, Rigshospitalet, Copenhagen, Denmark
Pawlik, G., Max-Planck-Institute of Neurological Research, University of Cologne, Cologne, Germany
Petit, ML., PET Laboratory, Caen, France
Pickard, JD., University of Cambridge Neurosurgery Unit, Cambridge, UK
Piepgras, A., Department of Neurosurgery, Ludwig-Maximilians-University, Munich, Germany
Pietrzyk, U., Max-Planck-Institute of Neurological Research, University of Cologne, Cologne, Germany
Radü, EW., Department of Neuroradiology, University of Basel, Basel, Switzerland
Read, DH., Department of Neurosurgery, Frenchay Hospital, Bristol, UK
Reiche, W., Department of Nuclear Medicine, Technical University of Aachen, Aachen, Germany
Rem, JA., Department of Neurosurgery, University of Basel, Basel, Switzerland
Ringelstein, EB., Department of Neurology, Technical University of Aachen, Aachen, Germany
Rootwelt, K., Institute of Chemical Biochemistry, The National Hospital, University of Oslo, Oslo, Norway

Russel, D., Department of Neurology, The National Hospital, University of Oslo, Oslo, Norway

Rzesacz, EH., Department of Neurosurgery, Hannover Medical School, Hannover, Germany

Schmidt, J., Department of Neurology, Rigshospotalet, Copenhagen, Denmark

Schmiedek, P., Department of Neurosurgery, Ludwig-Maximilians-University, Munich, Germany

Schürer, L., Department of Neurosurgery, Ludwig-Maximilians-University, Munich, Germany

Stanley, JC., Wessex Neurological Center, Southampton General Hospital, Southampton, UK

Strachan, RD., Department of Neurosurgery, Newcastle General Hospital, Newcastle Upon Tyne, UK

Stummer, W., Institute for Surgical Research, Ludwig-Maximilians-University, Munich, Germany

Tuor, U., Wellcome Surgical Institute, University of Glasgow, Scotland

Unterberg, AW., Department of Neurosurgery, Free University of Berlin, Berlin, Germany

Viader, F., Department of Neurology, CHU Côte de Nacre, Caen, France

Vilringer, A., Department of Neurology, Ludwig-Maximilians-University, Munich, Germany

Vorstrup, S., Department of Neurology, Righospitalet, Copenhagen, Denmark

Wahl, M., Physiological Institute, Ludwig-Maximilians-University, Munich, Germany

Waldemar, G., Department of Neurology, Righospitalet, Copenhagen, Denmark

Weissenborn, K., Department of Neurology, Hannover Medical School, Hannover, Germany

Widder, B., Department of Neurology, University of Ulm, Ulm, Germany

Yonas, H., Department of Neurosurgery, University of Pittsburgh, Pittsburgh, U.S.A.

Mailing List of Authors

Batjer, H., Department of Neurological Surgery, University of Texas Southwestern Medical Center, 5323 Harry Hines Boulevard, Dallars, Texas 75235-8855, U.S.A.

Bishop, C.C.R., Department of Surgery, United Medical Schools, St. Thomas Hospital, London, UK

Buell, U., Department of Nuclear Medicine, Technical University of Aachen, Pauwelsstraße 30, 5100 Aachen, Germany

Carter, Ph., Department of Surgery, Section of Neurosurgery, University of Arizona Medical Center, 1501 North Campbell, Tucson, Arizona 85724, U.S.A.

Derlon, JM., Department of Neurosurgery, CHU Côte de Nacre, 14033 Caen, France

Friberg, L., Department of Clinical Physiology and Nuclear Medicine, Glostrup Hospital, 2600 Glostrup, Denmark

Haberl, R., Department of Neurology, Klinikum Großhadern, Ludwig-Maximilians-University, Marchioninistraße 15, 8000 Munich, Germany

Harders, AG., Department of Neurosurgery, Technical University of Aachen, Pauwelsstraße 30, 5100 Aachen, Germany

Holl, K., Department of Neurosurgery, Hannover Medical School, Konstanty-Gutschow-Straße 8, 3000 Hannover, Germany

Iadecola, C., Department of Neurology, University of Minnesota, Box 295 UMHC, 420 Delaware Street S.E., Minneapolis, MN, 55455, U.S.A.

Kempski, O., Institute for Neurosurgical Pathophysiology, Johannes Gutenberg-University of Mainz, Langenbeckstraße 1, 6500 Mainz, Germany

Kim, P., Department of Neurosurgery, University of Tokyo, 7-3-1 Hongo, Bunkyo-ku, Tokyo 113, Japan

Kleiser, B., Department of Neurology, University of Ulm, Steinhövelstraße 9, 7900 Ulm, Germany

Kuschinsky, W., Department of Physiology, University of Heidelberg, Im Neuenheimer Feld 326, 6900 Heidelberg, Germany

Kummer, v. R., Department of Neurology, University of Heidelberg, Im Neuenheimer Feld 326, 6900 Heidelberg, Germany

Leinsinger, G., Department of Radiology/Nuclear Medicine, Klinikum Großhadern, Ludwig-Maximilians-University, Marchioninistraße 15, 8000 Munich, Germany

Mendelow, AD., Department of Neurosurgery, Newcastle General Hospital, Westgate Road, Newcastle Upon Tyne NE4 6BE, UK

Nyberg-Hansen, R., Department of Neurology, Rikshospitalet, The National Hospital, University of Oslo, 0027 Oslo 1, Norway

Pawlik, G., Max-Planck-Institute of Neurological Research, University of Cologne, Gleueler Straße 50, 5000 Cologne 41, Germany

Pickard, JD., University of Cambridge Neurosurgery Unit, Level 4, A Block, Addenbrooke's Hospital, Hills Road, Cambridge, CB2 2QQ, UK

Piepgras, A., Department of Neurosurgery, KLinikum Großhadern, Ludwig-Maximilians-University, Marchioninistraße 15, 8000 Munich, Germany

Rem, JA., Department of Neurosurgery, University of Basel, Spitalstraße 21, 4031 Basel, Switzerland

Ringelstein, EB., Department of Neurology, Technical University of Aachen, Pauwelsstraße 30, 5100 Aachen, Germany

Schmiedek, P., Department of Neurosurgery, KLinikum Großhadern, Ludwig-Maximilians-University, Marchioninistraße 15, 8000 Munich, Germany

Unterberg, AW., Department of Neurosurgery, Rudolf Virchow Medical Centre, Free University of Berlin, Augustenburger Platz 1, 1000 Berlin 65, Germany

Vilringer, A., Department of Neurology, Klinikum Großhadern, Ludwig-Maximilians-University, Marchioninistraße 15, 8000 Munich, Germany

Vorstrup, S., Department of Neurology, Righospitalet, 9, Blegdamsvej, 2100 Copenhagen, Denmark

Wahl, M., Department of Physiology, Ludwig-Maximilians-University, Pettenkoferstraße 12, 8000 Munich 2, Germany

Yonas, H., Department of Neurosurgery, University of Pittsburgh, 3459 Fifth Avenue, Pittsburgh, PA 15213, U.S.A.

Contents

Preface XV

Chapter 1: Regulation of Cerebral Blood Flow

Regulation of Cerebral Blood Flow: A Brief Review
A. UNTERBERG and M. WAHL 3

Capillary Perfusion in the Brain
W. KUSCHINSKY 12

Intrinsic and Extrinsic Neural Regulation of the Cerebral Circulation
C. IADECOLA 19

Endothelium-Dependent Relaxations and Concentrations: Their Physiology in the Cerebral Arteries and Pathology in Experimental Cerebral Vasospasm
P. KIM 37

Mechanisms of Cerebral Vasodilatation During Neuronal Activation by Bicuculline: A Review
M. WAHL 50

Postischemic Hyperperfusion and Outcome: An Experimental Study
O. KEMPSKI, W. STUMMER, C. BAUER, L. SCHÜRER, and A. BAETHMANN 55

Chapter 2: Methods for the Measurement of Cerebral Blood Flow

Erythrocyte Flow in Cerebral Capillaries Under Resting and Stimulated Conditions
A. VILLRINGER, U. DIRNAGL, A. PIEPGRAS, P. SCHMIEDEK, and K.M. EINHÄUPL ... 61

Continuous Measurement of Acetazolamide Stimulated Cerebral Blood Flow by Laser Doppler Flowmetry
R.L. HABERL, M. BOERSCHEL, U. DIRNAGL, A. PIEPGRAS, P. SCHMIEDEK, and K.M. EINHÄUPL 66

Transcranial Doppler Ultrasound and Regional Cerebral Blood Flow Assessment of Cerebral Hemodynamics: The Acetazolamide Test
A. DAHL, R. NYBERG-HANSEN, D. RUSSELL, and K. ROOTWELT 71

Continuous Monitoring of Cortical Blood Flow and Intracranial Pressure in Severe Cerebral Trauma
L. CARTER and C.A. DICKMAN 79

Role of Cerebral Blood Flow Imaging in the Evaluation of Subarachnoid Hemorrhage and Intracranial Arteriovenous Malformations
H.H. BATJER 84

Hemodynamic Assessment of Carotid Artery Obstructive Lesions: Comparison of PET and SPECT
J.M. DERLON, G. BOUVARD, M.C. PETIT, F. VIADER, B. LECHEVALIER, P. MORIN, and J.P. HOUTTEVILLE 94

Cerebral Blood Flow to Cerebral Blood Volume Relationship as a Correlate to Cerebral Perfusion Reserve
U. BUELL, W. REICHE, H.J. KAISER, K. ISENSEE, R. BARES, C. ALTEHOEFER, and E.B. RINGELSTEIN 111

Positron Emission Tomography Activation Studies in Neurological Patients
G. PAWLIK, G.R. FINK, U. PIETRZYK, M. GROND, and W.-D. HEISS 121

Chapter 3: Stimulation of Cerebral Blood Flow

Methods for Manipulation of Regional Brain Perfusion, Intracranial Artery Diameter, and Cerebral Blood Volume
L. FRIBERG 141

Carbon Dioxide and Oxygen Reactivity in Cerebral Circulation
R. VON KUMMER and T. BACK 150

Noninvasive Testing of Vasomotor Reserve
E.B. RINGELSTEIN 158

Identification of Hemodynamic Patients for EC-IC Bypass Surgery
S. VORSTRUP, J. SCHMIDT, G. WALDEMAR, J. HAASE, and O.B. PAULSON 171

Effect of Blood Pressure on Cerebral Blood Flow and Infarct Size: Hemodynamic Considerations
A.D. MENDELOW, R.D. STRACHAN, P.J. KANE, I. CHAMBERS, W. FITCH, D.I. GRAHAM, and U. TOUR 175

Effects of Acetazolamide on EEG and Intracranial Pressure
K. HOLL, H.E. HEISSLER, E.H. RZESACZ, K. WEISSENBORN, M.N. NEMATI, M.R. GAAB, B. HAUBITZ, and H. DIETZ 186

Mental Activity and Changes in Cerebral Blood Flow Evaluated by Transcranial Doppler Sonography
A.G. HARDERS, G. LABORDE, and D.W. DROSTE 200

Chapter 4: Clinical Application of Stimulated Cerebral Blood Flow Studies

Natural History of Patients Defined by Assessment of Cerebral Blood Flow Reserves
H. YONAS, S.R. DURHAM, and H.A. SMITH 215

Aspects of Cerebrovascular Autoregulation Following Subarachnoid Haemorrhage
J.D. PICKARD, R.J. NELSON, A.H.J. LOVICK, R.W.B. COULL, J.C. STANLEY, D.H. READ, J. HERBETKO, and M. CAMPBELL 220

Doppler CO_2 Test in Internal Carotid Artery Occlusions: Prospective and Retrospective Results
B. KLEISER and B. WIDDER 226

Changes in CBF After Carotid Endarterectomy: Follow-up in Neurologically Asymptomatic Patients
J.A. Rem, O. Gratzl, H.R. Müller, J. Müller-Brand, and E.W. RADÜ 232

Effect od Stenosis and Endarterectomy on Internal Carotid Artery Blood Flow
C.R. BISHOP 237

Cerebrovascular Reserve Capacity Measured with 133-Xenon Dynamic SPECT Before and After Carotid Endarterectomy
G. LEINSINGER, H. FÜRST, P. SCHMIEDEK, K. EINHÄUPL, and C.M. KIRSCH 250

Extra-Intracranial Bypass Surgery in Patients with Hemodynamic Cerebral Ischemia
P. SCHMIEDEK, A. PIEPGRAS, G. LEINSINGER, K. EINHÄUPL, and C.M. KIRSCH 257

Follow-up Studies of Cerebrovascular Reserve Capacity in Patients with Cerebrovascular Disease
A. PIEPGRAS, P. SCHMIEDEK, G. LEINSINGER, R.L. HABERL, C.M. KIRSCH, and K.M. EINHÄUPL 263

Subject Index 268

Preface

In view of the already abundant literature on cerebral blood flow one might wonder whether publishing yet another volume on this subject is justified. Admittedly, this was of some concern to us as well. We tought, however, that this book containing the proceedings of an international symposium on stimulated cerebral blood flow represents a worthwhile compilation of contributions on a rather special aspect of cerebral blood flow, namely its study under stimulated conditions.

Cerebral blood flow studies under stimulated conditions have already been reported in the literature in some detail. It has been known, for example, that cerebral blood flow through its physiological coupling to neuronal activity can be increased by various mental stimulations. Another approach to measuring stimulated cerebral blood flow is to assess the cerebrovasculature's ability to counteract a sudden drop in perfusion pressure using functional tests autoregulation or cerebrovascular reserve capacity. These tests are of great clinical interest for the whole field of cerebral ischemia and have an important impact on therapeutic concentrations, as is made clear in the final section of this book. Our own experience with the DIAMOX test over the last years in numerous patients with cerebral ischemia, subarachnoid hemorrhage, and cerebral sinus thrombosis provides further evidence that these studies are of definitive clinical relevance.

It was this experience and also the encouragement given by other groups working in this field which finally led to the plan to organize a meeting on stimulated cerebral blood flow, thus providing an oppertunity for an up-to-date and in-depth discussion of the topic. This, however, could only be achieved by limiting the number of participants and by inviting some acknowledged experts with a special interest in this field, including both basic scientists and those clinical interests. For those who could not attend the meeting, this volume will provide useful insights into the various aspects of stimulated blood flow.

The meeting and also the publication of this proceedings volume would not have been possible without the generous financial support of the Lederle Company. We would like to express our special gratitude to Mr. N. Lienau, who has been of invaluable help during the long process of planning and preparing the meeting. We gratefully acknowledge the organisational support provided by Mrs. Brauweiler zur Nieden during the meeting. We are indebted to the members of the Neurovascular Laboratory and to our young colleages who never failed to offer their help. We are also extremely grateful for the efforts of the contributors to this volume. Finally, we would like to thank Mr. V. Oehm and Mrs. U. Hilpert of Springer-Verlag for their constant assistance during the careful preparation of this proceedings volume.

Munich, October 1991

P. Schmiedek *K.M. Einhäupl* *C.M. Kirsch*

Chapter 1
Regulation of Cerebral Blood Flow

Regulation of Cerebral Blood Flow: A Brief Review

A. Unterberg and M. Wahl

Introduction

Under physiological conditions, global cerebral blood flow (CBF) is held very constant in contrast to blood flow of other organs. There are, however, significant changes in blood flow in various brain regions depending on neuronal function and metabolism (Kuschinsky and Wahl 1978; Lassen et al. 1978). These regional variations in flow are caused by changes in vascular resistance, which is mainly regulated by changes in arteriolar diameter (Edvinsson and MacKenzie 1977; Kuschinsky and Wahl 1978; Wahl 1985a).

Various mechanisms regulate CBF under physiological conditions. There are four different principles of regulation of cerebrovascular resistance in the brain:

1. Local chemical, metabolic factors
2. Vascular innervation and transmitters
3. Circulation hormones and autacoids
4. Endothelial factors

Local Chemical, Metabolic Factors Regulating Cerebrovascular Resistance

Regulation of cerebrovascular resistance by local chemical factors is based on the fact that vasoactive substances are released by neurons into the interstitial space depending on their metabolic activity (Kuschinsky and Wahl 1978; Roy and Sherrington 1890; Wahl 1985a). These vasoactive substances then cause changes in vascular contractility. To estimate the significance of local chemical factors one should know which vasomotor effects are caused by these factors, whether there are effective concentrations of these substances in the interstitial space under stimulated conditions, and whether there are interactions between the various factors.

Table 1 lists the most important local chemical factors and their effects. The micropuncture technique of studying the pial vessels during the microapplication of various substances was most helpful in the study of these effects. This technique varies the perivascular milieu of the superficial pial arteries and simultaneously monitors changes in vascular diameter (Wahl et al. 1970). Microapplication of alkaline solutions causes vasoconstriction whereas application of acid CSF induces dilation (Kuschinsky et al. 1972). These effects are also seen in intraparenchymal vessels. The well-known

Table 1. Local chemical factors and regulation of cerebrovascular restistance

Factor	Effect(s)			
pH (CO_2)	pH ↑	Constriction	pH ↓	Dilation
K^+	< 3 mM > 20 mM	Constriction	3–20 mM	Dilation
Ca^{2+}	Ca^{2+} ↑	Constriction	Ca^{2+} ↓	Dilation
Adenosine				Dilation
ATP				Dilation
Osmolarity	↓	Constriction	↑	Dilation

effect of CO_2 on CBF is also caused by local changes in hydrogen ion activity (Kuschinsky and Wahl 1978).

A reduction in the perivascular concentration of potassium below 3 mM causes constriction, whereas in increase up to 20 mM causes dilation of the pial arteries (Kuschinsky et al. 1972). Potassium concentrations above 20 mM constrict cerebral arteries, but are only reached under pathological conditions.

A significant reduction in the calcium concentration, which can be achieved, e.g., by ethylenediaminetetraacetic acid (EDTA), causes arterial dilation, and a significant increase leads to constriction (Wahl et al. 1970). Perivascular application of adenosine causes concentration-dependent dilations. ATP-induced dilations are even more remarkable (Wahl and Kuschinsky 1976). Cerebral arteries also react to changes in perivascular osmolarity. An increase in osmolarity induces dilation while vasoconstriction is observed during hypotonicity in the perivascular space (Wahl et al. 1973).

The various local chemical factors differ considerably in regard to their significance, and their interactions also have to be taken into consideration. The effect of potassium ions dominates the effect of hydrogen ions if the concentrations of both ions are simultaneously changed within a physiological range. Hydrogen ion induced vasodilation is stronger than dilation caused by adenosine. Changes in vascular diameter by calcium ions are quite moderate. This ion seems to modulate the effect of other local chemical factors: a decrease in calcium ion activity augments the dilatory effect of increased hydrogen and potassium ion activity, or the constrictive effect of reduced hydrogen ion activity (Kuschinsky and Wahl 1978).

Cortical or *neuronal activation* is associated with changes in concentrations of various factors in the extracellular space, and these local chemical factors are at least in part responsible for the coupling of flow and metabolism under these conditions. To summarize briefly, moderate neuronal activation is associated with an increase in potassium ions and a decrease in calcium ions, while strong neuronal activation is also associated with acidosis and a release of adenosine. Hyperemia associated with cortical activation is mediated by multiple factors, and potassium ions seem to be the most significant (Kuschinsky and Wahl 1978; Leniger-Follert and Lübbers 1976; Urbanics et al. 1978).

During hypoxia and ischemia there is also an increase in the extracellular potassium and hydrogen ion activity and release of adenosine (Kuschinsky and Wahl 1978).

Cerebrovascular Innervation

During recent years various systems of cerebrovascular innervation have been detected (Table 2), which has been made possible by the development of new immunohistochemical methods. It is hypothesized that regulation of CBF is achieved by vascular nerves and their transmitters, especially if flow and metabolism are not directly coupled (Edvinsson and MacKenzie 1977; Edvinsson and McCulloch 1987; Kuschinsky and Wahl 1978). Meanwhile it is clear that cerebral arteries regulating resistance have a sympathetic innervation (Edvinsson and Owman 1974; Edvinsson et al. 1976, Edvinsson and MacKenzie 1977; Kuschinsky and Wahl 1978; Wahl et al. 1972). The transmitter norepinephrine binding to α-receptors leads to contraction of cerebral arteries. Furthermore, stimulation of the cervical sympathetic ganglion induces constriction of pial arteries. The sympathetic innvervation of cerebral vessels does not seem to play a major role in the regulation of CBF under physiological conditions. It does, however, modulate cerebral autoregulation: a reduction in the sympathetic activity shifts the lower limit of autoregulation to lower perfusion pressures and an increased sympathetic activity is responsible for the constancy of CBF even at higher ranges of perfusion pressure. Thereby, an increase in sympathetic activity prevents the so-called "breakthrough" (Edvinsson and MacKenzie 1977; MacKenzie et al. 1979).

Cerebral vessels are also innervated by parasympathetic cholinergic nerves (Table 2). Perivascular application of acetylcholine dilates arteries, an effect which is mediated by postjunctional muscarine receptors (Kuschinsky et al. 1974). Coupling of flow and metabolism by collateral innervation of neurons and resistance vessels within cortical circuits might be a physiological role of the cholinergic innervation (Edvinsson and MacKenzie 1977; Edvinsson and McCulloch 1987; MacKenzie and Scatton 1987).

Table 2. Cerebrovascular innervation and regulation of CBF

1. Sympathetic innervation	Norepinephrine	Contraction	Modulation of autoregulation Protection of bbb
	Neuropeptide Y	Conctraction	
2. Parasympathetic, cholinergic innervation	Acetylcholine	Relaxation	Coupling of flow and metabolism
3. Serotoninergic innervation	Serotonin	Dilation	Connection: brain stem – cortex
4. Peptidergic innervation	Substance P	(Dilation)	
	CGRP	Dilation	Axon – reflex
	VIP	Dilation	
	Opioid peptides (Dynorphin/ Enkephalin)	No effect	

Besides a sympathetic and parasympathetic innervation there is also a serotonergic innervation of cerebral vessels, which projects from the brain stem. Whereas serotonin contracts isolated cerebral arteries, pial arteries in situ dilate on perivascular application of serotonin (Edvinsson et al. 1977; MacKenzie and Scatton 1987). Serotonin may be released by nerves, mast cells, and thrombocytes. Coupling of the brain stem and the mesencephalon with cortical neurons and blood vessels could be the functional significance of the serotonergic innervation (MacKenzie and Scatton 1987). Peptideric innervation of cerebral vessels has also been detected during the past few years. Trigeminal fibers, for example, release substance P (SP) and calcitonin-gene-related peptide (CGRP), like an axon reflex. Today, there is much speculation about the physiological role of these systems (Edvinsson and McCulloch 1987). Furthermore, opioid peptides, such as dynorphin and enkephalin, have been found to be related to cerebral vessels. These peptides do not appear to have vasoactive properties (Edvinsson and McCulloch 1987).

Regulation of Cerebrovascular Resistance by Hormones and Autacoids

Circulating hormones are of minor importance in regard to the regulation of cerebral microcirculation under physiological conditions, since most of the hormones do not penetrate the blood-brain barrier. Autacoids are, however, of great interest, especially under pathological conditions, where they are released in great amounts within the brain tissue (Baethmann et al. 1988; Wahl et al. 1988).

Various autacoids have an influence on the diameter of cerebral vessels, not only of arteries but also of veins, and, in addition, they affect cerebrovascular permeability (Wahl et al. 1988). Histamine, which is a neurotransmitter released by mast cells and by perivascular nerves, causes a dose-dependent dilation of arteries, which can be blocked by the addition of an H_2 receptor antagonist, such as cimetidine. Thus the dilatory effect of histamine is mediated by H_2 receptors (Wahl and Kuschinsky 1979a). The peptide bradykinin is released in considerable amounts under pathological conditions. Like histamine, bradykinin induces a dose-dependent dilation in arteries; while it has no short-term effect on cerebral veins but induces moderate constriction with longer exposure (Unterberg et al. 1984). Both bradykinin and histamine are substances which strongly affect the cerebrovascular permeability. They are therefore considered to be interesting mediator candidates of brain edema (Wahl et al. 1988). Eicosanoids, e.g. prostanoids and leukotrienes, as well as their precursor arachidonic acid are released after trauma, ischemia, hypoxia, etc. They are formed in the parenchyma as well as in vessels. Reports on the vasomotor effects of arachidonic acid are contradictory (Unterberg et al. 1987). Prostanoids exert various vasomotor effects, e.g., thromboxane constricts and prostacyclin dilates cerebral arteries like arteries of other organs (Pickard 1981). Leukotrienes induce a marked arterial constriction. More interestingly, leukotrienes also constrict veins (Unterberg et al. 1991).

Endothelial Factors and Regulation of Cerebrovascular Resistance

Regulation of resistance and blood flow in peripheral organs by endothelial factors has been intensively studied during the past few years. It is not surprising that endothelial factors are also involved in the regulation of cerebrovascular resistance. Meanwhile it has been demonstrated that cerebral vessels are also affected by endothelial-derived relaxing (EDRF) and constricting (EDCF) factors (Nakagomi et al. 1987; Harder et al. 1989).

Some substances dilating cerebral arteries are EDRF dependent, such as acetylcholine and bradykinin, whereas others are independent of EDRF, such as histamine or vasoactive intestinal polypeptide (VIP). There are also reports about EDCF in cerebral vessels (Harder et al. 1989). An example is endothelin, which is a potent vasoconstrictor peptide produced by endothelial cells (Kobayashi et al. 1990).

In pial vessels endothelin induces a strong arterial and venous constriction even in a nanomolar range (Hardebo et al. 1989; Robinson and McCulloch 1990). It is not yet clear under which conditions endothelin is mainly formed, but there are already reports that the sensitivity to endothelin is increased after subarachnoid hemorrhage (Alafaci et al. 1990).

Autoregulation

The constancy of CBF over a wide range of perfusion pressure is caused by the capability of cerebral arteries and arterioles to "autoregulate," a phenomenon of utmost importance for the brain. Some time ago, it was speculated that local chemical factors were responsible for "autoregulation." This hypothesis, however, could not be supported (Wahl 1985a).

Over a wide range of arterial blood pressure there are no significant changes in perivascular pH or perivascular potassium ion activity (Wahl and Kuschinsky 1979b). Furthermore, there are no changes in adenosine concentration in the autoregulatory range (Wahl 1985a). Therefore, autoregulation is probably achieved by myogenic mechanisms and is independent of local chemical factors. Recently, Harder (1985) studied the relation between membrane potential and transmural pressure of isolated cerebral vessels. Harder found that increasing transmural pressure caused depolarization. Based on this finding, Harder (1985) postulated that a myogenic electrical mechanism is responsible for autoregulation. Further studies revealed that the cerebral endothelium is of great importance in this context (Harder 1987). If the vessels studied in vitro had an intact endothelium, a depolarization was found with increasing transmural pressure. After destruction of the endothelium by perfusion with collagenase, this effect disappeared. Thus, it was concluded that endothelial cells play an important role in cerebral autoregulation. However, contradictory findings have recently been reported (McCarron et al. 1989).

Subarachnoid Hemorrhage and "Vasospasm"

An important dysregulation of CBF is the "cerebral vasospasm," seen especially after subarachnoid hemorrhage. There are hundreds of experimental and clinical studies and findings concerning this complication. Figure 1 puts together time course, neuropathological findings, and some putative mechanisms (Unterberg and Marguth 1988).

Subarachnoid hemorrhage may cause narrowing of the intracranial arteries, or "early vasospasm" within minutes after the bleeding (Brawley et al. 1969). At that time the only neuropathological finding is blood in the subarachnoid space. Putative mechanisms causing this early spasm are humoral factors, e.g., catecholamines, or a reflectory constriction (Svendgaard et al. 1985; Wahl 1985b). This early spasm is reversible. It may be speculated, however, that it is the basis for alterations leading to late, chronic vasospasm. To begin with in late vasospasm, which is the relevant clinical problem, endothelial lesions can be seen electron microscopically and there is opening of the blood-brain barrier (Kassell and Sasaki 1987). Barrier opening is the basis for extravasation of plasma-containing constricting mediators. Again catecholamines are interesting substances in this context (Wahl 1985b). Endothelial lesions are associated with reduced release of dilatory factors such as EDRF. Moreover, there are reports about changes in cerebrovascular sensitivity. In the early phase of chronic vasospasm cerebral arteries are hypersensitive to vasoconstrictor agents and less sensitive to dilating stimuli. Finally, smooth muscle cells are permenently contracted. Furthermore, endothelial lesions might explain why inflammatory and degenerative

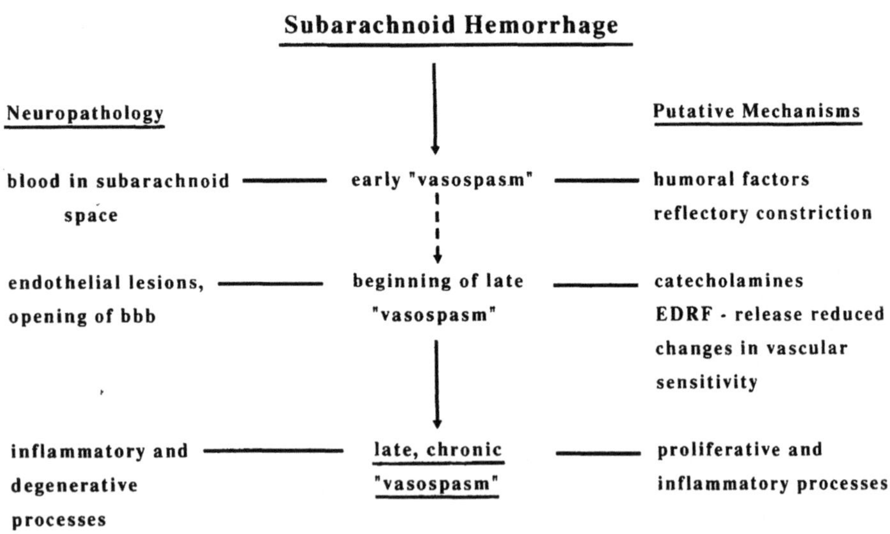

Fig. 1. Development of "cerebral vasospasm" following subarachnoid hemorrhage. A synopsis of putative mechanisms

changes are seen in late chronic vasospasm associated with adhesion of thrombocytes, aggregation of neutrophils, infiltration of the muscle layer with inflammatory cells, and finally necrosis of smooth muscle cells (Kassell and Sasaki 1987). It becomes obvious that numerous mechanisms are involved in this life-threatening complication and that a rational therapy is far away.

Conclusions

Regulation of vascular resistance in the brain is achieved by the same principles as in other organs. There are, however, remarkable differences in importance of the various factors involved. Much work is still needed to explore further the physiological and pathological mechanisms of CBF to improve the therapy of the major diseases and finally to develop more rational forms of treatment.

Acknowledgments: The excellent secretarial and technical assistance of Ms. Anita Riede and Ms. U. Goerke is highly appreciated.

References

Alafaci A, Jansen J, Arbab MAR, Shiokawa Y, Svendgaard NAA, Edvinsson L (1990) Enhanced vasoconstrictor effect of endothelin in cerebral arteries from rats with subarachnoid hemorrhage. Acta Physiol Cand 138:317–319

Baethmann A, Maier-Hauff K, Kempski O, Unterberg A, Wahl M, Schürer L (1988) Mediators of brain edema and secondary brain damage. Crit Care Med 16:972–978

Brawley BW, Strandness DE, Kelly WA (1968) The biphasic response of cerebral vasospasm in experimental subarachnoid hemorrhage. J Neurosurg 28:1–8

Edvinsson L, MacKenzie ET (1977) Amine mechanisms in the cerebral circulation. Pharmacol Rev 28:275–348

Edvinsson L, McCulloch J (eds) (1987) Peptidergic mechanisms in the cerebral circulation. Horwood, Chichester

Edvinsson L, Owman C (1974) Pharmacological characterization of adrenergic alpha and beta receptors mediating the vasomotor responses of cerebral arteries in vitro. Circ Res 35:835–849

Edvinsson L, Owman C, Siesjö BD (1976) Physiological role of cerebrovascular sympathetic nerves in the autoregulation of cerebral blood flow. Brain Res 117:519–523

Edvinsson L, Hardebo JE, MacKenzie ET, Stewart M (1977) Dual action of serotonin on pial arterioles in situ and the effect of propranolol on the response. Blood Vessels 14:366–371

Hardebo JE, Kahrström J, Owman C, Salford LY (1989) Endothelin is a potent constrictor of human intracranial arteries and veins. Blood Vessels 26:249–253

Harder DR (1985) A cellular mechanism for myogenic regulation of cat cerebral arteries. Ann Biomed Eng 13:335–339

Harder DR (1987) Pressure-induced myogenic activation of cat cerebral arteries is dependent on intact endothelium. Circ Res 60:102–107

Harder DR, Sanchez-Ferrer C, Kauser K, Stekiel WJ, Rubanyi GM (1989) Pressure releases a transferrable endothelial contractile factor in cat cerebral arteries. Circ Res 65:193–198

Kassell NF, Sasaki T (1987) Pathogenesis of cerebral vasospasm. In: Kikuchi H, Fukushima T, Watanabe K (eds) Intracranial aneurysms. Surgical timing and techniques. Nishimura, Tokyo, pp 250–256

Kobayaski H, Hayashi M, Kobayashi S, Kabuto M, Honda Y, Kewando H (1990) Effect of endothelin on the canine basilar artery. Neurosurgery 27:357–361

Kuschinsky W, Wahl M (1978) Local chemical and neurogenic regulation of cerebral vascular resistance. Physiol Rev 58:656–689

Kuschinsky W, Wahl M, Bosse O, Thurau K (1972) Perivascular potassium and pH as determinants of local pial arterial diameter in cats. A microapplication study. Circ Res 31:240–247

Kuschinsky W, Wahl M, Neiss A (1974) Evidence for cholinergic dilatatory receptors in pial arteries of cats. A microapplication study. Pflügers Arch 347:199–208

Lassen NA, Ingvar DH, Skinhoj E (1978) Brain function and blood flow. Sci Am 239:62–71

Leniger-Follert E, Lübbers DW (1976) Behaviour of microflow and local pO_2 of the brain cortex during and after direct electrical stimulation. A contribution to the problem of metabolic regulation of microcirculation in the brain. Pflügers Arch 366:39–44

MacKenzie ET, Scatton B (1978) Cerebral circulatory and metabolic effects of perivascular neurotransmitters. Crit Rev Clin Neurobiol 2:357–419

MacKenzie ET, McGeorge AP, Graham DI, Fitch W, Edvinsson L, Harper AM (1979) Effects of increasing arterial pressure on cerebral blood flow in the baboon: influence of the sympathetic nervous system. Pflügers Arch 378:189–195

McCarron JG, Osol G, Halpern WC (1989) Myogenic responses are independent of the endothelium in rat pressurized posterior cerebral arteries. Blood Vessels 26:315–319

Nakagomi T, Kassell NF, Sasaki T, Fujiwara S, Lehmann MR, Joshita H, Nazar GB, Torner JC (1987) Effect of subarachnoid hemorrhage on endothelium-dependent vasodilation. J Neurosurg 66:915–923

Pickard JD (1981) Role of prostaglandins and arachidonic acid derivatives in the coupling of cerebral blood flow to cerebral metabolism. J Cereb Blood Flow Metab 1:361–384

Robinson MJ, McCulloch J (1990) Contractile responses to endothelin in feline cortical vessels in situ. J Cereb Blood Flow Metab 10:285–289

Roy CW, Sherrington CS (1890) On the regulation of the blood supply of the brain. J Physiol 11:85–108

Svendgaard NA, Brismar J, Delgado TJ, Rosengren E (1985) Subarachnoid haemorrhage in the rat – effect of the development of vasospasm of selective lesions of the catecholamine systems in the lower brain stem. Stroke 16:602–608

Unterberg A, Marguth F (1988) Aktuelle Konzepte zur Pathogenese und Therapie des zerebralen Vasospasmus. MMW 130:543–544

Unterberg A, Wahl M, Baethmann A (1984) Effects of bradykinin on permeability and diameter of pial vessels in vivo. J Cereb Blood Flow Metab 4:574–585

Unterberg A, Wahl M, Hammersen F, Baethmann A (1987) Permeability and vasomotor response of cerebral vessels during exposure to arachidonic acid. Acta Neurapathol (Berl) 73:209–219

Unterberg A, Schmidt W, Wahl M, Ellis E, Marmarou A, Baethmann A (1991) Evidence against leukotrienes as mediators of brain edema. J Neurosurg 74:773–780

Urbanics R, Leniger-Follert E, Lübbers DW (1978) Time course of changes of extracellular H^+ and K^+ activities during and after direct electrical stimulation of the brain cortex. Pflügers Arch 378:47–53

Wahl (1985a) Local chemical, neural and humoral regulation of cerebrovascular resistance vessels. J Cardiovasc Pharmacol [Suppl 3] 7:S36–S46

Wahl M (1985b) A review of neurotransmitters and hormones implicated in mediating cerebral vasospasm. In: Voth D, Glees P (eds) Cerebral vascular spasm. de Gruyter, Berlin, pp 223–230

Wahl M, Kuschinsky W (1976) The dilatatory action of adenosine on pial arteries of cats and its inhibition by theophylline. Pflügers Arch 362:55–59

Wahl M, Kuschinsky W (1979a) The dilating effect of histamine on pial arteries of cats and its mediation by H_2 receptors. Circ Res 44:161–165

Wahl M, Kuschinsky W (1979b) Unimportance of perivascular H^+ and K^+ activities for the adjustment of pial arterial diameter during changes of arterial blood pressure in cats. Pflügers Arch 382:203–208

Wahl M, Deetjen P, Thurau K, Ingvar DH, Lassen NA (1970) Micropuncture evaluation of the importance of perivascular pH for the arteriolar diameter on the brain surface. Pflügers Arch 316:152–163

Wahl M, Kuschinsky W, Bosse O, Olesen J, Lassen NA, Ingvar DH, Michaelis J, Thurau K (1972) Effect of *l*-norepinephrine on the diameter of pial arterioles and arteries in the cat. Circ Res 31:248–256

Wahl M, Kuschinsky W, Bosse O, Thurau K (1973) Dependency of the pial arterial and arteriolar diameter on perivascular osmolarity in the cat. A microapplication study. Circ Res 32:162–169

Wahl M, Unterberg A, Baethmann A, Schilling L (1988) Mediators of blood-brain barrier dysfunction and formation of vasogenic brain oedema. J Cereb Blood Flow Metab 8:621–634

Capillary Perfusion in the Brain

W. Kuschinsky

Introduction

The perfusion mode of cerebral capillaries is still a matter of controversy. Whereas the interrelationships between the density of perfused capillaries, local glucose utilization, and local blood flow in the brain are well known (Klein et al. 1986), the question of the normal perfusion pattern of brain capillaries and of recruitment of capillaries under conditions of high blood flow is still open. The present investigation therefore aimed to test the normal perfusion pattern of brain capillaries by fluorescent staining of capillaries and of their contents. Another question posed by this study was whether drastic increases in cerebral blood flow (CBF) induced by CO_2 are accompanied by increases in the number of perfused capillaries. Experiments were performed on awake rats to avoid an influence of anesthesia on capillary perfusion. Since the results of such investigations are critically dependent on the method used to mark the perfused capillaries, additional studies were performed to verify the applicability of the fluorescence method used in the present and the previous (Klein et al. 1986) study. In one series of experiments the densities of perfused capillaries were compared with fluoresceinisothiocyanate (FITC) coupled to globulin, as used in the present study, or to dextran, as applied in studies by Weiss and his group (Buchweitz and Weiss 1986; Francois-Dainville et al. 1986; Grover et al. 1986; Weiss et al. 1982), who came to different conclusions about capillary perfusion from their data; another series of experiments investigated the question of whether the anesthesia, which preceded all the experiments (for placing the catheters), could have influenced the results of the capillary density measurements. To this end, FITC-globulin was injected into a tail vein in naive, untreated control rats and the density of perfused capillaries measured. In the last series of experiments, the capillary structures were stained using fluorescent antibodies against the basal membrane constituent fibronectin. The counts obtained were compared with those obtained with intravascular fluorescent markers. The results showed the validity of the method used and a continuous perfusion of all the capillaries during both normocapnia and hypercapnia.

Methods

The experiments were performed on male Sprague-Dawley rats. The animals were anesthetized by a gas mixture of halothane (1%–1.5%), N_20 (70%–80%), and O_2 (remainder). Body temperature was maintained at 37°–37.5°C with the use of a temperature-controlled heating pad. The arterial blood pressure was measured in the right femoral artery by a Statham pressure transducer. Substances were applied via a catheter in the right femoral vein. After surgery, the animals were placed in a rat restrainer. Three hours were allowed for recovery from the effects of anesthesia. The coupled fluorescent dye was then injected for staining of perfused capillaries. To identify the perfused capillaries, the fluorochrome (FITC) bound to bovine γ-globulin or FITC-dextran was used, as described previously (Klein et al. 1986). Anesthesia was not induced in the experimental group in which the fluorescent marker was given by tail vein injection.

Experimental Procedures

In a control group of eight conscious rats, FITC-globulin (0.3 ml/100 g body wt.) was applied via the femoral vein and allowed to circulate for 1 min. In four additional conscious rats FITC-dextran (100 mg/kg dissolved in 1 ml saline) was used in the same manner. After decapitation the brain was rapidly removed and frozen in 2-methylbutane chilled to –40° to –50°C with dry ice, stored in plastic bags at –70°C, and embedded and directly cut into 5-µm coronal sections in a cryomicrotome at –21°C. The sections were transferred to slides coated with pure alcohol and precooled in liquid nitrogen as described by Vetterlein et al. (1982). The preparations were kept at –21°C until the alcohol had thawed and impregnated the tissue. The sections were floated with alcohol at room temperature and embedded in an artificial medium (Entellan).

Another ten awake rats were allowed to inhale a water vapor saturated gas mixture containing 6.3%–8.3% CO_2, 21% O_2, the remainder N_2 for 15 min. This treatment resulted in a marked, noncompensated respiratory acidosis, as was evident from the arterial acid base status. FITC-globulin was given i.v. 1 min before the end of the experiment as a bolus injection. the brains were processed as described above for the control experiments.

In order to exclude the preceding anesthesia influencing the observed results of perfused capillaries, four additional rats received no pretreatment or anesthesia. They obtained FITC-globulin (0.3 ml/100 g body wt.) via a tail vein after the tail was placed in warm water for 5 min. One minute after injection of the dye the animals were decapitated and the brains processed as described above for the control experiments. In these animals blood pressure or acid base status could not be determined.

The effect of changes in the arterial PCO_2 on local CBF (LCBF) was investigated in an additional 15 rats, 9 of which were exposed to a water vapor saturated gas mixture containing 6.3%–8.3% CO_2, 21% O_2, the remainder N_2 for 15 min. The density of perfused capillaries and LCBF was measured as described previously (Klein et al. 1986). Details have been published elsewhere (Göbel et al. 1989).

In another seven conscious rats the density of capillaries detectable on morphological examination was determined using a newly developed fluorescent fibronectin antibody method. The animals were killed by decapitation and the brains were processed as described above. The brains were cut into 6 µm sections at –21°C in a cryomicrotome. The frozen sections were transferred to glass slides, air dried, and then fixed with acetone at –21°C for 3 min. Excess acetone was allowed to evaporate at room temperature. Thereafter the indirect immunofluorescent technique was performed as follows: The polyclonal anti-human-fibronectin antibody, developed in rabbit (Code A 245, Dakopatts, Glostrup, Denmark), and diluted 1:100 in phosphate-buffered saline (PBS, pH 7.4), was used as primary antibody. Each section was overlaid with 70 μl antibody solution and incubated in a humid chamber at room temperature for 30 min. Slides were dipped briefly in PBS and then washed three times in PBS for 5 min (using a fresh PBS bath in each case and resulting in a washing time of 15 min). The margins of the prepared sections were wiped dry and the wet sections were overlaid with 70 μl of the FITC-conjugated anti-rabbit-immunoglobulin antibody, developed in swine (Code F 205, Dakopatts, Glostrup, Denmark), as secondary antibody. Before use, this antibody was diluted 1:60 in PBS and centrifuged at 12 000 rpm for 5 min. The supernatant was taken. The prepared sections were allowed to incubate for 30 min in a humid chamber at room temperature. The slides were washed in PBS as described above, observed, and photographed (x 40 objective) by fluorescent microscopy without coverslips using PBS as an immersion medium. Details have been published elsewhere (Göbel et al. 1990).

Results

Validation of Method of Intravascular Fluorescent Staining

The local densities of perfused capillaries were compared using three application methods in each of the ten brain structures investigated: (a) injection of FITC-globulin, (b) injection of FITC-dextran, both into a femoral vein, and (c) injection of FITC-globulin into a tail vein of naive rats with no catheters implanted. There was no statistical difference ($p<0.05$) between the three respective density values of perfused capillaries in any of the structures tested. The congruity of the FITC-globulin and FITC-dextran values shows that both markers of perfused capillaries are interchangeable and can be used equally for the detection of perfused capillaries; the congruity of these results with those obtained after tail vein injection demonstrates that pretreatment of the animals with transient N_2O-halothane anesthesia (for placing the catheters) did not influence the densities of perfused capillaries.

Density of Perfused Capillaries and CBF During Hypercapnic Hyperemia

The dependency of CBF and density of perfused capillaries on the arterial PCO_2 are shown in Fig. 1, which gives the mean values of CBF and density of perfused capillaries obtained from the mean of the local values found in each rat. Each point thus represents the mean value of one rat. The upper part of Fig. 1 shows that hypercapnia induced the expected increases in CBF whereas the lower part demonstrates that these CBF increases were not paralleled by increases in the density of perfused capillaries. The correlation coefficients obtained for the correlations between arterial PCO_2 values and CBFs were not significantly different from zero, indicating a lack of dependency of both global and local densities of perfused capillaries on arterial PCO_2. It follows that, in spite of a strong hypercapnic hyperemia, there is no recruitment of perfused capillaries in the rat brain.

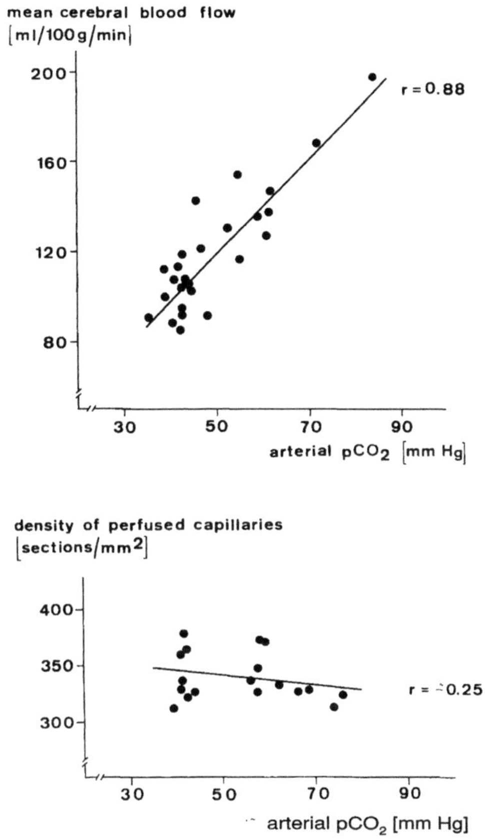

Fig. 1. Dependency of CBF and density of perfused capillaries on the arterial pCO_2. The well-known increase in CBF was found during hypercapnia (upper part). On the other hand, there was no change in the density of perfused capillaries under comparable experimental conditions (lower part). These data show a lack of capillary recruitment during hypercapnic hyperemia in the brain

Fluorescent Staining of the Capillary Morphology

The capillary structures were stained using antibodies against the basement membrane constituent, fibronectin, and marking of the antibodies by fluorochrome-coupled anti-antibodies. Capillary structures could be photographed through a fluorescent microscope in complete analogy with the detection of the intravascular fluorescent dyes. As found for the intravascular fluorescent markers, capillary density varied depending on the brain structure investigated. Structures which had previously been found to have a high metabolic rate for glucose, a high blood flow, and a high density of perfused capillaries also showed a high density of capillaries detectable on morphological examination and vice versa. This is shown in Fig. 2. Comparison of the number of existing capillaries with that of perfused capillaries yielded highly congruent results in all brain structures investigated.

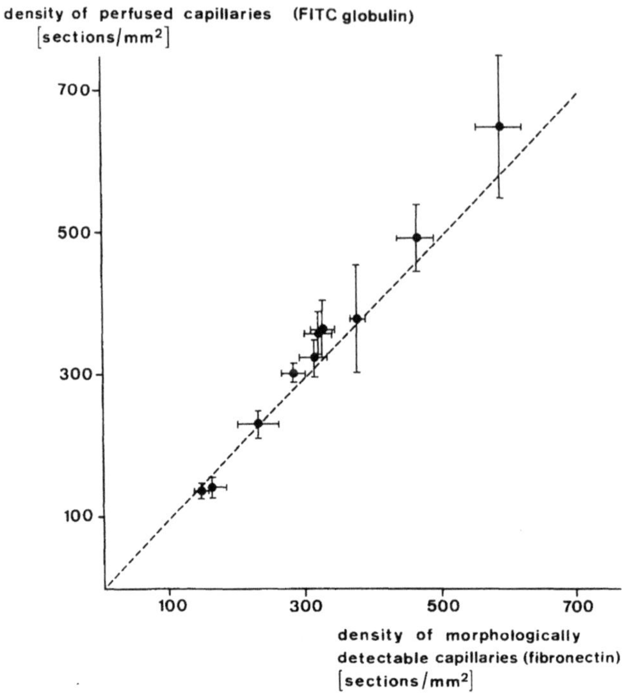

Fig. 2. Density of morphologically detectable capillaries in relation to the density of perfused capillaries. The density of morphologically existing capillaries was determined by a fibronectin-antibody immunofluorescent method whereas the number of perfused capillaries was determined after intravenous injection of fluorochrome-coupled globulin. The measured values are close to the line of identify indicating the perfusion of all capillaries in all brain structures. Means ± SE

Discussion

The present study shows a high congruence of existing and perfused capillaries in normal, awake rats and the lack of capillary recruitment during hypercapnia, which is a typical high flow situation. The issue of capillary recruitment is controversial for the brain. A prerequisite for capillary recruitment is the existence of reserve capillaries which are not or only intermittently perfused during conditions of normal flow. Our previous and the present experiments using antibodies against the vessel wall constituent, fibronectin, gave no indication of the existence of reserve capillaries in the rat brain. The density of perfused capillaries was not different when the circulation times of the fluorescent intravascular marker varied from 10 s to 30 min (Klein et al. 1986). These previous findings of our group have already strongly indicated that all or the majority of capillaries are permanently perfused in the brain. The present experiments support this conclusion since no reserve capillaries could be found which are perfused during hypercapnic hyperemia only. Our results are in accordance with conclusions drawn from experiments in rhesus monkeys during hyper- and hypocapnia (Eichling et al. 1974; Raichle et al. 1976), in which isotope extractions varied inversely and linearly with flow, which is congruent with a constant permeability-surface area product under these conditions. With a significant amount of capillary recruitment, permeability-surface area product should change in parallel. On the other hand, capillary recruitment in the brain has also been reported, based on studies of extraction fractions (Pardridge and Fierer; 1985; Phelps et al. 1981), use of indicator dilution techniques (Bolwig et al. 1977; Hertz and Paulson 1982), and fluorescent microscopic studies (Buchweitz and Weiss 1986; Francois-Dainville et al. 1986; Grover et al. 1986; Weiss 1988). The fluorescent microscopic studies by Weiss and coworkers may not have been sensitive enough to detect all perfused capillaries, since air drying of the tissue leads to a loss of fluorescent spots. Concerning the measurements of permeability-surface area product, such studies may allow conclusions about capillary recruitment only as long as the permeability is unchanged. This may not be the case for all experimental conditions. For the pathophysiological condition of streptozotocin-induced diabetes, Moos Knudsen et al. (1986) showed that the permeability-surface area product was decreased for Na^+, but unchanged for sucrose and Cl^-. These data can be interpreted to indicate a decrease in permeability for Na^+ on an unchanged surface area, as indicated by the unaltered permeability-surface area product for sucrose and Cl^-. This unchanged surface area would point to an unchanged capillary perfusion. Whether changes in permeability with an unchanged capillary surface area occur under more physiological conditions remains to be established.

The data obtained during hypercapnia demonstrate a lack of capillary recruitment during hypercapnia, although CBF was markedly increased. These data do not completely rule out the existence of capillary recruitment during alternative states of hyperemia in the brain. Such a possibility was excluded by additional experiments employing antibody staining of capillary structures, showing convincingly that identical counts could be found for morphologically existing and for perfused capillaries in all brain structures investigated. From these experiments it is concluded that all capillaries are perfused all the time in the brains of conscious rats. There is nothing to indicate the existence of reserve capillaries. These conclusions are further supported by double staining experiments, in which we visualized both existing and perfused capillaries in the same brain section using fluorescent microscopy (Göbel et al. 1990).

Acknowledgment. This study was supported by a grant from the Deutsche Forschungsgemeinschaft.

References

Bowling TG, Hertz MM, Paulson OB, Spotoft H, Rafaelsen OJ (1977) The permeability of the blood-brain barrier during electrically induced seizures in man. Eur J Clin Invest 7:87–93

Buchweitz E, Weiss HR (1986) Alterations in perfused capillary morphometry in awake vs. anesthetized brain. Brain Res 377:105–111

Eichling JO, Raichle ME, Grubb RL, Ter-Pogossian MM (1974) Evidence of the limitations of water as a freely diffusible tracer in brain of the rhesus monkey. Circ Res 35:358–364

Francois-Dainville E, Buchweitz E, Weiss HR (1986) Effect of hypoxia on percent of arteriolar and capillary beds perfused in the rat brain. J Appl Physiol 60:270–288

Göbel U, Klein B, Schröck H, Kuschinsky W (1989) Lack of capillary recruitment in the brains of awake rats during hypercapnia. J Cereb Blood Flow Metab 9:491–499

Göbel U, Theilen H, Kuschinsky W (1990) Congruence of total and perfused capillary network in rat brains. Circ Res 66:271–281

Grover GJ, Francois-Dainville E, Buchweitz E, Weiss HR (1986) Effect of hemorrhage on regional morphometric indexes of cerebral capillarity. J Appl Physiol 61:1712–1719

Hertz MM, Paulson OB (1982) Transfer across the human blood-brain barrier: evidence for capillary recruitment and for a paradox glucose permeability increase in hypocapnia. Microvasc Res 24:364–376

Klein B, Kuschinsky W, Schröck H, Vetterlein F (1986) Interdependency of local capillary density, blood flow and metabolism in rat brains. Am J Physiol 251:H1330–H1340

Moos Knudsen G, Jakobsen J, Juhler M, Paulson OB (1986) Decreased blood-brain barrier permeability to sodium in early experimental diabetes. Diabetes 35:1371–1373

Pardridge WM, Fierer G (1985) Blood-brain barrier transport of butanol and water relative to *N*-isopropyl-*p*-iodoamphetamine as the internal reference. J Cereb Blood Flow Metab 5:275–281

Phelps ME, Huang SC, Hoffman EJ, Selin C, Kuhl CE (1981) Cerebral extraction of N-13 ammonia: its dependence on cerebral blood flow and capillary permeability – surface area product. Stroke 12:607–619

Raichle ME, Eichling JO, Straatmann MG, Welch MJ, Larson KB, Ter-Pogossian MM (1976) Blood-brain barrier permeability of ^{11}C-labeled alcohols and ^{15}O-labeled water. Am J Physiol 230:543–552

Vetterlein F, Dal Ri H, Schmidt G (1982) Capillary density in rat myocardium during timed plasma staining. Am J Physiol 242:H133-H141

Weiss HR (1988) Measurement of cerebral capillary perfusion with a fluorescent label. Microvasc Res 36:172–180

Weiss HR, Buchweitz E, Murtha TJ, Auletta M (1982) Quantitative regional determination of morphometric indices of the total and perfused capillary network in the rat brain. Circ Res 51:494–503

Intrinsic and Extrinsic Neural Regulation of the Cerebral Circulation

C. IADECOLA

Introduction

Throughout the early 1900s the concept of regulation of the cerebral circulation was dominated by the Monro-Kelly doctrine (Friedland and Iadecola 1991), which stated that the cerebral blood content cannot change since the brain is enclosed in the rigid skull. This concept led to the erroneous assumption that also cerebral blood flow (CBF) had to be constant as cerebral vessels had no room to expand and contract (e.g., Bayliss and Hill 1895). While the work of Donders (1849), Mosso (1881), and Roy and Sherrington (1890) challenged this assumption, this interpretation of the Monro-Kelly doctrine received emphatic support by others (e.g., Hill 1896) and remained in vogue until the early 1900s.

It is now well established that CBF is dynamically regulated at the local level. Thus, an increase in cerebral activity can evoke rapid changes in flow (< 1 s) that can be highly restricted to the regions in which cellular activity incrases (e.g., Schmidt and Hendrix 1938; Olesen 1971; Moskalenko 1975; Greenberg 1979; Leniger-Follert and Hossmann 1979; Frostig et al. 1990). Thus, the brain has the capacity to regulate its own blood flow with considerable spatial and temporal precision.

How does cerebral activation produce such changes in CBF? For the past several decades the prevailing view has been that originally proposed by Roy and Sherrington in 1890. These authors suggested that neuronal activity releases vasoactive substances that, by diffusion, reach local vessels producing changes in vascular diameter (metabolic hypothesis) (Roy and Sherrington 1890; Cobb 1938; Schmidt 1950; Sokoloff 1959; Rosenblum 1965; Kuschinsky and Wahl 1978; Wahl 1985). This hypothesis is supported by the evidence that neuronal and glial activity releases a variety of vasoactive substances in the extracellular space (Lou et al. 1987). However, as discussed in detail elsewhere (Iadecola and Raichle 1992), a "metabolic" mechanism based on Fickian diffusion of agents in the extracellular space cannot explain the rapidity and spatial confinement of the change in CBF reported experimentally. Thus, it is unlikely that a metabolic mechanism is the only factor influencing CBF during neuronal activity.

Another aspect of the regulation of the cerebral circulation which has long been studied relates to the role of neurogenic factors. Most of the initial experimental efforts were focused on the role of the sympathetic and parasympathetic innervation of the cerebral blood vessels (i.e., extrinsic nerves, see below) [see Purves (1972) for an historical review]. However, due to limitations of techniques and experimental approaches used, the influence of these factors on CBF has been considered negligible (Hill

1896; Schmidt 1950; Sokoloff 1959; Heistad and Marcus 1978). The recent expansion of the neurosciences has led to the reexamination of the neurogenic regulation of the cerebral vessels in light of contemporary neurobiological concepts and techniques. In particular, anatomical and physiological studies have explored the possibility that intrinsic neural pathways, i.e., pathways originating and terminating within the brain, can also influence the cerebral vasculature (Reis and Iadecola 1991). These studies have indeed shown that there are intrinsic neural networks that have a powerful influence on the cerebral circulation. In this paper some of these neural systems will be reviewed and hypotheses regarding their functional role will be discussed.

Intrinsic and Extrinsic Neurogenic Regulation of CBF

Extrinsic Neural Systems

It has long been known that the cerebral vessels are innervated by nerve fibers originating from cranial autonomic ganglia (Purves 1972). These fibers form a dense perivascular plexus and innervate vascular smooth muscles through varicose terminals resembling autonomic synapses (Nielsen et al. 1971). This innervation, termed extrinsic to emphasize its peripheral origin, is mostly confined to extraparenchymal vessels (MacKenzie and Scatton 1987). A brief description of the major extrinsic systems is presented in Table 1. Pertinent references can be found in recent reviews on this subject (MacKenzie and Scatton 1987; Moskowitz 1986; Uddman and Edvinsson 1989; Owman 1990). While the chemical anatomy of this innervation and the effects of activation and lesions have been extensively studied, the role of extrinsic pathways in the regulation of CBF has not been fully elucidated. Some of these pathways may act to protect the brain from the consequence of hypertension (Heistad and Kontos 1983; Sakas et al. 1989), vasospasm (McCulloch et al. 1986), or seizures (Sakas et al. 1989). They have also been implicated in the pathogenesis of migraine and vascular headaches (Goadsby and Lance 1988; Moskowitz 1984).

Intrinsic Neural Systems

That intrinsic neural pathways may participate in the regulation of the cerebral circulation is supported by three lines of evidence. First, there are nerve fibers and terminals that are in "close association" with intracerebral arterioles and capillaries (Table 2). Second, cerebral microvessels are endowed with receptors for a wide variety of neurotransmitters and neuromodulators (Harik 1984). Third, excitation of intrinsic neural pathways can modulate CBF independently of local cerebral metabolic activity and via different transmitter systems. While it remains unclear whether the "close associations" between neural processes and capillaries have functional significance in CBF regulation, the biochemical and physiological evidence more convincingly indicates that these systems can have powerful effects in CBF. Collectively, these studies suggest that there might be widespread central neural networks dedicated to the regulation of CBF and metabolism (Reis 1984; Lou et al. 1987; Iadecola and Raich 1992).

A brief synopsis of the cerebrovascular actions of these neural systems is presented in Table 3. A more detailed description of some of them has been provided in recent

Table 1. Major sources of extrinsic innervation of the cerebral blood vessels

Nerve system	Major pathway	Primary target vessels	Transmitters	Effect of activation	Effect of lesion
Superior cervical ganglion	Sympathetic trunk, perivascular plexus	Extra-parenchymal vessels	norepinephrine neuropeptide Y, dopamine, serotonin (?), GABA	Vasoconstriction; expanded upper limit of autoregulation	Transient vasodilation or no effect on CBF; vascular atrophy
Trigeminal ganglion	Trigeminal nasociliary nerve, perivascular plexus	Extra-parenchymal vessels	Substance P, neurokinin A, calcitonin gene related peptide, galanin	Vasodilation; increased permeability of dural vessels	No effect on resting CBF, attenuation of CBF increases in seizures, hyperten-sion or after ischemia; enhanced vasoconstric-tion nore-pinephrine
Sphenopala-tine and otic ganglia	Ethmoidal nerve, perivascular plexus	Extra-parenchymal vessels	Acetylcholine, vasoactive intestinal polypeptide, peptide histidine isoleucine, neuropeptide Y	Vasodilation	No effect on resting CBF and on hypoxic and hypercapnic vasodilation

See text for references. GABA: γ-aminobutyric acid

Table 2. Some ultrastructural evidence of innervation of cerebral capillaries

Author	Species and brain region	Transmitter and technique	Target	Morphology of neurovascular contacts
Rennels and Nelson (1975)	Cat; anterior hypothalamus	Dense and clear core vesicles (?monoamines)	Capillary basal lamina; pericytes	Terminals with mitochondria and vesicles; no intervening glial membranes; no specializations in capillary basal lamina
Swanson et al. (1977)	Rat with chronic cervical sympathectomy; paraventricular hypothalamus	5-OHDA-induced dense core vesicles prevented by reserpine (monoamines?)	Capillaries, basal lamina; pericytes	Same as above

Table 2. continuation

Itakura et al. (1977)	Rat with chronic cervical sympathectomy; cerebral cortex	Clear core (acetylcholine?) and dense core (monoamines?) vesicles	Capillaries, basal lamina	Terminals with vesicles; no intervening glial processes
Hendry et al. (1983)	Monkey, rat; cerebral cortex	CCK-8; immuno-cytochemistry	Capillaries, basal lamina, arterioles, venules	Immunoreactive somata or processes; no basal lamina specializations
Eckenstein and Baughman (1984)	Rat; cerebral cortex	VIP, acetylcholine; VIP/CAT immuno-cytochemistry	Capillary basal lamina and "larger vessels"	Same as above
Kapadia and de Lanerolle (1984)	Cat, monkey; dorsal raphe and interpeduncular nucleus	Substance P, met-enkephalin, serotonin; immuno-cytochemistry	Capillary basal lamina	Dendrites with or without intervening glia
Obata-Tsuto et al (1984)	Cat; arcuate nucleus	VIP; immuno-cytochemistry	Capillary basal lamina	Immunoreactive processes; no basal lamina specializations
Armstrong (1986)	Rat; amygdala and nucleus of the diagonal band	Acetylcholine; CAT immuno-cytochemistry	Capillary basal lamina	Somata and dendrites; with or without intervening glia; no basal membrane specializations
Milner et al. (1987)	Rat; rostral ventrolateral medulla	Epinephrine; PNMT immuno-cytochemistry	Capillary basal lamina	Dendrites, somata, and axons; with intervening glia; no basal lamina specializations
Papadopulos et al. (1989)	Rat; visual cortex	Norepinephrine; immuno-cytochemistry	Capillary basal lamina in cortical laminae II–IV	Immunoreactive profiles; with or without intervening glia
Aoky and Pickel (1989)	Rat; caudate nucleus and cerebral cortex	Neuropeptide Y; immuno-cytochemistry	Capillary basal lamina	Immunoreactive terminals often with intervening glia

Unless otherwise specified, immunocytochemistry was performed using antibodies raised against the transmitter studied. *Abbreviations:* CAT, choline acetyltransferase; CCK-8, cholecystokinin; PNMT, phenylethanolamine *N*-methyltransferase; VIP, vasoactive intestinal polypeptide; 5-OHDA, 5-hydroxydopamine.

Table 3. Central neural systems influencing the cerebral microcirculation

Region	Neural elements involved	Effects of stimulation	Effects of lesion	Target	Pathways	Transmitter
Nucleus of the solitary tract	Neurons *and/or* passing fibers	Vasodilation	Abolish autoregulation	Whole brain	Efferent projections (?)	?
Rostral ventro-lateral medulla	Cl area neurons (?)	Vasodilation	Reduce hypoxic vasodilation	Whole brain	?	?
Dorsal medullary reticular formation	Neurons *and/or* passing fibers	Vasodilation	?	Whole brain	Efferent projections (?)	In Part, epinephrine released from adrenals
Cerebellar fastigial nucleus	Passing fibers	Vasodilation	No effect on resting CBF	Whole brain	Through RVL and basal forebrain	Acetyl-choline
	Local neurons	Vaso-constriction	No effect on resting CBF	Whole brain	?	?
Para-brachial nucleus	Neurons *and/or* passing fibers	Vasodilation or vaso-constiction[a]	?	Especially cerebral cortex	Efferent cortical projections (?)	?
Locus cerculeus	Noradren-ergic neurons (?)	Vaso-constriction; decreased BBB perme-ability to water	In rat no effect on resting CBF or on CBF rise in hypercapnia	Cerebral cortex	Efferent cortical micro-vascular projections	Norepin-ephrine (?)
Dorsal raphe	Neurons *and/or* passing fibers	Vasodilation or vaso-constriction[b]	?	Mostly whole brain	Efferent micro-vascular projections (?)	Serotonin (?)
Thalamus para-fascicular complex	Neurons *and/or* passing fibers	Vasodilation	?	Especially cerebral cortex	Thalamo-cortical projections (?)	In Part, adrenal catechol-amines
Basal forebrain	Cholin-ergic neurons (?)	Vasodilation	Decrease in resting CBF, no effect on CBF rise with hypercapnia	Cerebral cortex	Cholinergic cortical projection system (?)	Acetyl-choline

[a] Stimulation of the parabrachial nucleus can both increase and decrease CBF depending on the subnucleus activated.

[b] Dorsal raphe stimulation increases CBF in awake rats and decreases CBF in chloralose – anesthetized rats. See text for references

reviews (Seylaz et al. 1986; Goadsby and Lance 1988; Reis and Iadecola 1991). Two of these networks have been studied in greater depth with respect to the pathways and transmitters involved in their cerebral vascular actions. These systems involve a region of the dorsal medullary reticular formation (DMRF) and the cerebellar fastigial nucleus (FN).

Dorsal Medullary Reticular Formation: A System for Neural and Humoral Regulation of Cerebral Metabolism

Electrical stimulation of a region of the DMRF, largely comprising the dorsal portion of the nucleus parvocellularis, elevates CBF globally throughout the brain and maximally in the cerebral cortex (up to 2.4-fold) (Iadecola et al. 1983a). The inceases in flow are associated with corresponding increases in local cerebral glucose utilization (CGU) (Iadecola et al. 1983b), indicating that the vasodilatation is probably a consequence of increased metabolic activity. Interestingly, stimulation of the DMRF does not produce desynchronization on the electroencephalogram (Iadecola et al. 1983a). Since the primary action of the DMRF is on cerebral metabolism, the cerebrovasodilation has been termed *secondary vasodilation* to emphasize its dependence on local metabolic activity (Iadecola et al. 1983b). DMRF stimulation also increases spinal cord blood flow, a finding indicating that its effects are not only restricted to the brain but involve the entire neuraxis (Iadecola et al. 1989).

A distinctive feature of the cerebrovasodilation elicited from the DMRF is that the increases in metabolism and flow are abolished in some regions and greatly reduced in others by acute adrenalectomy (Iadecola et al. 1987b, c). This observation indicates that humoral factors released from the adrenals participate in the vasodilation. The adrenal factors appear to be catecholamines, mostly epinephrine, which are released in large quantity by DMRF stimulation (Lacombe et al. 1990). Thus the vasodilatation evoked from the DMRF has *catecholamine-dependent* (humoral) and *catecholamine-independent* (neural) components and, as such, is not entirely mediated by factors intrinsic to the brain.

Neural Pathways and Transmitters. The neural pathways mediating the cerebral vascular actions of the DMRF have not been fully elucidated. Since electrical stimulation activates both neurons and passing fibers the response may be due to stimulation of local reticular formation neurons and/or axons passing through the area. Of interest is the observation that a large portion of the axons traversing the DMRF originates from the rostral ventrolateral medulla (RVL), a region including the adrenergic neurons of the C1 group of Hökfelt (Hökfelt et al. 1974). These neurons have monosynaptic connections with the preganglionic sympathetic neurons of intermediolateral column of the thoracic spinal cord (Ruggiero et al. 1989). Therefore excitation of their axons could be responsible for the massive elevation in plasma catecholamines elicited by stimulation of the DMRF. Since excitation of neurons in the RVL increases CBF globally (Underwood 1988), RVL axons could also participate in the adrenal-independent component of the cerebrovasodilation. However, the increases in CBF elicited from stimulation of the RVL are not associated with elevations in cerebral glucose utilization (Underwood 1988), and, as such, they differ from those elicited by DMRF stimulation. Another possibility is that the adrenal-independent component is mediated by excitation of local neurons of the parvocellular reticular formation and/or passing fiber of the central tegmental tract. This hypothesis, however, remains to be tested experimentally.

In cerebral cortex the elevations in CBF have a significant catecholamine-independent component (Iadecola et al. 1987b). The neural pathways mediating the cortical response have not been identified. Since the cortical cerebrovasodilation is not affected by spinal cord transection or transection of the cervical sympathetic trunk, the pathways are likely to be intrinsic to the brain (Iadecola et al. 1983a, 1987b). It has been proposed that the cortical vasodilation is mediated by activation of nonspecific thalamocortical projections arising from the medline thalamus, a region which receives monosynaptic projections from the DMRF (Iadecola et al. 1983b). This hypothesis is supported by the observation that stimulation of the intralaminar thalamus (parafascicular-centromedian complex) increases cortical CBF, an effect that is attenuated by acute adrenalectomy (Mraovitch et al. 1986). However, the increases in cortical CBF elicited by stimulation of the intralaminar nuclei differ from those elicited by the DMRF in that they are not associated with corresponding elevations in CGU (Mraovitch and Seylaz 1987). Thus, the DMRF and intralaminar thalamus may influence cortical CBF via different mechanisms. Nevertheless, considering that the DMRF projects directly to the midline thalamus and that the cortical metabolic activation elicited by DMRF stimulation involves predominantly lamina IV (Iadecola et al. 1983b), the possibility that thalamocortical projections participate in the response remains highly likely.

Local mechanisms of cerebrovasodilation. The mechanisms by which the plasma catecholamines participate in the adrenal-dependent component of the increases in CBF are poorly understood. It is well established that circulating catecholamines do not influence CBF and CGU as long as the blood-brain barrier (BBB) is intact [see Edvinsson and MacKenzie (1977) for review]. However, when the BBB is bypassed these substances can increased CBF by presumably increasing cerebral metabolic activity (Edvinsson et al. 1978). It is unlikely that plasma catecholamines enter the brain because of a gross disruption of the BBB occurring during DMRF stimulation, since the blood-brain transfer of aminoisobutyric acid, a nonspecific marker of BBB permeability, appears not to be increased during DMRF stimulation (Iadecola et al. 1987b). One possible explanation is that catecholamines act on brain sites that are devoid of BBB, such as the circumventricular organs. Coactivation of these sites by both catecholamines and DMRF stimulation would then mediate the increases in CBF via their efferent projections (Iadecola et al. 1987b).

The local mechanisms of the adrenal-independent component of the vasodilation in cerebral cortex also remain to be elucidated. In particular, whether the incoming pathways act directly on local blood vessels or whether there are local cortical neurons or astrocytes interposed remains to be established.

Cerebellar Fastigial Nucleus: An Intrinsic System for Primary Cholinergic Cerebrovasodilation

Electrical stimulation of the rostral pole of the FN in rat, as in other species, increases CBF globally [see Reis and Iadecola (1991) for references]. The increases are greatest in the cerebral cortex (up to 230% of control) and are mediated by central neural pathways (Nakai et al. 1982; Iadecola et al. 1983c, 1987a). In many regions of the brain, including mostly areas which do not receive direct (monosynaptic) projections from the FN such as the cerebral cortex and hippocampus, the increases in local CBF are not associated with an increase in CGU, as determined by the 2-deoxyglucose (2DG) method (Nakai et al. 1983). This phenomenon has been termed *primary vasodilatation* (Nakai et al. 1983) to emphasize its independence from local metabolism and is in contrast to the increases in CBF elicited from the DMRF which are a consequence of increased local metabolic activity *(secondary vasodilatation)* (Iadecola et al. 1983b). Furthermore, the cerebrovasodilation appears to be mediated via cholinergic mechanisms as it is globally abolished by systemic administration of the muscarinic cholinergic receptor antagonist atropine (Iadecola et al. 1986; Iadecola and Reis 1990).

Neural Pathways. The source and the precise course of the neural pathways mediating the cerebrovasodilation are now beginning to be elucidated (Iadecola et al. 1983c; Chida et al 1989, 1990). Recent studies have discovered that both the elevations in arterial pressure and CBF elicited from the FN originate not from local neurons in FN but from fibers passing through the area (Chida et al. 1986, 1989). The exact source of these neural processes remains unknown. Since lesions of the C1 area abolish the cerebrovasodilation, the axons mediating the response must involve both the FN and C1 (Chida et al. 1990). Thus, it has been proposed these processes could be collateral axons of neurons lying in the dorsolateral portion of the parabrachial nucleus of the pons (PBNd) (Fig. 1) (Chida et al. 1990). This hypothesis is supported by the following observations. First, this region is likely to be the site of origin of the pressor response elicited from the FN (Miura and Takayama 1988), which, in the medulla, shares its pathways with the cerebrovascular response (Chida et al. 1990). Second, neurons in this area tend to have divergent axon collaterals (Dietrichs 1985). Third, some neurons in PBNd are cholinergic (Armstrong et al. 1983). Fourth, stimulation within the PBNd produces global increases in CBF (Mraovitch et al. 1985). Interestingly, excitation of local neurons in FN was found to *decrease* CBF, an effect which is associated with a concomitant decrease in CGU (Chida et al. 1989). Thus, the FN is associated with two neural systems which can exert opposite influences on the cerebral circulation: a system for primary vasodilation and a system for secondary vasoconstriction.

The ascending neural pathways mediating the cerebrovasodilation elicited by FN stimulation have not been entirely clarified. A hypothetical model of these pathways is presented in Fig. 1. Since electrolytic lesions of the RVL abolish the cerebrovasodilation (Chida et al. 1990), it is likely that the pathways mediating the response terminate into or pass through the RVL (Fig. 1). Indeed excitation of RVL neurons increases CBF globally and independently of CGU (primary vasodilation), thereby resembling the vasodilation elicited from FN stimulation (Underwood 1988). Thus, RVL neurons may be involved in the response. However, the efferent projections of the RVL are restricted to selected brain stem nuclei and do not reach the cerebral cortex (Underwood 1988). Therefore, the projections mediating the global cerebrovasodilation are likely to be polysynaptic and, perhaps, involve the locus ceruleus (Fig. 1). This region is a likely candidate for the following reasons: (a) it receives a major input from the RVL (Ennis and Aston-Jones 1988, and (b) it has widespread efferent connections, including most regions of the cerebral cortex (Aston-Jones et al. 1986).

Fig. 1. Schematic representation of the possible neural pathways mediating the elevations in cerebral blood flow (CBF) elicited by electrical stimulation of the cerebellar fastigial nucleus (FN). The CBF response originates not from local FN neurons but from neural processes traversing the area. Evidence presented in the text suggest that these processes could be collateral branches of axons originating from an unknown brain stem site, possibly the dorsolateral portion of the parabrachial nucleus, and terminating within the FN. The pathways then involve the C1 area of the rostral ventrolateral medulla (RVL). Whether they terminate on neurons of the RVL or traverse the area is not known. It has been established that the pathways reach the cerebral cortex through the basal forebrain (BF). The pathways could reach the BF and the cerebral cortex via the widespread efferent connections of the locus ceruleus, a nucleus which receives a substantial projection from C1. Whether the pathways traverse the BF or whether they have synaptic contacts with the local BF neurons remains to be established. In the cerebral cortex the vasodilation is mediated by local neurons, possibly a restricted group of cortical interneurons

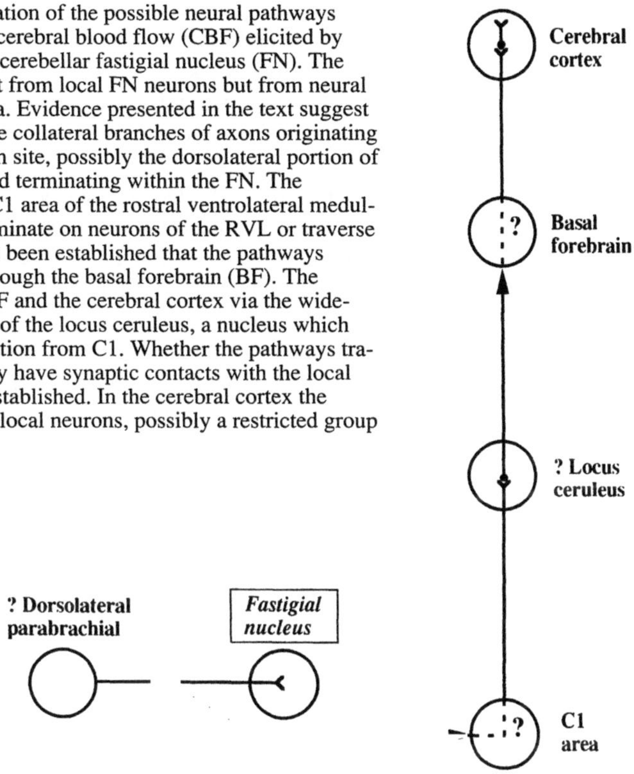

How do the cerebrovasodilatory pathways involving the FN reach the cerebral cortex? As stated above these are likely to be polysynaptic. It has been established that the pathways reach the cerebral cortex via the basal forebrain (BF) (Iadecola et al. 1983c) (Fig. 1). However, whether these axons have a synaptic connection with local BF neurons or whether they pass through the BF remains to be established. The question has been raised as to whether the basal forebrain cholinergic neurons participate in the cerebrovasodilation (Iadecola et al. 1983c). Indeed these neurons may have terminals closely associated with cortical microvessels (Eckenstein and Baughman 1984) and their activation releases acetylcholine (ACh) in cerebral cortex and increases cortical CBF (Arneric 1989; Biesold et al. 1989; Kurosawa et al. 1989a, b). Since the increases in CBF elicited by FN stimulation are also cholinergically mediated, it is conceivable that this pathway participates in the cortical cerebrovasodilation. However, whether the cholinergic neurons of the basal forebrain initiate the increases in cortical CBF elicited by FN stimulation remains to be demonstrated.

Local Mechanisms of Cortical Vasodilatation. In the cerebral cortex the increases in CBF are mediated by local neurons which, presumably, receive inputs from incoming axons originating or passing through the basal forebrain (Iadecola et al. 1987a). Indirect evidence suggests that these neurons are likely to be a restricted group. First, FN stimulation does not produce EEG changes consistent with widespread cortical activation (Iadecola et al. 1986, 1990; Arneric et al. 1987). Second, FN stimulation does not increase CGU in most cortical regions (Nakai et al. 1983). The latter observation indicates that these neurons and their processes are sparsely distributed throughout the cortex and/or that their number is small, so that their activation does not increase CGU as assessed by the 2DG method. Third, stimulation of the FN produces elevations in interstitial K^+ concentration that are restricted to selected cortical laminae (Iadecola and Kraig 1991). Since increases in interstitial K^+ usually reflect synaptic activity (Walz and Hertz 1983), the finding indicates that the cortical neural activity evoked by FN stimulation is highly restricted. Thus FN could activate a group of cortical neurons dedicated to the local regulation of blood flow.

The mechanisms whereby these neurons mediate the increase in cortical CBF have not been elucidated. Three possible models, not mutually exclusive, are illustrated in Fig. 2. First, local neurons may contact cerebral microvessels and release vasoactive transmitters directly into the perivascular space (possibility *1* in Fig. 2). Second, local neurons may influence cortical flow by releasing vasoactive factors into the interstitium (possibility *2* in Fig. 2). These factors would then reach the local microvasculature by simple diffusion determining the changes in flow. Third, vasoactive factors released from local neurons could be conveyed, or "siphoned," into the perivascular space through the astroglial end-feet. This possibility, indicated in Fig. 2 as "K^+ siphoning," is explained in greater detail below.

The recent observation that the increases in cortical CBF elicited by FN stimulation have a slow time course, reaching their peak in 50–60 s, indicates that the vasodilation

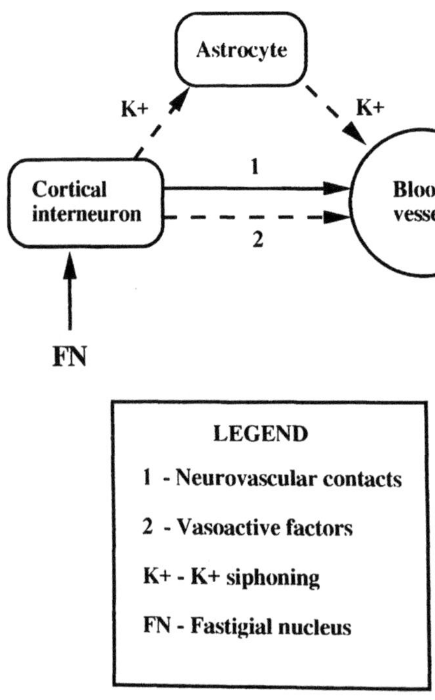

Fig. 2. Three hypothetical mechanisms mediating the local cortical vasodilation elicited by stimulation of the fastigial nucleus *(FN)*. First (possibility *1* in the figure), local cortical neurons could mediate the vasodilation via direct vascular projections onto blood vessels. Second (possibility *2*), these neurons could release vasoactive agents into the interstitial space. These agents (e.g., K^+, H^+, adenosine, nitric oxide, neurotransmitters, or neuropeptides) could then diffuse into the perivascular space and produce relaxation of vascular smooth muscles. Third (K^+ siphoning), K^+ ions and possibly other agents could act on local blood vessels through astrocytes. This possibility is explained in greater detail in the text

is likely to be mediated by the interstitial release of vasoactive factors rather than by direct neurovascular associations (Iadecola and Reis 1990). Since the cortical vasodilation is largely cholinergically mediated (Arneric et al. 1987) ACh could be one of the vasoactive factors involved. ACh could be released at the microvascular level from cholinergic interneurons (Eckenstein and Baughman 1984), or from endothelial cells (Parnavelas et al. 1985). ACh may act directly on vascular smooth muscles, by stimulating the production of the endothelium-derived relaxing factor (EDRF) (Furchgott and Zawadzky 1980; Ignarro 1989) (see below) or indirectly by promoting the release of another vasoactive substance, for example a peptide. In addition, vasoactive intestinal polypeptide (VIP), a potent cerebrovasodilator peptide colocalized with ACh in cortical interneurons (Eckenstein and Baughman 1984), could be coreleased and participate in the cerebrovasodilation.

Among the other diffusible vasoactive factors which may be released interstitially and participate in the vasodilatation are K^+ ions. K^+ is a powerful cerebrovasodilator at certain concentrations (Wahl 1985) and has long been considered to be involved in local blood flow regulation (Lou et al. 1987). That indeed K^+ may be involved in the increases in cortical CBF is suggested by the observation that FN stimulation increases cortical interstitial K^+ concentration (Iadecola and Kraig 1991). K^+ ions may influence vascular smooth muscles either directly or through intervening astroglia (Fig. 2). Astrocytes, which are responsible for the K^+ homeostasis in the extracellular space (ECS), could participate in this process by "siphoning" K^+ to the perivascular space (Paulson and Newman 1987). K^+ when released into the ECS by active neurons enters

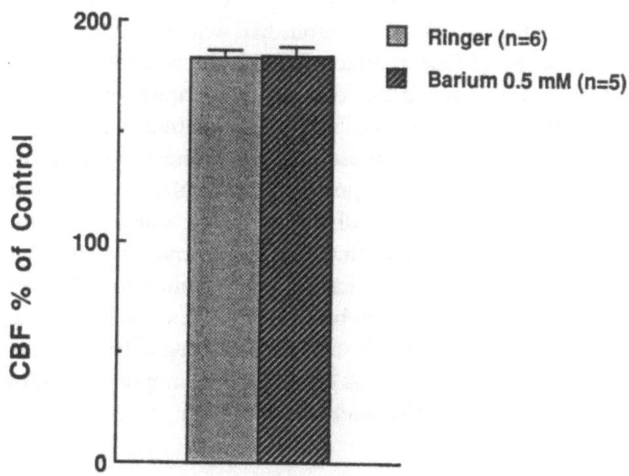

Fig. 3. Effect of the K^+ channel blocker barium chloride on the increases in cortical CBF elicited by FN stimulation. Rats were anesthetized with halothane (1–3%) and artificially ventilated. Blood gases were controlled. The FN was stimulated electrically (100 μA; 50 Hz; 1 s on/1 s off). To prevent the elevations in arterial pressure associated with FN stimulation, the spinal cord was transected at the first cervical segment and arterial pressure maintained by continuous infusion of phenylephrine. CBF was monitored continuously in parietal cortex by using a laser-doppler flowmeter. The site of CBF monitoring was superfused either with normal Ringer or with Ringer containing barium chloride (0.5 m*M*). Note that superfusion with barium did not affect the magnitude of the elevations in CBF elicited by FN stimulation ($p>0.05$; *t*-test)

into astrocytes and through an outward current is then redistributed to distant areas via the glial syncytium (spatial buffering). Since most of the K^+ conductance of astrocytes is located at the foot processes abutting the cerebral microvessels, the outward current carrying K^+ would flow out of the cell largely through the end-feet (*K^+ siphoning*). The perivascular K^+ concentration would thus increase, producing relaxation of the vascular smooth muscles. Since glial cells are functionally coupled with each other, focal K^+ changes produced by the local neurons could be spread out to involve larger cortical areas. Whether K^+ acts on vascular smooth muscles directly or through intervening astroglia is now being investigated. In preliminary experiments we have studied whether topical application barium chloride, a K^+ channel blocker that inhibits K^+ syphoning, influences the cortical vasodilation elicited by FN stimulation. As shown in Fig. 3, topical application of barium chloride does not affect the magnitude of the increases in CBF elicited by FN stimulation. Thus, these preliminary results do not support the hypothesis that K^+ syphoning participate in the cortical cerebrovasodilation. However, further studies will be required to establish this point more firmly.

Another powerful vasodilating agents that could be involved in the cerebrovasodilation is nitric oxide (NO). NO has many of the biological characteristics of EDRF and mediates the vascular dilatation elicited by ACh (Ignarro, 1989). Recent data suggest that NO plays an important role in CBF regulation as it participates in fundamental responses of the cerebral circulation such as the cerebrovasodilation elicited by hypercapnia (Iadecola, 1992). We have begun to investigate whether NO also participates in the increases in CBF elicited by FN stimulation (Iadecola, 1991). NO produces relaxation of vascular smooth muscles by stimulating soluble guanylyl cyclase (GC). We studied whether inhibition of GC by methylene blue (MB) attenuates the increases in CBF elicited by FN stimulation. MB was topically superfused on the parietal cortex and neocortical CBF monitored at the site of application by a laser-Doppler probe (see legend to Fig. 3 for further details). Application of MB (1 mM) dramatically attenuated the CBF increase elicited by FN stimulation (Fig. 4; $p < 0.01$). We next sought to determine whether inhibition of NO synthesis by L-nitroarginine (L-NA) would also affect the vasodilation. Application of L-NA (1 mM) attenuated the increases in CBF substantially ($p < 0.01$), while D-NA, the inactive stereoisomer of nitroarginine, had no effect (Fig. 4). These findings demonstrate that arginine-derived NO participates in the cerebrovasodilation elicited by FN stimulation. However, the cellular source(s) of NO and the site of the cerebral vasculature on which NO acts remain to be determined. These issues are currently being investigated. Irrespective of the source of NO, these findings support the notion that NO is an important biological mediator involved also in the regulation of the cerebral circulation.

Biological Significance

The biological significance of these neural networks is far from being clear. In contrast to the abundant data showing that activation of these pathways modulates CBF, little is known about their role in cerebrovascular regulation in physiological and pathological conditions. However, on the basis of some of the characteristics of the CBF changes elicited by excitation of these systems, some hypothesis about their functional role can be made.

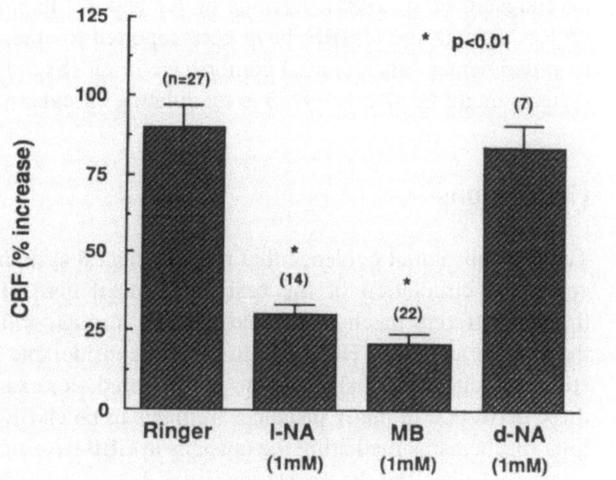

Fig. 4. Effect of L-nitroarginine (L-NA), D-nitroarginine (D-NA) or methylene blue (MB) on the increases in CBF elicited by FN stimulation in halothane anesthetized rat. A brief description of the methods is provided in the legend to figure 3. During superfusion with Ringer FN stimulation increased CBF by about 90%. Superfusion with L-NA or MB attenuated the CBF increases substantially ($p < 0.01$; analysis of variance and Tukey's test). In contrast, D-NA, the inactive stereoisomer of L-NA, had no effect on the response ($p > 0.05$)

Fastigial Nucleus

The role of the FN in the regulation of CBF has not been investigated systematically. However, the FN has little or no role in the maintenance of resting CBF (Chida et al. 1989). The initial suggestion that FN may be involved in rapid, "anticipatory" increases in CBF designed to increase delivery of substrates in preparation for brain activation (Nakai et al. 1983) seems less plausible in view of the slow time course of the vasodilation (Iadecola and Reis 1990). Furthermore, the global character of the cerebrovasodilation suggests that this system is unlikely to participate in the regulation of CBF when the changes in flow are anatomically restricted. However, the FN might be involved in situations in which CBF changes in a more diffuse and stereotyped fashion, such as during anxiety (Reiman et al. 1989), exercise (Thomas et al. 1989), or sleep (Sawaya and Ingvar 1989). Recent studies suggest that the FN may also play a role in the reaction of the brain to injury. Electrical stimulation of the FN reduces by about 40% the size of the infarct resulting from occlusion of the middle cerebral artery in rat (Reis et al. 1989). Thus, this network is able to protect the brain from cerebral ischemia. Whether this protective effect is a consequence of the increase in cortical CBF or whether it is due to the local release of endogenous protective agents remains to be established.

Dorsal Medullary Reticular Formation

As discussed above, this system is able to influence the metabolism of the entire neuraxis through neural and humoral factors. Similar widespread metabolic effects that are in part mediated by adrenal catecholamines have been reported during stress and hypoglycemia (Bryan 1990). Therefore it has been proposed that the DMRF may represent the neural substrate through which these effects are mediated (Iadecola et al. 1987b; Bryan 1990). That intrinsic neural pathways associated with the DMRF may also participate in the vasospasm after subarachnoid hemorrhage has also been suggested

(Svendgaard et al. 1985). Lesions of A1 and A2 monoaminergic cell groups, which project through the DMRF, have been reported to attenuate the vasospasm secondary to experimental subarachnoid hemorrhage in rat (Svendgaard et al. 1985). Thus, these systems might be also involved in modulating vascular tone in pathological conditions.

Conclusions

There is substantial evidence that intrinsic neural system can exert a powerful influence on the circulation of the brain and spinal cord. These systems modulate CBF through different mechanisms and they act through widespread networks that involve the brain at all levels. However, in spite of considerable progress in this field, there are still many questions that remain to be answered. For example, the chemical anatomy of these networks, in many instances, remains to be clarified. Furthermore, the local cellular mechanisms mediating the changes in CBF have not been fully elucidated. In particular, whether the "close associations" between neurons and cerebral microvessels represent a true neurovascular effector system or whether nonneuronal cells, such as astroglia, endothelium, and pericytes, participate in regulating microvascular tone remains to be established. Also, the mechanisms by which intrinsic networks gate circulating catecholamines and other humoral factors through the BBB to control cerebral metabolism remains to be elucidated. Finally and most importantly, the biological significance of these networks and the specific role that they play in the complex mechanisms regulating brain function remains obscure. Further studies will be necessary to answer these challenging questions.

Supported by Grants-in-Aid by the American Heart Association (Minnesota) and the Minnesota Medical Foundation.

References

Aoki C, Pickel VM (1989) Neuropeptide Y in the cerebral cortex and the caudate-putamen nuclei: ultrastructural basis for interactions with GABAergic and non-GABAergic neurons. Neurosci 9(12):4333–4354

Armstrong D (1986) Ultrastructural characterization of choline acetyltransferase-containing neurons in the basal forebrain of rat: evidence for a cholinergic innervation of intracerebral blood vessels. J Comp Neurol 250:81–92

Armstrong D, Saper C, Levey A, Wainer B, Terry R (1983) Distribution of cholinergic neurons in rat brain: demonstrated by the immunocytochemical localization of choline acetyltransferase. J Comp Neurol 216:53–68

Arneric S (1989) Basal forebrain neurons modulate cortical blood flow: increases by nicotinic cholinergic mechanisms. J Cereb Blood Flow Metab [Suppl 1] 9:S502

Arneric S, Iadecola C, Underwood M, Reis D (1987) Local cholinergic mechanisms participate in the increase in cortical cerebral blood flow elicited by electrical stimulation of the fastigial nucleus in rat. Brain Res 411:212-225

Aston-Jones G, Ennis M, Pieribone V, Nickell W, Shipley M (1986) The brain nucleus locus coeruleus: restricted afferent control of a broad efferent network. Science 234:734–737

Bayliss W, Hill L (1895) On intracranial pressure and the cerebral circulation. J Physiol (Lond) 18:334–362

Biesold D, Inanami O, Sato A, Sato Y (1989) Stimulation of the nucleus basalis of Meynert increases cerebral cortical blood flow in rats. Neurosci Lett 98:39–44

Bryan R JR (1990) Cerebral blood flow and energy metabolism during stress. Am J Physiol 259:H269–H280

Chida K, Iadecola C, Reis DJ (1990) Lesions of rostral ventrolateral medulla abolish some cardio- and cerebrovascular components of the cerebellar pressor and depressor responses. Brain Res 508:93–104

Chida K, Iadecola C, Reis JD (1989) Global reduction in cerebral blood flow and metabolism elicited from intrinsic neurons of fastigial nucleus. Brain Res 500:177–192

Chida K, Iadecola C, Underwood M, Reis D (1986) A novel vasodepressor response elicited from the rat cerebellar fastigial nucleus: the fastigial depressor response. Brain Res 370:378–382

Cobb S (1938) Cerebral circulation. Res Publ Assoc Res Nerv Ment Dis 18:719–752

Dietrichs E (1985) Divergent axon collaterals to cerebellum and amygdala from neurons in the parabrachial nucleus, the nucleus locus coeruleus and some adjacent nuclei. A fluorescent double label study using rhodamine labelled latex and fast blue as retrograde tracers. Anat Embryol (Berl) 172:375–382

Donders F (1849) De bewegingen der hersenen en de veranderingen der vaatvulling van de pia mater, ook bij gesloten onuitzet-beren schedel regtstreeks onderzocht. Onderzoek Ged Inh Physiol Lab Utrecht Hoogeoch 2:97–128

Eckenstein F, Baughman R (1984) Two types of cholinergic innervation in the cortex, one colocalized with vasoactive intestinal polypeptide. Nature 309:153–155

Edvinsson L, MacKenzie E (1977) Amine mechanisms in the cerebral circulation. Pharmacol Rev 28:275–348

Edvinsson L, Hardebo J, MacKenzie E, Owman C (1978) Effect of exogenous noradrenaline on local cerebral blood flow after osmotic opening of the blood-brain barrier in the rat. J Physiol (Lond) 274:149–156

Ennis M, Aston-Jones G (1988) Activation of locus coeruleus from nucleus paragigantocellularis: a new excitatory amino acid pathway in brain. J Neurosci 8:3644–3657

Friedland R, Iadecola C (1991) Roy and Sherrington (1890) A centennial reexamination of "On the regulation of the blood-supply of the brain". Neurology 41:10–14

Frostig RD, Lieke EE, Ts'o DY, Grinvald A (1990) Cortical function architecture and local coupling between neuronal activity and the microcirculation revealed by in vivo high-resolution optical imaging of intrinsic signals. Proc Natl Acad Sci USA 87:6082–6086

Furchgott R, Zawadzky J (1980) The obligatory role of endothelial cells in the relaxation of arterial smooth muscles by acetylcholine. Nature 228:373–376

Goadsby P, Lance J (1988) Brain stem effects on intra- and extracerebral circulations. Relation to migraine and cluster headache. In: Olesen J, Edvinsson L (eds) Basic mechanisms of headache. Elsevier, Amsterdam, pp 413–427

Greenberg J (1979) Localized metabolic-flow couple during functional activity. Acta Neurol Scand 72:12–13

Harik SI (1984) Neurotransmitter receptors in cerebral microvessels. In: MacKenzie ET, Seylaz J, Bes A (eds) Neurotransmitters and the cerebral circulation. Raven, New York, pp 1–7

Heistad D, Kontos H (1983) Cerebral circulation. In: Abbound F, Shephard J (eds) Handbook of physiology: the cardiovascular system. American Physiological Society, Bethesda, pp 137–182

Heistad D, Marcus M (1978) Evidence that neural mechanisms do not have important effects on cerebral blood flow. Circ Res 42:295–302

Hendry S, Jones, E, Beinfeld M (1983) Cholecystokinin-immunoreactive neurons in rat and monkey cerebral cortex make symmetric synapses and have intimate association with blood vessels. Proc Natl Acad Sci USA 80:2400–2404

Hill L (1896) The physiology and pathology of the cerebral circulation: an experimental research. Churchill, London.

Hökfelt T, Fuxe K, Goldstein M, Johansson O (1974) Immunohistochemical evidence for the existence of adrenaline neurons in rat brain. Brain Res 66:235–251

Iadecola C (1991) EDRF participates in the neocortical vasodilation elicited by stimulation of the fastigial nucleus. Soc Neurosci Abstr 17, 27

Iadecola C (1992) Does nitric oxide mediate the cerebrovasodilation elicited by hypercapnia? Proc Natl Acad Sci USA (in press)
Iadecola C, Kraig RP (1991) Focal elevations in neocortical interstitial K^+ produced by stimulation of the fastigial nucleus in rat. Brain Res 563: 273–277
Iadecola C, Raichle ME (1992) Local regulation of the cerebral microcirculation: toward a neurobiological understanding. Trends Neurosci (in press)
Iadecola C, Reis DJ (1990) Continuous monitoring of cerebrocortical blood flow during stimulation of the cerebellar fastigial nucleus: a study by laser-Doppler flowmetry. J Cereb Blood Flow Metab 10:608–617
Iadecola C, Nakai M, Arbit E, Reis D (1983a) Global cerebral vasodilation elicited by focal electrical stimulation within the dorsal medullary reticular formation in anesthetized rat. J Cereb Blood Flow Metab 3:270–279
Iadecola C, Nakai M, Mraovitch S, Ruggiero DA, Tucker LW, Reis DJ (1983b) Global increase in cerebral metabolism and blood flow produced by focal electrical stimulation of dorsal medullary reticular formation in rat. Brain Res 272:101–114
Iadecola C, Mraovitch S, Meeley M, Reis D (1983c) Lesions of the basal forebrain in rat selectively impair the cortical vasodilation elicited from cerebellar fastigial nucleus. Brain Res 279:41–52
Iadecola C, Underwood M, Reis D (1986) Muscarinic cholinergic receptors mediate the cerebrovasodilation elicited by stimulation of the cerebellar fastigial nucleus in rat. Brain Res 368:375–379
Iadecola C, Arneric S, Baker H, Tucker L, Reis D (1987a) Role of local neurons in the cerebrocortical vasodilation elicited from cerebellum. Am J Physiol 252:R1082–R1091
Iadecola C, Lacombe P, Ishitsuka T, Underwood M, Reis D (1987b) Role of adrenal catecholamines in the cerebrovasodilation evoked from the brain stem. Am J Physiol 252:H1183–H1191
Iadecola C, Chida K, Lacombe P, Underwood M, Sved A, Reis D (1987c) Adrenal catecholamines participate in the cerebrovasodilation elicited from the dorsal medullary reticular formation by increasing cerebral metabolism. J Cereb Blood Flow Metab 7:S281
Iadecola C, Chida K, Lacombe PM, Underwood MD, Reis DJ (1989) Global increase in spinal cord blood flow elicited from the dorsal medullary reticular formation in rat. J Cereb Blood Flow Metab 9:S480
Iadecola C, Springston ME, Reis DJ (1990) Dissociation by chloralose of the cerebrovascular and cardiovascular responses evoked from the cerebellar fastigial nucleus. J Cereb Blood Flow Metab 10:375–382
Ignarro LJ (1989) Biological actions and properties of endothelium-derived nitric oxide formed and released from artery and vein. Circ Res 65:1–21
Itakura T, Yamamoto K, Tohyama M, Shimuzu N (1977) Central dual innervation of arterioles and capillaries in the brain. Stroke 8:360–365
Kapadia SE, de Lanerolle NC (1984) Immunohistochemical and electron microscopic demonstration of vascular innervation in the mammalian brain stem. Brain Res 292:33–39
Kurosawa M, Sato A, Sato Y (1989a) Stimulation of the nucleus basalis of Meynert increases acetylcholine release in the cerebral cortex in rats. Neurosci Lett 98:45–50
Kurosawa M, Sato A, Sato Y (1989b) Well-maintained responses of acetylcholine release and blood flow in the cerebral cortex to focal electrical stimulation of the nucleus basalis of Meynert in aged rats. Neurosci Lett 100:198–202
Kuschinsky W, Wahl M (1978) Local chemical and neurogenic regulation of cerebral vascular resistance. Physiol Rev 58(3):656–689
Lacombe PM, Iadecola C, Underwood MD, Sved AF, Reis DJ (1990) Plasma epinephrine modulates cerebrovasodilation evoked from brain stem. Brain Res 506:93–100
Leniger-Follert E, Hossmann KA (1979) Simultaneous measurement of microflow and evoked potentials in the somato-motor cortex of the cat during specific sensory activation. Pflugers Arch 380:85–89
Lou HC, Edvinsson L, MacKenzie ET (1987) The concept of coupling blood flow to brain function: revision required? Ann Neurol 22:289–297
MacKenzie ET, Scatton B (1987) Cerebral circulatory and metabolic effects of perivascular neurotransmitters. CRC Crit Rev Clin Neurobiol 2:357–419

McCulloch J, Uddmann R, Kingman T, Edvinsson L (1986) Calcitonin gene-related peptide: functional role in cerebrovascular regulation: Proc Natl Acad Sci USA 83:5731–5735
Milner TA, Pickel VM, Park DH, Joh TH, Reis DJ (1987) Phenylethanolamine *N*-methyltransferase-containing neurons in the rostral ventrolateral medulla of the rat. I. Normal ultrastructure. Brain Res 411:28–45
Miura M, Takayama K (1988) The site of origin of the so-called fastigial pressor response. Brain Res 473:352–358
Moskalenko Y (1975) Regional cerebral blood flow and its control during increased functional activity. In: Ingvar D, Lassen N (eds) Brain work. The coupling of function, metabolism and blood flow in the brain. Munksgaard, Copenhagen, pp 343–352
Moskowitz M (1984) The neurobiology of vascular head pain. Ann Neurol 16:157–168
Moskowitz M (1986) The anatomy and neurochemistry of trigeminovascular neurons. In: Owman C, Hardebo J (eds) Neural regulation of brain circulation. Elsevier, Amsterdam, pp 393–405
Mosso A (1881) Ueber den Kreislauf des Blutes im menschlichen Gehirn. Veit, Leipzig
Mraovitch S, Seylaz J (1987) Metabolism-independent cerebral vasodilation elicited by electrical stimulation of the centromedian-parafascicular complex in rat. Neurosci Lett 83:269–274
Mraovitch S, Iadecola C, Ruggiero D, Reis D (1985) Widespread reduction in cerebral blood flow and metabolism elicited by electrical stimulation of the parabrachial nucleus in rat. Brain Res 341:283–296
Mraovitch S, Lasbennes F, Calando Y, Seylaz J (1986) Cerebrovascular changes elicited by electrical stimulation of the centromedian-parafascicular complex in rat. Brain Res 380:42–53
Nakai M, Iadecola C, Reis D (1982) Global cerebral vasodilation by stimulation of rat fastigial cerebellar nucleus. Am J Physiol 243:H226–H235
Nakai M, Iadecola C, Ruggiero D, Tucker L, Reis D (1983) Electrical stimulation of cerebellar fastigial nucleus increases cerebrocortical blood flow without change in local metabolism: evidence for an intrinsic system in brain for primary vasodilation. Brain Res. 260:35–49
Nielsen K, Owman C, Sporrong B (1971) Ultrastructure of the autonomic innervation apparatus in the main pial arteries of rats and cats. Brain Res 27:25–32
Obata-Tsuto H, Tsuto T, Okamura H, Kubo T, Fukui F, Yanaihara N, Ibata Y (1984) The fine structures of the VIP-like immunoreactive neurons in the cat hypothalamus. Brain Res Bull 12:315–321
Olesen J (1971) Contralateral focal increase of cerebral blood flow in man during arm work. Brain 94:635–646
Owman C (1990) Peptidergic vasodilator nerves in the peripheral circulation and in the vascular beds of the heart and brain. Blood Vessels 27:73–93
Papadopoulos G, Parnavelas J, Buijs R (1989) Light and electron microscopic immunocytochemical analysis of the noradrenaline innervation of the rat visual cortex. J Neurocytol 18:1–10
Parnavelas J, Kelley W, Burnstock G (1985) Ultrastructural localization of choline acetyltransferase in vascular endothelial cells in rat brain. Nature 316:724–725
Paulson OB, Newman EA (1987) Does the release of potassium from astrocyte endfeet regulate cerebral blood flow? Science 237:896–898
Purves M (1972) The physiology of the cerebral circulation. Cambridge University Press, Cambridge
Reiman E, Fusselman M, Fox P, Raichle M (1989) Neuroanatomical correlates of anticipatory anxiety. Science 243:1071–1074
Reis D (1984) Central neural control of cerebral circulation and metabolism. In: MacKenzie ET, Seylaz J, Bes A (eds) Neurotransmitters and the cerebral circulation. Raven, New York, pp 91–119
Reis D, Iadecola C (1991) Intrinsic central regulation of cerebral blood flow and metabolism in relation to volume transmission. In: Fuxe K, Agnati L (eds) Volume transmission in the brain. Raven, New York, pp 523–538
Reis D, Underwood MD, Berger SB, Kayata M, Zaiens N III (1989) Fastigial nucleus stimulation reduces the volume of cerebral infarction produced by occlusion of the middle cerebral artery in rat. In: Seylaz J, MacKenzie ET (eds) Neurotransmission and cerebrovascular function I. Elsevier, Amsterdam, pp 401–404

Rennels M, Nelson E (1975) Capillary innervation in the mammalian central nervous system: an electron microscope demonstration (1). Am J Anat 144:233–241
Rosenblum W (1965) Cerebral microcirculation: a review emphasizing the interrelationship of local blood flow and neuronal function. Angiology 16:485–507
Roy C, Sherrington C (1890) On the regulation of the blood-supply of the brain. J Physiol (Lond) 11:85–108
Ruggiero D, Cravo S, Arango V, Reis D (1989) Central control of the circulation by the rostral ventrolateral reticular nucleus: anatomical substrates: In: Ciriello J, Caverson M, Polosa C (eds) Progress in brain research. Elsevier, Amsterdam, pp 49–79
Sakas D, Moskowitz M, Wei E, Kontos H, Kano M, Ogilvy C (1989) Trigeminovascular fibers increase blood flow in cortical gray matter by axon reflex-like mechanisms during acute severe hypertension. Proc Natl Acad Sci USA 86:1401–1405
Sawaya R, Ingvar DH (1989) Cerebral blood flow and metabolism in sleep. Acta Neurol Scand 80:481–491
Schmidt C (1950) The cerebral circulation in health and disease. Thomas, Springfield
Schmidt C, Hendrix J (1938) Action of chemical substances on cerebral blood vessels. Res Publ Assoc Res Nerv Ment Dis 18:229-276
Seylaz J, Pinard E, Mraovitch S (1986) Influence of specific intracerebral structures on the regulation of cerebral circulation. In: Owman C, Hardebo J (eds) Neural regulation of brain circulation. Elsevier, Amsterdam, pp 148–167
Sokoloff L (1959) The action of drugs on the cerebral circulation. Pharmacol Rev 11:1–85
Svendgaard N, Brismar J, Delgado T, Rosengren E (1985) Subarachnoid haemorrhage in the rat: effect on the development of vasospasm of selective lesions of the catecholamine systems in the lower brain stem. Stroke 16:602–608
Swanson L, Connelly M, Hartman B (1977) Ultrastructural evidence for central monoaminergic innervation of blood vessels in the paraventricular nucleus of the hypothalamus. Brain Res 136:166–173
Thomas SN, Schroeder T, Secher NH, Mitchell JH (1989) Cerebral blood flow during submaximal and maximal dynamic exercise in humans. J Appl Physiol 67(2):744–748
Uddman R, Edvinsson L (1989) Neuropeptides in the cerebral circulation. Cerebrovasc Brain Metab Rev 1:230–252
Underwood M (1988) Control of the cerebral circulation and metabolism by the rostral ventrolateral medulla: possible role in the cerebrovascular response to hypoxia. PhD Dissertation, Cornell University, New York
Wahl M (1985) Local chemical, neural, and humoral regulation of the cerebrovascular resistance vessels. J Cardiovasc Pharmacol [Suppl 3] 7:S36–S46
Walz W, Hertz L (1983) Functional interactions between neurons and astrocytes. II. Potassium homeostasis at the cellular level. Prog Neurobiol 20:133–183

Endothelium-Dependent Relaxations and Concentrations: Their Physiology in the Cerebral Arteries and Pathology in Experimental Cerebral Vasospasm

P. KIM

The physiological control and pathological alterations of the cerebral circulation are still not fully understood. Mechanisms underlying well-known phenomena such as pressure autoregulation, adjustment with metabolic demand, and chronic arterial spasm have not been fully explained. In the past decade, the physiology and pharmacology of blood vessels have been dramatically revised with new concepts. One of the major breakthroughs in this respect is undoubtedly the recognition of the interaction between the endothelium and the smooth muscle (Fig. 1). Endothelium works not simply as a selective barrier, but modifies the tone of the underlying smooth muscle in response to chemical and physical signals in the blood stream. The location of endothelium is certainly most advantageous for this function. The specific mode of signal transduction from endothelium to smooth muscle has been studied extensively, is now being observed

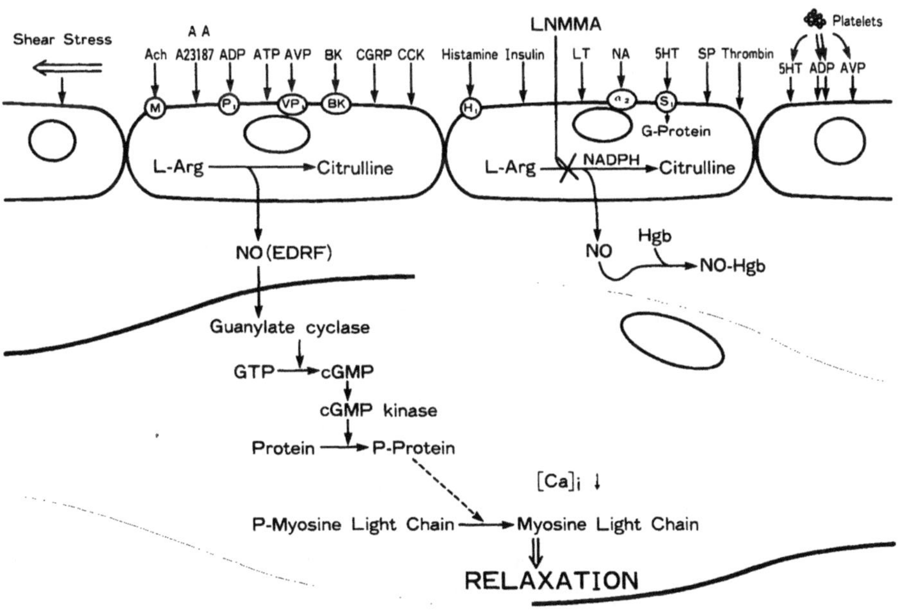

Fig. 1. Summary of the signal transduction from endothelial cells *(above)* to smooth muscle *(below)* in endothelium-dependent relaxations. (With permission, Kim and Vanhoutte 1990)

outside blood vessels, and may open new vistas in general physiology. In the present chapter, current knowledge concerning endothelium-dependent relaxations and contractions is reviewed, and our findings in the cerebral arteries and alterations in experimental cerebral vasospasm are summarized.

Endothelium-Dependent Relaxations

Furchgott and Zawadzki (1980) first described the obligatory role of endothelium in vascular relaxations. Its presence was mandatory for isolated arterial preparation for relaxation in response to acetylcholine. The discovery reconciled the previous enigmatic discrepancy between responses to acetylcholine recorded in vitro and those observed in vivo. Endothelium dependency was soon recognized in the actions of other various physiological substances, such as arachidonic acid, ATP, ADP, argine vasopressin, bradykinin, calcitonin gene-related peptide, cholecystokinin, histamine, insulin, leukotrienes, norepinephrine, serotonin, substance P, and thrombin (for review see Furchgott and Vanhoutte 1989). The phenomenon was first studied in the isolated arterial preparations but subsequently its importance was demonstrated in intract animals; endothelium-dependent vasodilatation in response to acetylcholine and substance P was observed in the femoral artery of dog using sonometry (Angus et al. 1983); acetylcholine and bradykinin caused endothelium-dependent relaxations in mouse pial arterioles in vivo (Rosenblum 1986); release of a diffusible relaxing factor from the cortical vessels was demonstrated in the cranial window in cats (Kontos et al. 1988); and an increase in the intraluminal flow caused endothelium-dependent relaxations of the coronary artery in conscious dogs (Holtz et al. 1984).

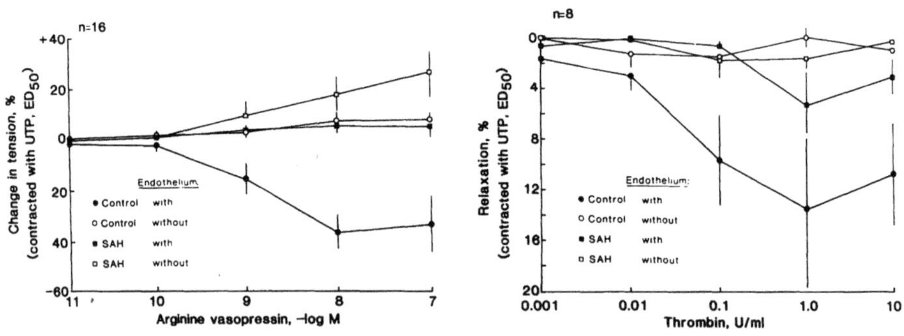

Fig. 2. Concentration-response curve of arginine vasopressin *(left)* and thrombin *(right)* in canine basilar arteries with and without endothelium. The arterial rings were contracted with individual ED_{50} of uridine triphosphate *(UTP)*. The relaxations were expressed as percentages of the maximal relaxations to papaverine. In the control groups, relaxations were observed in rings with endothelium but not in those without (endothelium dependent). The relaxations were significantly impaired in the subarachnoid hemorrhage group. Values shown are means ± SEMs for 16 (arginine vasopressin) and 8 (thrombin) specimens, 2 preparations from each of 8 animals. (With permission, Kim et al. 1988)

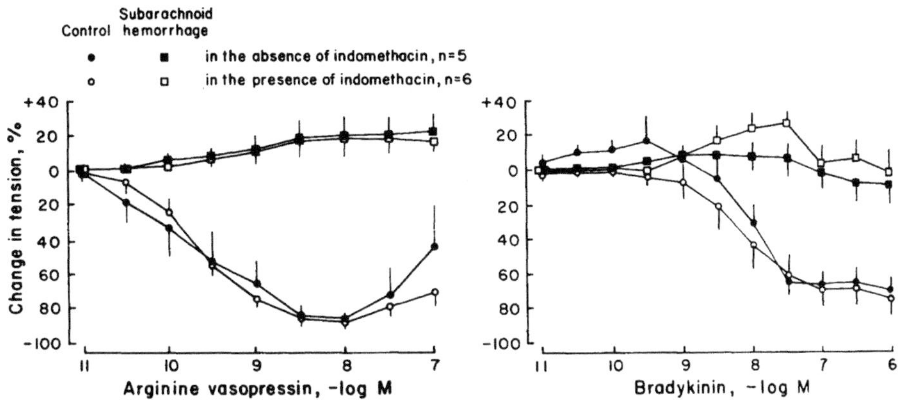

Fig. 3. Endothelium-dependent response in the absence and presence of indomethacin responses to arginine vasopressin *(left)* and bradykinin *(right)* of canine basilar artery with endothelium. The arterial rings were contracted with uridine triphosphate ($3x10^{-6}M$). Responses are expressed as percentages of the maximal relaxation of each ring to papaverine ($10^{-4}M$). (With permission, Kim et al. 1989, Figs. 3, 5, 6)

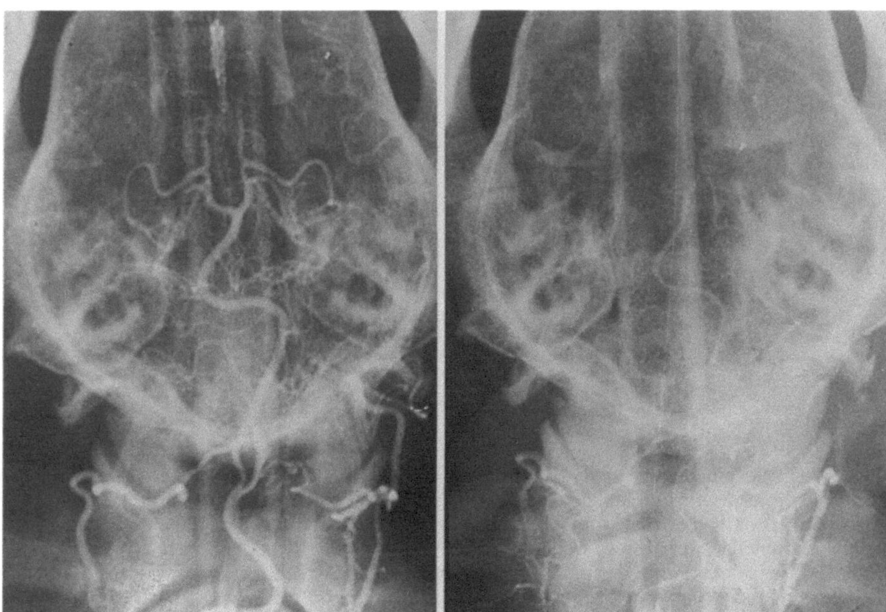

Fig. 4. Angiograms of the canine basilar artery, taken prior to injections of autologous blood *(left)* and 7 days after the initial injection *(right)*

Endothelium-dependent relaxations were elicited in the isolated canine basilar artery by arginine vasopressin, thrombin, and bradykinin (Figs. 2, 3) (Katusic et al. 1984; Kim et al. 1988). The relaxations were not affected by the presence of indomethacin, indicating vasodilator prostanoids are not involved in the responses (Fig. 3) (Kim et al. 1989). Chronic vasospasm of the canine basilar artery was induced by two injections of autologous blood (8–12 ml) into the cisterna magna (Fig. 4). In the spastic basilar arteries obtained 8 days after the subarachnoid hemorrhage, endothelium-dependent relaxations were abolished (Kim et al. 1988).

Release of the Relaxing Factor EDRF

Diffusion of a vasodilatory substance from the endothelium was first demonstrated by a "sandwich" experiment; relaxations were restored by reconstituting the contact between detached layers of the intima and the media (Furchgott and Zawadzki 1980). The substance was named endothelium-derived relaxing factor (EDRF) (Furchgott 1983). Release of EDRF from a segment of intact artery (Griffith et al. 1984; Rubanyi et al. 1985) or cultured endothelial cells (Cocks et al. 1985) was demonstrated by bioassays, where the activity of EDRF was detected by relaxations of the arterial strips free of endothelium. EDRF is spontaneously released without stimulation ("basal release") and a larger amount is released upon stimulation by vasodilator agonists. The factor

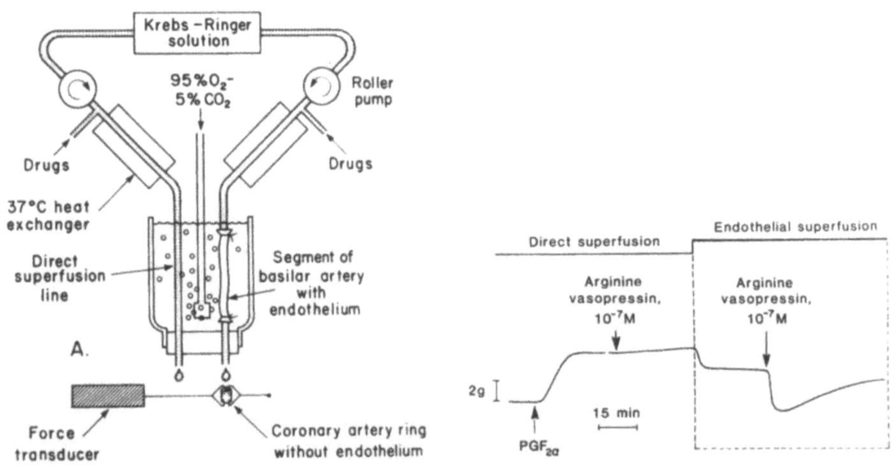

Fig. 5. *Left:* Schematic representation of the bioassay system for analysis of EDRF released from the basilar artery. Drugs to induce release of the factor were injected upstream of the arterial segment. Effects of the perfusate through a metal line (direct superfusion) and that through the intact artery (endothelial superfusion) were compared.
Right: A typical recording during a bioassay experiment. A coronary artery ring without endothelium (bioassay ring) was contracted with prostaglandin F_{2a} ($4\times10^{-6}M$). When the contraction reached a plateau, arginine vasopressin was given during direct superfusion. After the perfusion was switched to the arterial line (endothelial superfusion), arginine vasopressin was added to the perfusate upstream of the basilar artery.

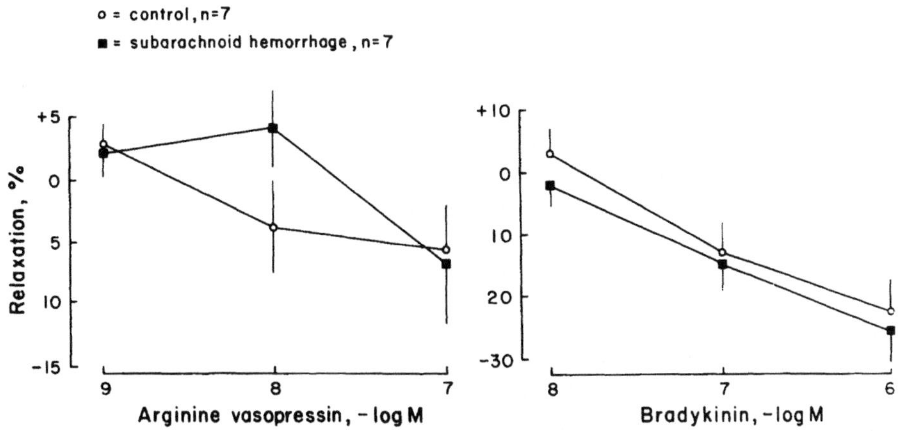

Fig. 6. Release of EDRF from the canine basilar arteries measured under the bioassay conditions. The relaxations of the bioassay ring are expressed as percentages of the response to sodium nitroprusside ($10^{-6}M$).

has very short half-life in the bioassay conditions, as demonstrated by changing the transit time of the perfusion pathway, and is susceptible to oxidation and protected by superoxide dismutase (Rubanyi and Vanhoutte 1986).

Release of EDRF from the canine basilar artery was measured by a bioassay setup using coronary artery without endothelium as the detector tissue (Kim et al. 1989) (Fig. 5, left). A generous amount of basal release was observed, as well as an induced release in response to bradykinin and arginine vasopressin (Fig 5, right). The release of the factor was concentration-dependent on the agonists. Contrary to our expectation, the release was not impaired in the basilar arteries in chronic vasospasm (Fig. 6).

Formation of Cyclic GMP and Effect of Hemoglobin

The effect of EDRF is mediated by the activation of guanylate cyclase and formation of cyclic GMP (Rapoport and Murad 1983; Diamond and Chu 1983; Furchgott et al. 1984; Ignarro et al. 1984). Nitrovasodilators such as sodium nitroprusside and glyceryl trinitrate had been known to activate the enzyme of vascular smooth muscle (Schultz et al. 1977). The relaxations caused by EDRF and nitrovasodilators are commonly blocked by oxyhemoglobin and methylene blue (Murad et al. 1978; Martin et al. 1985). The heme moiety of guanylate cyclase has a high affinity to nitric oxide and the binding increases the activity of the enzyme (Murad et al. 1978). Hemoglobin in the ferrous form (oxygemoglobin) competes for EDRF with guanylate cyclase and blocks endothelium-dependent relaxations. It also binds with nitric oxide (Gibson and Roughton 1957), which is probably the reactive intermediate of the nitrovasodilators, and thus inhibits relaxations to the group of agents. Methylene blue oxidizes guanylate cyclase and inhibits relaxations (Ignarro et al. 1984; Martin et al. 1985). The mechanisms of the cyclic GMP causing relaxations in the smooth muscle are not yet fully understood. Cyclic GMP-dependent protein kinase is activated and may cause a cascade of changes in protein phosphorylation, resulting in dephosphorylation of myosin light chain and thus leading to relaxation (Rapoport et al. 1983). There are reports of suppression of intracellular Ca^{2+} by cyclic GMP; it increases Ca^{2+} extrusion by activation of Ca^{2+} ATPase (Itoh et al. 1985; Rashatwar et al. 1987), decreases membrane influx of Ca^{2+}, and inhibits intracellular Ca^{2+} release (Collins et al. 1986; Twort and van Breemen 1988); hydrolysis of phosphatidylinositol, which causes Ca^{2+} mobilization subsequent to agonist-receptor binding, is also reduced by cyclic GMP (Rapoport 1986).

In the canine basilar artery, cyclic GMP content was measured using radioimmunoassay (Kim et al. 1992). Levels of cyclic GMP were higher in rings with endothelium than in those without (Table 1), reflecting the effect of basal release of EDRF. A potent increase in the levels of cyclic GMP was observed in response to EDRF relea-

Table 1. Basal levels of cyclic GMP in rings with and without endothelium of the canine basilar artery

Endothelium	With	Without
Cyclic GMP (pmol/mg protein)		
Control	13.6	1.6
SAH	5.3	1.5

SAH, subarachnoid hemorrhage

Table 2. Cyclic GMP formation induced by bradykinin ($10^{-7}M$, rings with endothelium) in the canine basilar artery

Incubation time	0 s	60 s	120s
Cyclic GMP (pmol/mg protein)			
Control	13.6	59.7	41.2
SAH	5.3	32.1	20.1

SAH, subarachnoid hemorrhage

Table 3. Responses of cGMP evoked by NO ($10^{-6}M$, rings without endothelium) in the canine basilar artery

Incubation time	0 s	60 s	120s
Cyclic GMP (pmol/mg protein)			
Control	1.6	99	5.7
SAH	1.5	24	8.9

SAH, subarachnoid hemorrhage

sed by stimulation with bradykinin (Table 2), as well as to authentic nitric oxide (Table 3). In the spastic canine basilar artery after subarachnoid hemorrhage, the formation of cyclic GMP was significantly impaired. A membrane-permeable cyclic GMP analogue, 8-Br-cyclic GMP, caused comparable relaxations in the arteries of the control and subarachnoid hemorrhage groups (Kim et al. 1992).

Identity of EDRF: Nitric Oxide

The common characteristics shared by relaxations to nitrovasodilators and those mediated by endothelium lead to the speculation that the reactive intermediate of the nitrovasodilators, nitric oxide (NO), is likely to be EDRF (Furchgott 1988; Ignarro et al. 1988). The short half-life, action of activating guanylate cyclase, inactivation by ferrous hemoglobin, sensitivity to superoxide, and protection by superoxide dismutase are all shared between the two. Measurement of chemiluminescence generated in reaction with ozone demonstrated release of NO in the perfusate of cultured endothelial cells when stimulated by bradykinin (Palmer et al. 1987), presenting direct evidence for the identity of EDRF as NO. Absorbance of hemoglobin combined with EDRF showed an identical pattern to that of hemoglobin combined with NO (Ignarro et al. 1987). Recent studies by the group of Moncada et al. showed NO is derived from L-arginine (Palmer et al. 1988a). Release of EDRF/NO was enhanced by infusion of L-arginine but not D-arginine. Treatment with *N*-monomethyl-L-arginine (LNMMA), which replaces the L-arginine pool competitively, inhibited release of EDRF and endothelium-dependent relaxations. Mass spectrometric analysis showed the origin of NO to be the terminal guanidino nitrogen of the amino acid (Palmer et al. 1988b). Administration of LNMMA in vivo resulted in systemic hypertension in rabbits (Rees et al. 1989).

Nitric oxide caused relaxations in the canine basilar artery, which was abolished in the presence of hemoglobin. The relaxations were significantly impaired after subarachnoid hemorrhage (Table 4), as well as the formation of cyclic GMP stimulated by the radical (Table 3) (Kim et al. 1992).

Table 4. Responses to NO in rings (without endothelium) of canine basilar arteries

NO (log[*M*])	–8	–7	–6
Relaxation (% to maximal relaxation)			
Control	–5.6	–45	–87
(+HgB	0	0	–1.8)
(+MB	0	0	–0.82)
SAH	–1.8	–34	–48

Relaxations were measured during contraction to UTP (3×10^{-6} *M*), and expressed as a percentage of the maximal relaxation to papaverine (3×10^{-4} *M*) plus diltiazem (10^{-4} *M*). The effects of hemoglobin (HgB 10^{-5} *M*) or methylene blue (MB 10^{-5} *M*) were measured in the control group after incubation for 20 min.

SAH, subarachnoid hemorrhage

Other Functions of Nitric Oxide

Endothelium-derived relaxing factor released from rabbit aorta inhibited platelet aggregation caused by arachidonic acid (Azuma et al. 1986). The anti-aggregating activity of EDRF was mediated by cyclic GMP and the effect of EDRF was synergistic with prostacyclin (Radomski et al. 1987). Neutrophils release a factor with identical characteristics to EDRF, which relaxes vascular smooth muscle (Rimele et al. 1988). Nitric oxide was detected from human neutrophils, when stimulated by platelet-activating factor, leukotriene B_4, or chemotactic peptide (Schmidt et al. 1989). Cytotoxicity of macrophage is suppressed by exposure to LNMMA. Macrophages, activated by bacterial lipopolysaccharide or by interferon, synthesize NO from L-arginine (Hibbs et al. 1988), which causes inhibition of DNA synthesis and mitochondrial respiration.

Endothelium-Dependent Contractions

Arachidonic acid augmented contractions to norepinephrine in canine veins (De Mey and Vanhoutte 1982), and the effect was inhibited by indomethacin, a blocker of cyclooxygenase. Under quiescent conditions, arachidonic acid, the calcium ionophore A23187, ADP, and acetylcholine (ACh) (when exposure is repeated) evoked endothelium-dependent contractions in the canine basilar artery (Figs. 7, 8) (Katusic et al. 1988; Kim et al. 1988). These contractions were suppressed by indomethacin, by inhibitors of thromboxane synthetase, and by thromboxane receptors. Mechanical stretch induces sustained increase in the tension in the canine basilar artery and the response is endothelium dependent (Katusic et al. 1987). The responses were also inhibited by indomethacin, indicating the factor released from the endothelium is a cyclooxygenase product. In the isolated feline cerebral artery, elevation of perfusion pressure resulted in reduction of diameter, which was endothelium dependent and associated with depolarization of smooth muscle (Harder et al. 1989). The contractions elicited by mechanical stimuli may contribute to pressure autoregulation in the cerebral circulation. Anoxia causes endothelium-dependent contraction which is not a result of inhibition of spontaneous release of EDRF, since it is not affected by inhibitors of EDRF (Rubanyi and Vanhoutte 1985; Katusic and Vanhoutte 1986). Unlike endothelium-dependent contractions elicited by other stimuli, the response to hypoxia is not blocked by indomethacin. Endothelium-dependent contractions to hypoxia could be reproduced by "sandwiching" the intimal layer and the medial layer, suggesting the presence of a diffusible substance mediating the process (Rubanyi and Vanhoutte 1985). However, attempts to bioassay the substance have never been successful in various arterial preparations including the canine basilar artery. The nature of the endothelium-derived contracting factor released by hypoxia is not clear. It is a diffusible substance, but not a product of arachidonic acid metabolism. The onset is rapid and the contraction is readily reversible when hypoxic conditions cease to exist. The time course suggests the contraction is not mediated by endothelin, or peptides released from the hypoxic endothelial cells. Cultured bovine aortic endothelial cells release a peptide which contracts vascular smooth muscle (Hickey et al. 1985). Yanagisawa et al. identified a 21-residue peptide, endothelin, from culture media of endothelial cells, which is a potent constric-

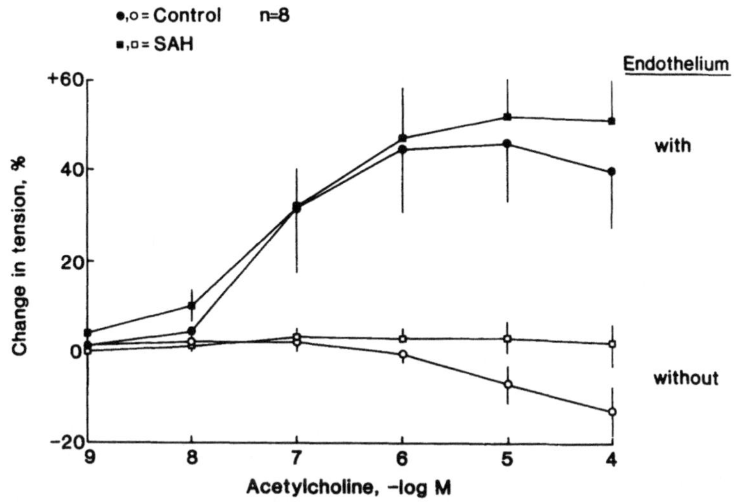

Fig. 7. Concentration-response curve to acetylcholine in quiescent rings of basilar arteries from the control and subarachnoid hemorrhage groups. Contractions were expressed as percentages of the maximal contractions to uridine triphosphate. In both groups, acetylcholine caused contractions only in rings with endothelium (endothelim dependent). Data are shown as means ± SEMs for eight animals. (With permission, Kim et a. 1988, Figs. 7–10)

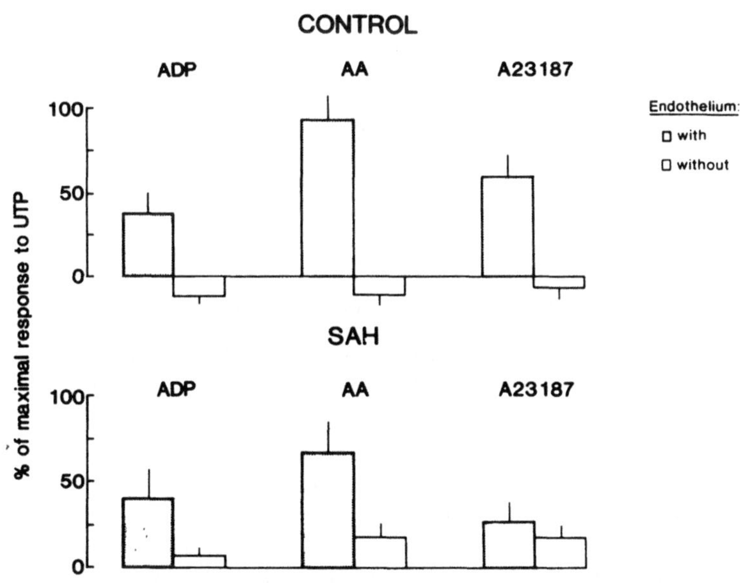

Fig. 8. Summary of the endothelium-dependent contractions to adenosine diphosphate (ADP, $10^{-4}M$), arachidonic acid (AA, ($10^{-5}M$), and the calcium ionophore A23187 ($10^{-6}M$). The maximal response for each agent is shown. Contractions are expressed as percentages of the maximal response to uridine triphosphate. *n*=8

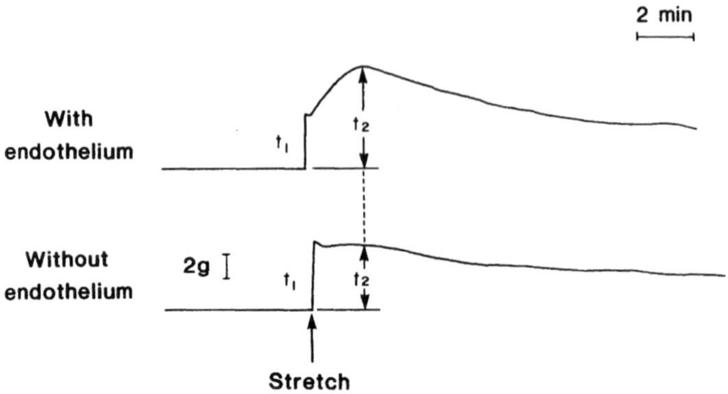

Fig. 9. Isometric tension recordings in response to rapid stretch. Stretching to the optimal length caused subsequent development of tension in rings with endothelium *(upper traces),* but not in rings without *(lower trace).* The ratio between the peak tension developed (t_2) and the tension required to reach the optimal length (t_1) was measured. In rings without endothelium, t_2 was measured as the tension at the same time point as the peak was obtained in the paired rings with endothelium.

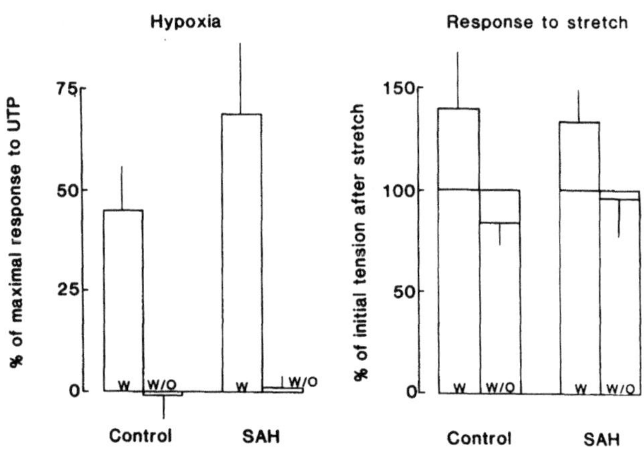

Fig. 10. Endothelium-dependent contractions to hypoxia *(left)* and stretch *(right)* in the control and SAH groups. Switching the gas mixture from 95% O_2–5% CO_2 to 95% N_2–5% CO_2 caused subsequent development of tension in rings with endothelium, but not in rings without. Responses to hypoxia are expressed as percentages of the maximal contraction to UTP.

tor (Yanagisawa et al. 1988). The effect is suppressed by calcium antagonists and by elimination of extracellular calcium. The physiological or pathological role of the peptide remains to be established in intact animals.

Endothelium-dependent contractions were elicited in the canine basilar arteries by mechanical stretch, anoxia, arachidonic acid, ADP, the calcium ionophore A23187, and acetylcholine. In spastic basilar arteries after subarachnoid hemorrhage, the contractions, as expressed as a percentage of the maximal contractions to KCl, remained comparable to those in the control group after subarachnoid hemorrhage (Figs. 7, 10) (Kim et al. 1988).

References

Angus JA, Campbell GR, Cocks TM, et al. (1983) Vasodilatation by acetylcholine is endothelium-dependent: a study by sonomicrometry in canine femoral artery in vivo. J Physiol (Lond) 344:209-222

Azuma H, Ishikawa M, Sakizaki S (1986) Endothelium-dependent inhibition of platelet aggregation. Br J Pharmacol 88:411-415

Cocks TM, Angus JA, Campbell JH, et al. (1985) Release and properties of endothelium-derived relaxing factor (EDRF) from endothelial cells in culture. J Cell Physiol 123:310–320

Collins P, Griffith TM, Henderson AH, Lewis MJ (1986) Endothelium-derived relaxing factor alters calcium fluxes in rabbit aorta: a cyclic guanosine monophosphate-mediated effect. J Physiol (Lond) 381:427–437

De Mey JG, Vanhoutte PM (1982) Heterogeneous behavior of the canine arterial and venous wall: importance of the endothelium. Circ Res 51:439–447

Diamond J, Chu EWS (1983) Possible role for cyclic GMP in endothelium-dependent relaxation of rabbit aorta by acetylcholine. Comparison with nitroglycerin. Res Commun Pathol Pharmacol 41:369–381

Furchgott RF (1983) Role of endothelium in response of vascular smooth muscle. Circ Res 53:557–573

Furchgott RF (1988) Studies on relaxation of rabbit aorta by sodium nitrate: basis for the proposal that the acid-activatable component of the inhibitory factor from retractor penis is inorganic nitrate and the endothelium-derived relaxing factor is nitric oxide. In: Vanhoutte PM (ed) Mechanisms of vasodilation. Raven, New York, pp 401–414

Furchgott RF, Vanhoutte PM (1989) Endothelium-derived relaxing and contracting factors. FASEB J 3:2007–2018

Furchgott RF, Zawadzki JV (1980) The obligatory role of endothelial cells in the relaxation of arterial smooth muscle by acetylcholine. Nature 288:373–376

Furchgott RF, Cherry PD, Zawadzki JV (1984) Endothelial cells as mediators of vasodilatation of arteries. J Cardiovasc Pharmacol [Suppl 2] 6:S336–S344

Gibson QH, Roughton FJW (1957) The kinetics and equilibria of the reactions of nitric oxide with sheep haemoglobin. J Physiol (Lond) 136:507–526

Griffith TM, Edwards DH, Lewis MJ, et al. (1984) The nature of endothelium-derived relaxant factor. Nature 308:645–647

Harder DR, Sanchez-Ferrer C, Kauser K, et al. (1989) Pressure release a transferable endothelial contractile factor in cat cerebral arteries. Circ Res 65:193–198

Hibbs JB Jr, Taintor RR, Vavrin Z, et al. (1988) Nitric oxide: a cytotoxic activated macrophage effector molecule. Biochem Biophys Res Commun 157:87–94

Hickey KA, Rubanyi G, Paul RJ, et al. (1985) Characterization of a coronary vasoconstrictor produced by cultured endothelial cells. Am J Physiol 248:C550-C556

Holtz J, Forstermann U, Pohl U, Giesler M, Bassenge E (1984) Flow-dependent, endothelium-mediated dilation of epicardial coronary arteries in conscious dogs: effects of cyclooxygenase inhibition. J Cardiovasc Pharmacol 6:1161–1169

Ignarro LJ, Burke TM, Wood KS, Wolin MS, Kadowitz PJ (1984) Association between cyclic GMP accumulation and acethylcholine-elicited relaxation of bovine pulmonary artery. J Pharmacol Exp Ther 228:682–690

Ignarro LJ, Byrns, RE, Buga GM, Wood KS (1987) Endothelium-derived relaxing factor from pulmonary artery and vein possesses pharmacological and chemical properties that are identical to those for nictric oxide radical. Circ Res 61:866–879

Ignarro LJ, Byrns RE, Wood KS (1988) Biochemical and pharmacological properties of endothelium-derived relaxing factor and its similarity to nitric oxide radical. In: Vanhoutte PM (ed) Mechanisms of vasodilation. Raven, New York, pp 427–435

Itoh T, Kanmura Y, Kuriyama H, Sasaguri T (1985) Nitroglycerine- and isoprenaline-induced vasodilatation: assessment from the actions of cyclic nucleotides. Br J Pharmacol 84:393–406

Katusic ZS, Vanhoutte PM (1986) Anoxic contractions in isolated canine cerebral arteries. Contribution of endothelium-derived factors, metabolites or arachidonic acid and calcium entry. J Cardiovasc Pharmacol 8:S97–S101

Katusic ZS, Shepherd JT, Vanhoutte PM (1984) Vasopressin causes endothelium-dependent relaxation of the canine basilar artery. Circ Res 55:575–579

Katusic ZS, Shepherd JT, Vanhoutte PM (1987) Endothelium-dependent contraction to stretch in canine basilar arteries. Am J Physiol 252:H671–H673

Katusic ZS, Shepherd JT, Vanhoutte PM (1988) Endothelium-dependent contraction to calcium ionophore A23187, arachidonic acid and acetylcholine in canine basilar arteries. Stroke 19:476–479

Kim P, Vanhoutte PM (1990) Endothelium-dependent relaxations and contractions. In: Sano K et al. (ed) Cerebral vasospasm – Proceedings of the Vth International Conference on Cerebral Vasospasm, Tokyo 1990. University of Tokyo Press, Tokyo, pp 221–226

Kim P, Sundt TM, Vanhoutte PM (1988) Alterations in endothelium-dependent responsiveness of the canine basilar artery after subarachnoid hemorrhage. J Neurosurg 69:239–246

Kim P, Lorenz R, Sundt TM, Vanhoutte PM (1989) Release of endothelium-derived relaxing factor after subarachnoid hemorrhage. J Neurosurg 70:108–114

Kim P, Schini V, Sundt TM Jr, Vanhoutte PM (1992) Reduced production of cyclic GMP underlies the loss of endothelium-dependent relaxations in the canine basilar artery after subarachnoid hemorrhage. Circ Res (in press)

Kontos HA, Wei EP, Marshall J (1988) In vivo bioassay of endothelium-derived relaxing factor. Am J Physiol 255:H1259–H1262

Martin W, Villani GM, Jothianandan D, et al. (1985) Selective blockade of endothelium-dependent and glyceryl trinitrate-induced relaxation by hemoglobin and by methylene blue in the rabbit aorta. J Pharmacol Exp Ther 232:708–716

Murad F, Mittal CK, Arnold WP, et al. (1978) Guanylate cyclase activation by azide, nitrocompounds, nitric oxide, and hydroxyl radical and inhibition by hemoglobin and myoglobin. Adv Cyclic Nucleotide Res 9:145–158

Palmer RMJ, Ferrigo AG, Moncada S (1987) Nitric oxide release accounts for the biological activity of endothelium-derived relaxing factor. Nature 327:524–525

Palmer RMJ, Ashton DS, Moncada S (1988a) Vascular endothelial cells synthesize nitric oxide from L-arginine. Nature 333:664–666

Palmer RMJ, Rees DD, Ashton DS, et al. (1988b) L-arginine is the physiological precursor for the formation of nitric oxide in endothelium-dependent relaxation. Biochem Biophys Res Commun 153:1251–1256

Radomski MW, Palmer RMJ, Moncada S (1987) Comparative pharmacology of endothelium-derived relaxing factor, nitric oxide and prostacyclin in platelets. Br J Pharmacol 92:181–187

Rapoport RM (1986) Cyclic guanosine monophosphate inhibition of contraction may be mediated through inhibition of phosphatidylinositol hydrolysis in rat aorta. Circ Res 58:407–410

Rapoport RM, Draznin MB, Murad F (1983) Endothelium-dependent relaxation in rat aorta may be mediated through cyclic GMP-dependent protein phosphorylation. Nature 306:174–176

Rashatwar SS, Cornwell TL, Lincoln TM (1987) Effects of 8-Bromo-cGMP on CA^{2+} levels in vascular smooth muscle cells: possible regulation of Ca^{2+}-ATPase by cGMP-dependent protein kinase. Proc Natl. Acad Sci USA 84:5685–5689

Rees DD, Palmer RMJ, Moncada S (1989) Role of endothelium-derived nitric oxide in the regulation of blood pressure. Proc Natl Acad Sci USA 86:3375–3378

Rimele TJ, Sturm RJ, Adams LM, et al. (1988) Interaction of neutrophile with vascular smooth muscle: identification of a neutrophil-derived relaxing factor. J Pharmacol Exp Ther 245:102–111

Rosenblum WI (1986) Endothelial dependent relaxation demonstrated in vivo in cerebral arterioles. Stroke 17:494–497

Rubanyi GM, Vanhoutte PM (1985) Hypoxia releases a vasoconstrictor substance from the canine vascular endothelium. J Physiol (Lond) 364:45–56

Rubanyi GM, Vanhoutte PM (1986) Oxygen-derived free radicals, endothelium, and responsiveness of vascular smooth muscle. Am J Physiol 250:H815–H821

Rubanyi GM, Lorenz RR, Vanhoutte PM (1985) Bioassay of endothelium-derived relaxing factor. Am J Physiol 215:H1077–H1080

Schmidt HHHW, Seifert R, Bohme E (1989) Formation and release of nitric oxide from human neutrophils and HL-60 cells induced by a chemotactic peptide, platelet activating factor and leukotriene B_4. FEBS Lett 244:357–360

Schultz KD, Schultz K, Schultz G (1977) Sodium nitroprusside and other smooth muscle-relaxants increase cyclic GMP levels in rat ductus deferens. Nature 265:750–751

Twort CH, van Breemen C (1988) Cyclic guanosine monophosphate-enhanced sequestration of Ca^{2+} by sarcoplasmic reticulum in vascular smooth muscle. Circ Res 62:961–964

Yanagisawa M, Kurihara H, Kimura S, et al. (1988) A novel potent vasoconstrictor peptide produced by vascular endothelial cells. Nature 332:411–415

Mechanisms of Cerebral Vasodilatation During Neuronal Activation by Bicuculline: A Review

M. Wahl

Bicuculline-induced seizure is an established experimental model of increased neuronal activity. Bicuculline is a plant alkaloid that blocks the inhibitory action of γ-aminobutyric acid (GABA) at postsynaptic sites (Curtis and Johnston 1974). In cerebral arteries the GABA receptor antagonist does not exert vasomotor effects in a concentration range of 10^{-11} to 10^{-4} *M* as shown by perivascular microapplication (Kuschinsky and Wahl 1979). However, after bicuculline-induced neuronal activation a tremendous increase in cerebral blood flow (CBF), up to six to seven fold, has been found (Meldrum and Nilsson 1976; Chapman et al. 1977; Mueller et al. 1979). The increase in CBF is due to an increase in the perfusion pressure and to a fall in vascular resistance. Several mechanisms which appear to be involved in the mediation of the decrease in cerebrovascular resistance during neuronal activation will be discussed in the following article. In particular, the role of local-chemical factors, prostanoids, and free radicals as well as of trigeminovascular nerves will be reviewed briefly.

Local Factors

Several ions such as K^+, H^+, and Ca^{2+} have been found to induce strong vasomotor reactions of extraparenchymal arteries when their concentrations in the perivascular space are changed by micropuncture technique. A pH increase leads to vasoconstriction whereas a pH decrease induces vasodilatation (Wahl et al. 1970, 1987; Kuschinsky et al. 1972; Schneider et al. 1977; Wahl and Kuschinsky 1977). This has been confirmed in isolated intraparenchymal arteries (Dacey and Duling 1982). Similarly, a reduction in the perivascular K^+ concentration below normal and an increase in K^+ up to 20 m*M* elicit constriction and dilatation of pial arteries, respectively (Kuschinsky et al. 1972; Kuschinsky and Wahl 1977; Wahl and Kuschinsky 1977; Betz and Csornai 1978; Wahl et al. 1987). The dilating effect of K^+ is Ca^{2+} dependent, as at 1.5 m*M* Ca^{2+} the K^+-induced vasodilatation is twice as high as at 2.5 m*M* Ca^{2+} (Kuschinsky et al. 1972; Kuschinsky and Wahl 1977; Betz and Csornai 1978).

As these ions produced pronounced vasomotor effects, 10–15 years ago several groups investigated whether their concentrations changed in the interstitial space during neuronal activation. An immediate increase in K^+ activity was found during chemically (Astrup et al. 1976, 1978; Heuser 1978; Leniger-Follert 1984) and electrically (Heinemann et al. 1977; Urbanics et al. 1978) induced activation, which correlated well with the increase in CBF. During bicuculline seizure, divergent pH changes were found. Using semimicro-pH electrodes, Astrup et al. (1976, 1978) measured an initial alkaline shift 15 s in duration which was followed by acidosis. The alkaline shift was interpreted as evidence against a mediator role of hydrogen ions during neuronal activation. However, using micro-pH electrodes, thus minimizing tissue damage, Heuser (1978) and Kuschinsky and Wahl (1979) found an initial acidic shift in pH, which was later confirmed by others (Leniger-Follert 1984; Siesjö et al. 1985). Since the time course of the developing interstitial acidosis correlated well with vasodilatation and CBF increase (Heuser 1978; Kuschinsky and Wahl 1979; Leniger-Follert 1984) it was concluded that pH was one of the mediators reducing cerebrovascular resistance during neuronal activation. Furthermore, a decrease in the Ca^{2+} activity in the cortical interstitial space was detected during chemically and electrically induced neuronal activation (Heinemann et al. 1977; Heuser 1978). This would also facilitate vasodilatation.

Adenosine is another potent dilator of extraparenchymal cerebral arteries when administered from the perivascular side (Berne et al. 1974; Wahl and Kuschinsky 1976, 1977; Dora 1986; Morii et al. 1986; Wahl et al. 1987). This effect, which can also be elicited in isolated cerebral arteries (Hardebo and Edvinsson 1979), can be blocked by theophylline in situ (Wahl and Kuschinsky 1976; Dora 1986) and in vitro (Hardebo and Edvinsson 1979). The adenosine content of the brain has been demonstrated in increase during electrically and bicuculline-induced neuronal activation (Rubio et al. 1975; Schrader et al. 1980; Winn et al. 1980), but this could not be confirmed by others (Rehncrona et al. 1978). Recently, employing the microdialysis technique, an incease in the adenosine concentration in the interstitial fluid of the brain has also been detected (Park et al. 1987). These authors reported an enhancement of adenosine to concentrations which have been found to induce vasodilatation under control conditions (see above). A role for adenosine in the mediation of CBF increase during neuronal activation can also be deduced from data of Dora (1986) and Pinard et al. (1990). These authors found that the CBF increase during chemically induced neuronal activation was significantly reduced by local or systemic administration of theophylline. However, the reduction of flow in the presence of theophylline was rather small. This may indicate that adenosine does not produce such marked effects under neuronal acitivation as under control conditions.

One reason for the reduced dilating effect of adenosine during neuronal activation appears to be that interactions occur with other local factors, the concentrations of which are changed simultaneously. It has been found by Wahl and Kuschinsky (1977) that the dilating effect of adenosine is decreased under control conditions when the pH is decreased or the K^+ concentration is simultaneously increased in the perivascular space. From this and other studies (Kuschinsky et al. 1972; Betz and Csornai 1978), dealing with the interaction between H^+, K^+, and Ca^{2+} ions, the following conclusions can be drawn: (a) K^+ ion dominates H^+ ion and adenosine, (b) H^+ ion dominates adenosine, and (c) a reduction in Ca^{2+} ion enhances the dilatation induced by an increase in K^+ or H^+ ion.

Considering the concentration change in K^+, H^+, and Ca^{2+} ions and adenosine in the perivascular space during neuronal activation and their vasoactive effects, one may conclude that several local factors are involved in the mediation of vasodilatation during functional hyperemia. Of the interactions between these factors, K^+ appears to be the most important.

Prostanoids and Free Radicals

Besides the local factors, prostanoids and free radicals have been suggested to be involved in the increase in CBF during neuronal activation. Busija and Leffler (1989) found that the increase in CBF during bicuculline seizure was accompanied by an increase in prostaglandin E_2, 6-keto-prostaglandin $F_{1\alpha}$, thromboxane B_2, and prostaglandin $F_{2\alpha}$ in the fluid of the cortical subarachnoid space. Since the increase in CBF could be reduced by treatment with indomethacin, these authors concluded that prostanoids and/or their metabolites are involved in the mediation of CBF increase during neuronal activation. During the synthesis of prostanoids, superoxide radicals are generated which can be assayed by the reduction of nitroblue tetrazolium to nitroblue formazan. Indeed, Armstead et al. (1989) found an increase in the reduction of nitroblue tetrazolium during bicuculline seizure, indicating an increased formation of superoxide anion. These authors suggested that the increase in blood pressure during seizure activates phospholipase A_2 and increases, via the cyclooxygenase pathway, the formation of prostanoids and free radicals, which could thus participate in the mediation of the decrease of cerebrovascular resistance. However, the functional importance of these compounds mediating the CBF increase during neuronal activation is small for several reasons: (a) dilating and constrictor prostanoids are released simultaneously (Busija and Leffler 1989); (b) the increase in radical formation is small (Armstead et al. 1989); and (c) free radicals have only a weak dilating effect in cerebral resistance vessels (Unterberg et al. 1988).

Trigeminovascular Nerves

Recent data from Moskowitz's group show that trigeminovascular nerves are also involved in the mediation of the decrease in cerebrovascular resistance and the increase in CBF during neuronal activation by bicuculline (Sakas et al. 1989). These authors found that the increase in cortical gray matter flow was 30% less in the regions of the left hemisphere supplied by anterior middle and posterior cerebral arteries after left trigeminal ganglionectomy in comparison to the corresponding areas in the contralateral intact hemisphere. These are areas in which the arteries have a trigeminovascular innervation. Since there were no side differences in flow after left trigeminal rhizotomy, the authors concluded that the increase in flow is in part mediated by an axon-like reflex. They also suggested that the afferent fibers are activated by the increased interstitial K^+ concentration during bicuculline-induced neuronal activation.

Conclusions

1. Several local factors such as K^+, H^+, Ca^{2+}, and adenosine are involved in the mediation of vasodilation during neuronal activation. Considering the vasomotor effects, the interactions and concentration change in the perivascular space K^+ appears to be the most important factor.
2. Prostanoids, free radicals, and trigeminovascular axon-like reflexes may participate in the mediation of CBF increase during neuronal activation.

References

Armstead WM, Mirro R, Leffler CW, Busija DW (1989) Cerebral superoxide anion generation during seizures in newborn pigs. J Cereb Blood Flow Metab 9:175–179

Astrup J, Heuser D, Lassen NA, Nilsson B, Norberg K, Siesjö BK (1976) Evidence against H^+ and K^+ as the main factors in the regulation of cerebral blood flow during epileptic discharges, acute hypoxemia, amphetamine intoxication, and hypoglycemia. A microelectrode study. In: Betz E (ed) Ionic actions on vascular smooth muscle. Springer, Berlin Heidelberg New York, pp 110–115

Astrup J, Heuser D, Lassen NA, Nilsson B, Norberg K, Siesjö BK (1978) Evidence against H^+ and K^+ as main factors for the control of cerebral blood flow: a microelectrode study. In: Purves MJ (ed) Cerebral vascular smooth muscle and its control. Elsevier, Amsterdam, pp 313–332

Berne RM, Rubio R, Curnish RR (1974) Release of adenosine from ischemic brain. Effect on cerebral vascular resistance and incorporation into cerebral adenine mucleotides. Circ Res 35:262–271

Betz E (1976) Ionic interaction in pial vascular smooth muscles. In: Betz E (ed) Ionic actions on vascular smooth muscle. Springer, Berlin Heidelberg New York, pp 75–77

Betz E, Csornai M 81978) Action and interaction of perivascular H^+, K^+ and Ca^{++} on pial arteries. Pflügers Arch 374:67–72

Busija DW, Leffler CW (1989) Role of prostanoids in cerebrovascular responses during seizures in piglets. Am J Physiol 256:H120–H125

Chapman AG, Meldrum BS, Siesjö BK (1977) Cerebral metabolic changes during prolonged epileptic seizures in rats. J Neurochem 28:1025–1036

Curtis DR, Johnston GAR (1974) Amino acid transmitter in the mammalian central nervous system. Ergeb Physiol 69:1025–1039

Dacey RG, Duling BR (1982) A study of rat intercerebral arterioles: methods, morphology and reactivity. Am J Physiol 243:H598–H606

Dora E (1986) Effect of theophylline treatment on the functional hyperaemic and hypoxic responses of cerebrocortical microcirculation. Acta Physiol Hung 68:183–198

Hardebo JE, Edvinsson L (1979) Adenine compounds: cerebrovascular effects in vitro with reference to their possible involvement in magraine. Stroke 10:58–61

Heinemann U, Lux HD, Gutnick MJ (1977) Extracellular free calcium and potassium during paroxysmal activity in the cerebral cortex of the cat. Exp Brain Res 27:237–243

Heuser D (1978) The significance of cortical extracellular H^+, K^+ and Ca^{2+} activities for regulation of local cerebral blood flow under conditions of enhanced neuronal activity. In: Purves JM (ed) Cerebral vascular smooth muscle and its control. Elsevier, Amsterdam, pp 339–349

Kuschinsky W, Wahl M (1977) Interactions between perivascular norepinephrine and potassium or osmolarity on pial arteries of cats. Microvasc Res 14:173–180

Kuschinsky W, Wahl M (1979) Perivascular pH and pial arterial diameter during bicuculline induced seizures in cats. Pflügers Arch 382:81–85

Kuschinsky W, Wahl M, Bosse O, Thurau K (1972) Perivascular potassium and pH as determinates of local pial arterial diameter in cats. A microapplication study. Circ Res 31:240–247

Leniger-Follert E (1984) Mechanisms of regulation of cerebral microflow during bicuculline induced seizures in anaesthetized cats. J Cereb Blood Flow Metab 5:150–165
Meldrum BS, Nilsson B (1976) Cerebral blood flow and metabolic rate early and late in prolonged epileptic seizures induced in rats by bicuculline. Brain 99:523–542
Morii S, Ngai AC, Winn HR (1986) Reactivity of rat pial arterioles and venules to adenosine and carbon dioxide: with detailed description of the closed cranial window technique in rats. J Cereb Blood Flow Metab 6:34–41
Mueller SM, Heistad DA, Marcus ML (1979) Effect of sympathetic nerves on cerebral vessels during seizures. Am J Physiol 237:H178–H184
Park TS, van Wylen DGL, Rubio R, Berne RM (1987) Interstitial fluid adenosine and sagittal sinus blood flow during bicuculline-seizures in newborn piglets. J Cereb Blood Flow Metab 7:633-639
Pinard E, Riche D, Puiroud S, Seylaz J (1990) Theophylline reduces cerebral hyperaemia and enhances brain damage induced by seizures. Brain Res 511:303–309
Rehncrona S, Siesjö BK, Westerberg E (1978) Adenosine and cyclic AMP in cerebral cortex of rats in hypoxia, status epilepticus and hypercapnia. Acta Pyhsiol Scand 104:453–463
Rubio R, Berne RM, Bockman EL, Curnish RR (1975) Relationship between adenosine concentration and oxygen supply in rat brain. Am J Physiol 228:1896–1902
Sakas DE, Moskowitz MA, Wei EP, Kontos HA, Kano M, Ogilvy CS (1989) Trigeminovascular fibers increase blood flow in cortical gray matter by axon reflex-like mechanisms during acute severe hypertension or seizures. Proc Natl Acad Sci USA 86:1401–1405
Schneider W, Wahl M, Kuschinsky W, Thurau K (1977) The use of microelectrodes for measurement of local H^+ activity in the cortical subarachnoid space of cats. Pflügers Arch 372:103–107
Schrader J, Wahl M, Kuschinsky W, Kreutzberg GW (1980) Increase of adenosine content in cerebral cortex of the cat during bicuculline-induced seizure. Pflügers Arch 387:245–251
Siesjö BK, van Hanwehr R, Nergelius G, Nevander G, Ingvar M (1985) Extra- and intracellular pH in the brain during seizures and in the recovery period following the arrest of seizures activity. J Cereb Blood Flow Metab 5:47–57
Unterberg A, Wahl M, Baethmann A (1988) Effects of free radicals on permeability and vasomotor response of cerebral vessels. Acta Neuropathol (Berl) 76:238–244
Urbanics R, Leniger-Follert E, Lübbers DW (1978) Time course of changes of extracellular H^+ and K^+ activities during and after direct electrical stimulation of the brain cortex. Pflügers Arch 378:47–53
Wahl M, Kuschinsky W (1976) The dilatory action of adenosine on pial arteries of cats and its inhibition by theophylline. Pflügers Arch 362:55-59
Wahl M, Kuschinsky W (1977) Influence of H^+ and K^+ on adenosine-induced dilatation at pial arteries of cats. Blood Vessels 14:285–293
Wahl M, Deetjen P, Thurau K, Ingvar DH, Lassen NA (1970) Micropuncture evaluation of the importance of perivascular pH for the arteriolar diameter on the brain surface. Pflügers Arch 316:152–163
Wahl M, Lauritzen M, Schilling L (1987) Change of cerebrovascular reactivity after cortical spreading depression in cats and rats. Brain Res 411:72–80
Winn HR, Welsh JE, Rubio R, Berne RM (1980) Changes in brain adenosine during bicuculline-induced seizures in rats: effects of hypoxia and altered systemic blood pressure. Circ Res 47:568–577

Postischemic Hyperperfusion and Outcome: An Experimental Study

O. KEMPSKI, W. STUMMER, C. BAUER, L. SCHÜRER, and A. BAETHMANN

Introduction

The selective vulnerability of discrete brain regions after short episodes of cerebral ischemia is a phenomenon still unexplained. In the hippocampus in particular, nerve cell loss may become prominent after only 5 min of ischemia. Neurons appear intact during the initial 1–2 days of reperfusion, after which they succumb. In order to investigate the mechanisms involved in this "delayed neuronal death," and postischemic nerve cell damage in general, in a previous study we demonstrated that preischemic physical activity may protect experimental animals from damage in the gerbil forebrain ischemia model (in preparation; Weber et al. 1989). With 15 min of ischemia there was a dramatic enhancement of survival from 44% in controls to 85% in animals which had access to a "running wheel" before experiencing ischemia. Although the phenomenon is of much scientific interest in itself, it may serve as a tool to study the significance of pathophysiological parameters for outcome from an ischemic episode: With animals from conventional cages and those from cages with access to a running wheel, two groups of gerbils with a known and significantly different *prognosis* are available. Hence, it is possible to use these animals for short-term experiments where the final outcome of individual experiments cannot be assessed. The present investigation served to compare postischemic regional blood flow for the two groups. It is still an open question whether postischemic *hyper*perfusion or the delayed *hypo*perfusion contribute to postischemic damage, and which of these phases has worse consequences for outcome. Therefore, in short-term study regional cerebral blood flow (rCBF) was measured with the hydrogen clearance technique before and up to 3 h after a 15-min episode of forebrain ischemia. In a long-term model, histological outcome was evaluated, again for animals with and without previous access to voluntary running.

Methods

Male Mongolian gerbils with a body weight of 60–90 g were anesthetized with halothane (introduction, 4%; maintenance, 1.5%). Both common carotid arteries were exposed and carefully isolated from the surrounding tissue, using an operating microscope. Special care was taken not to damage peripheral nerve tissue. A 6–0 monofilament thread was looped around both arteries and was used simultaneously to occlude both carotids by attaching a 15-g weight to both ends of the thread. Halothane was reduced to 0.5% during ischemia. Forebrain ischemia was terminated after 15 min by cutting the ligature. During the surgical preparation, ischemia, and 30 min of recirculation after ischemia, body temperature was kept at 37°C by a feedback-controlled heating pad.

Short-Term Experiments

In order to evaluate short-term changes in rCBF during and after ischemia, cortical rCBF was measured using the hydrogen clearance technique. Animals from conventional cages as well as from cages equipped with running wheels were used. Cortical rCBF was evaluated by using Ag/AgC1 electrodes 75 µm in diameter and 750 µm in length. Measurements were taken at 15-min intervals beginning 1 h before onset of ischemia until 3 h postischemia; during ischemia no reliable data could be generated due to an instable baseline.

Long-Term Experiments

To study the effect of forebrain ischemia on histological outcome, the animals were allowed to recover from ischemia for 4 days, when they were killed perfusion fixed using phosphate-buffered 2% paraformaldehyde, and the brains processed for the morphometric evaluation of nerve cell loss in hippocampus, cortex, thalamus, and striatum. Animals were divided into three groups: (a) sham-operated animals without ischemia, (b) animals with 15-min forebrain ischemia, maintained in conventional cages and (c) gerbils which had had access to running wheels for 3 weeks prior to experiencing a 15-min episode of forebrain ischemia. Brains were embedded in paraffin and cut into sagittal sections. From each brain, cresyl-violet-stained sections from 1.6 mm rostral and 0.6 mm dorsal to the bregma were chosen for morphometric evaluation (Weber et al. 1988) of hippocampal sectors, striatum, and thalamus.

Results

Morphometric analysis of hippocampus and striatum revealed a marked protection of both structures by preischemic voluntary running (Table 1), except for the CA1 sector of the hippocampus. In the thalamus, in 7 out of 14 hemispheres from animals kept in conventional cages, small infarcts were found, as compared to 2 out of 16 hemispheres with infarcts in the "runner" group ($p<0.025$). The mean infarcted area in the sections taken from 0.6 mm posterior to the bregma was 2.24±1.1 mm^2 in "nonrunners" compared with 0.13±0.1 mm^2 in runners.

The preischemic cortical rCBF was identical in both groups at 44.5±1.4 ml/100 g min in runners and 45.6±1.7 ml/100 g min in nonrunners (Table 2). During recirculation an enhacement of rCBF – corresponding to the well-known postischemic hyperperfusion phase – was seen mainly in runners. In nonrunners, reperfusion began slowly, and reached a maximum rather late. In runners, hyperperfusion occurred earlier (27 ms. 62 min of recirculation, $p<0.05$), and was far more pronounced (159% vs. 104% of control, $p<0.05$). These differences could not be explained by changes in the systemic

Table 1. Mean nerve cell counts in hippocampal sectors, gyrus dentatus, and striatum from sham-operated animals as well as from gerbils killed 4 days after a 15-min episode of forebrain ischemia with and without prior access to running wheels (runners and nonrunners) (neurons/mm^2 ± SD)

	Hippocampus				Gyrus dentatus	Striatum
	CA1	CA2	CA3	CA4		
Shamoperated (n = 5)	3115 ± 9	1927 ± 88	1322 ± 43	1629 ± 67	5690 ± 186	844 ± 33
Nonrunners (n = 7)	90 ± 20	141 ± 24	123 ± 36	57 ± 13	3288 ± 631	92 ± 48
Runners (n = 8)	120 ± 15	286 ± 36	683 ± 175	286 ± 99	6136 ± 202	374 ± 82

Table 2. Postischemic rCBF (cortex) in gerbils from conventional cages (nonrunners) and with free access to running wheels (runners) after 15 min of bilateral occlusion of the carotid arteries

	Nonrunners	Runners
Early reflow (ml/100 g min)	15.9 ± 1.9	31.2 ± 6.7
Hyperperfusion (ml/100 g min)	47.0 ± 5.0	70.8 ± 7.4
Time after ischemia (min)	62.2 ± 12.3	27.4 ± 7.0
Hypoperfusion (ml/100 g min)	30.1 ± 2.4	29.0 ± 2.4
Time after ischemia (min)	97.3 ± 9.8	95.2 ± 11.0

arterial blood pressure, which was identical for both groups. Surprisingly, rCBF during the "delayed hypoperfusion phase," the minimum of which was seen at 80 min of recirculation, showed no differences between runners and nonrunners; in both groups, blood flow was reduced to 64%–69% of control.

Discussion

The result presented here confirm our earlier report (Weber et al. 1989) that physical exercise improves the outcome in gerbils after 15 min of forebrain ischemia. All brain regions studied so far were better preserved in the runner group. Besides, the observation of decreased nerve cell counts in various brain structures after 15 min of ischemia suggests that "selective vulnerability" is not an all-or-nothing phenomenon only found in the hippocampus. More likely there are varying thresholds for neural vulnerability throughout the brain, with the CA1 sector of the hippocampus being most sensitive, which has already been suggested by Crain et al. (1988). The current data point to the significance of a better and earlier reperfusion in exercising animals. Postischemic hypoperfusion, on the other hand, appears to be not affected and, therefore, is also less likely to be a detrimental event for the brain than previously believed. Postischemic hyperperfusion could well explain the better outcome of runners, which would be in line with reports that even long periods of ischemia up to 1 h may be survived, provided no reflow is prevented (Hossmann and Zimmermann 1974; Hossmann and Grosse Ophoff 1986). The better reperfusion could (a) help to wash out platelets (Hossmann et al. 1980; Turcani et al. 1988) and leukocytes (Hallenbeck et al. 1986) impeding blood flow after ischemia or (b) be explained by a reduced accumulation of such cellular elements during ischemia in runners. These hypotheses are favored by the observation of a reduced release of thromboxane into the CSF during the reperfusion phase of "runners" (data not shown). It is an open question, however, by what mechanism exercise affects the release of thromboxane or other mediator substances.

In conclusion, the current data support the assumption that nerve cell death is not an inevitable fate after an episode of cerebral ischemia, but evolves postischemically via mediator mechanisms which might be inhibited by specific treatment. In the gerbil model of forebrain ischemia, physical exercise offers the highest level of protection observed so far with any therapeutic regimen. The data point to a beneficial role of a fast and efficient reperfusion after ischemia. Although not supported by the current data, an additional, detrimental effect of the delayed hypoperfusion phase cannot be excluded.

Acknowledgement. The excellent secretarial services of Mrs. M. Westenhuber and the first-class technical assistance by Mrs. H. Leiner are gratefully acknowledged.

References

Crain BJ, Westerkam WD, Harrison AH, Nadler JV (1988) Selective neuronal death after transient forebrain ischemia in the Mongolian gerbil: a silver impregnation study. Neuroscience 27:387–402

Hallenbeck JM, Dutka AJ, Tanishima T, Kochanek PM, Kumaroo KK, Thompson C, Obrenovitch TP, Contreras TJ (1986) Polymorphonuclear leukocyte accumulation in brain regions with low blood flow during the early postischemic period. Stroke 17:246-253

Hossmann K-A, Grosse Ophoff B (1986) Recovery of monkey brain after prolonged ischemia. I. Electrophysiology and brain elektrolytes. J Cereb Blood Flow Metab 6:15–21

Hossmann K-A, Zimmermann V (1974) Resuscitation of the monkey brain after 1 h complete ischemia. I. Physiological and morphological observations. Brain Res 81:59–74

Hossmann V, Hossmann K-A, Takagi S (1980) Effect of intravascular platelet aggregation on blood recirculation following prolonged ischemia of the cat brain. J Neurol 222:159–170

Turcani P, Gotoh F, Ishihara N, Tanaka K, Gomi S, Takashima S, Mihara B (1988) Are blood platelets involved in the pathogenesis of ischemic brain edema in gerbils? Stroke 19:486–689

Weber K, Baethmann A, Kempski O (1988) Determinants of survival after forebrain ischemia in Mongolian gerbils. Metab Brain Dis 3:247–255

Weber K, Tranmer B, Schürer L, Baethmann A, Kempski O (1989) Physical activity determines survival of Mongolian gerbils from forebrain ischemia. In: Hartmann A, Kuschinsky W (eds) Cerebral ischemia and calcium. Springer, Berlin Heidelberg New York, pp 79–82

Chapter 2
Methods for the Measurement of Cerebral Blood Flow

Erythrocyte Flow in Cerebral Capillaries Under Resting and Stimulated Conditions

A. Villringer, U. Dirnagl, A. Piepgras, P. Schmiedek, and K. M. Einhäupl

Introduction

Due to the poor depth resolution of conventional light microscopy, most studies on the cerebral microcirculation in vivo have been limited to the observation of pial vessels on the brain surface. Anectodal reports on the visualization of deeper vascular structures such as capillaries (Rosenblum and Zweifach 1963; Ma et al. 1974; Ivanov et al. 1981; Pawlik et al. 1981) lack the precise definition of the depth beneath the brain surface (Rosenblum and Zweifach 1963; Ma et al. 1974; Ivanov et al. 1981; Pawlik et al. 1981), do not use a cranial window to maintain physiological intracranial pressure (ICP) (Ivanov et al. 1981; Pawlik et al. 1981), or are associated with impalement of brain tissue (Pawlik et al. 1981).

In previous reports (Villringer et al. 1990; Dirnagl et al. 1991), we demonstrated that confocal laser scanning microscopy (CLSM), a new light microscopic technique with far improved depth discrimination properties, permits the in vivo observation of fluorescein-filled blood vessels down to 250 μm beneath the brain surface in noninvasive optical sections. Based on adjacent planes 2 μm apart from each other, three-dimensional reconstructions of the microvascular architecture from the pial level to the capillary network 250 μm beneath the brain surface were obtained in vivo. In this communication, we demonstrate that in the same model intracapillary erythrocyte flow can be monitored continuously under baseline conditions and after stimulation of cerebral blood flow (CBF).

Animals, Material, and Methods

Ten male Wistar rats were anesthetized with thiobutabarbiturate (100 mg/kg body wt.), tracheotomized, artificially ventilated, and paralyzed (pancuronium bromide 0.1 mg/kg body wt.). The animals were equipped with a closed cranial window over the right parietal surface after the dura had been removed (Morii et al. 1986) and placed in a stereotactic frame beneath the confocal microscope. Arterial blood pressure, intracranial pressure, body temperature, and end expiratory CO_2 were monitored continuously, blood gases were measured serially, and hematocrit was measured at the beginning and at the end of each experiment.

We used a Bio-Rad MRC 600 CLSM system attached to a Nikon Optiphot microscope; the microscope objective was a x 40 water immersion objective (Zeiss, FRG) with a numerical aperture of 0.75 and a working distance of 1.6 mm. The light source

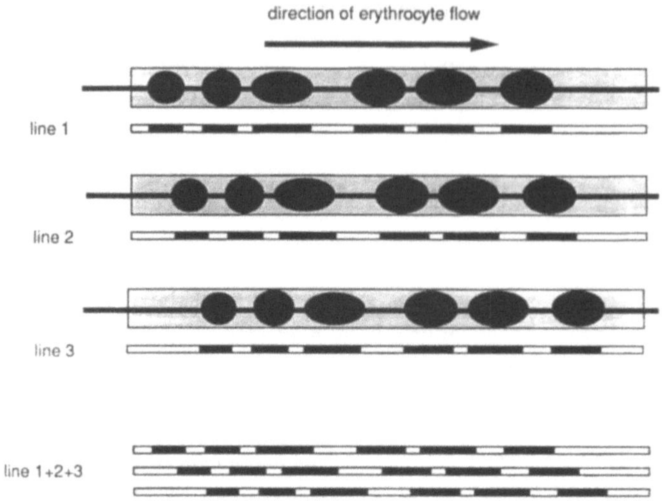

Fig. 1a, b. Principle of the single line method. **a** Instead of a two-dimensional image, a one-dimensional image, i.e., a single line, is imaged. Thus the time resolution is increased to 2 ms. The line is placed within the horizontal part of a capillary (see upper part of figure). The one-dimensional image obtained is displayed below, showing the pattern of erythrocytes in the capillary at this moment. Two milliseconds later the pattern has shifted to the right according to the direction of erythrocyte flow. The display of subsequent one-dimensional images in a space-time plot (vertical axis is time, horizontal axis is space) results in the visualization of single erythrocytes as oblique stripes.

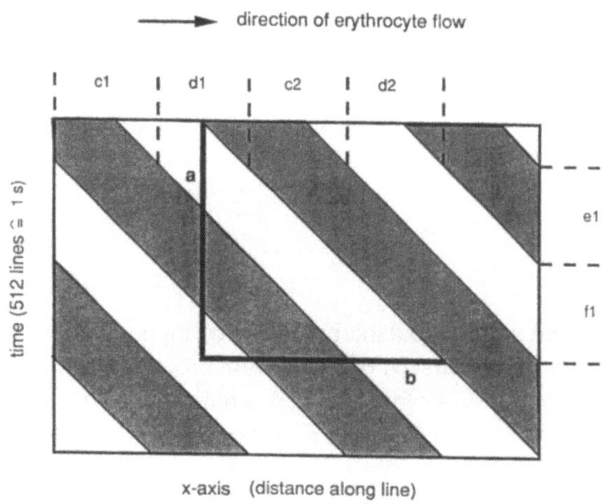

b. From such a space-time plot the following parameters can be determined: *b/a*, blood cell velocity; *c1+d1*, distance between blood cells; *e1+f1*, time distance between blood cells

was an argon laser with principal lines at 488 nm and 514 nm. Acquisition time for a two-dimensional image ranged from 1 s (768x512) to 1/16 s (168x128) and was 2 ms for a single line in the line scan mode. To reduce motion artifacts for the acquisition of three-dimensional data sets single frames were triggered to respiration. For fluorescein angiography 2 mg/100 g body wt. sodium-fluorescein in saline solution was injected i.v. as a bolus. More details regarding the three-dimensional reconstruction of the microvascular network are given by Dirnagl et al. (1991).

The time required for the data acquisition of a three-dimensional data set is on the order of several minutes and therefore too slow for dynamic studies. For these studies we used a one-dimensional approach. The data acquisition time for one horizontal line is 2 ms. If such a line is scanned repeatedly and subsequent acquisitions are displayed in a two-dimensional image a space (horizontal)-time (vertical) plot is obtained (Fig. 1). For studies of erythrocyte flow within cerebral capillaries, we placed the line within the horizontal part of a capillary. Figure 1 shows schematically why moving erythrocytes are seen as oblique stripes. From such an image one can calculate (Fig. 1b) the *velocity* of each erythrocyte *b/a*, the *erythrocyte supply rate* (n/s; *n*=number of stripes, s=second), i.e., the number of erythrocytes passing per second, and the *distance* between subsequent blood cells in space (*c1+d1* or *c2+d2*) and time (*e1+f1*). Space time images can be acquired continuously and video monitored in order to monitor changes in the above-mentioned parameters over time.

Results

An example of a three-dimensional reconstruction of a part of the microvascular network is given in Fig. 2. In a capillary within this network (see horizontal line), erythrocyte flow was studied with the single line approach (see "Methods"). The space time plot demonstrating erythrocyte flow is given in Fig. 3a. The number of stripes corresponds to the blood cells supply rate, the angle of the stripes is a measure of the erythrocyte velocity, the horizontal distance between subsequent stripes gives the distance in space, and the vertical distance between subsequent stripes gives the distance in time between the moving blood cell. The increase in erythrocyte volocity

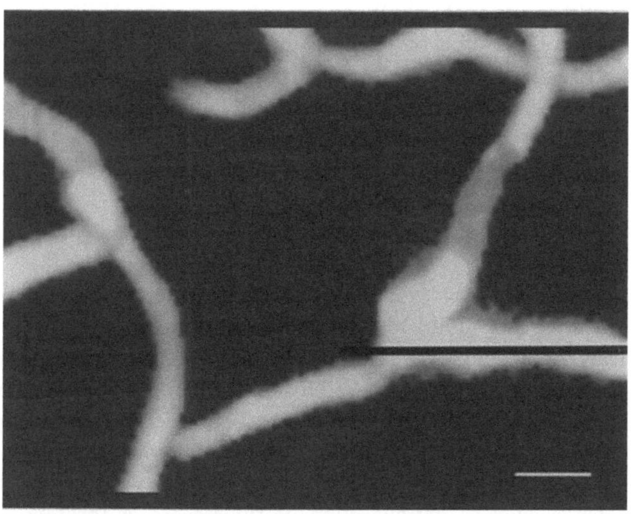

Fig. 2. Three-dimensional reconstruction of part of the capillary network 85–105 μm beneath the brain surface. The *scale bar (lower right)* is 10 μm. The *horizontal line* within the capillary on the right side of the image is the position chosen for continuous one-dimensional imaging (see Fig. 3)

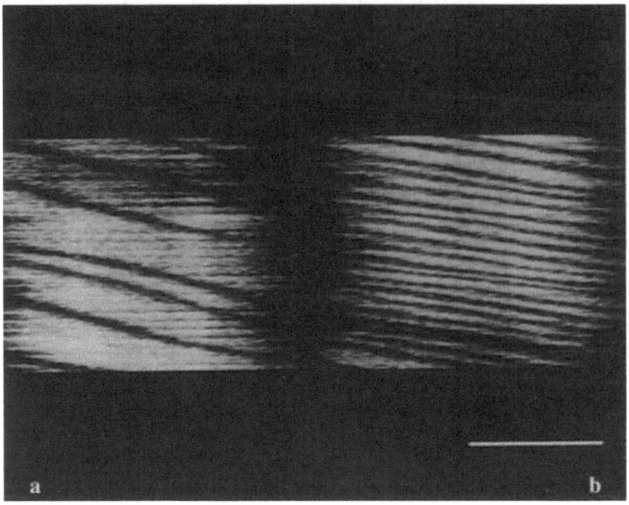

Fig. 3a, b. Example of single line method to assess erythrocyte flow within a single capillary before and after CO_2 stimulation. **a** Space time image of capillary indicated in Fig. 2 under normocapnia. Scale bar is 25 μm. Distance from top to bottom, 1 s. Erythrocyte velocities are between 150 and 200 μm/s. **b** Space time image of the same capillary under hypercapnia (ventilation with 5% CO_2). Erythrocyte velocities are between 250 and 300 μm/s. Scale bar is 25 μm. Distance from top to bottom is 1 s.

and supply rate during hypercapnia is demonstrated in Fig. 3b showing the same capillary as in Fig. 3a during ventilation of 5% CO_2.

Discussion

We have established a new approach for the study of the cerebral microcirculation in vivo using confocal laser scanning microscopy.

The method permits:
- The observation of superficial pial vessels under resting and stimulated conditions (Villringer et al. 1989).
- The observation of fluorescein-filled blood vessels down to a depth of 250 μm beneath the brain surface (Villringer et al. 1990, Dirnagl et al. 1991).
- Three-dimensional reconstructions of the microvascular network in vivo based on optical sections (Villringer et al. 1990, Dirnagl et al. 1991).
- The differentiation of plasma and blood cells within cerebral capillaries (Dirnagl et al. 1990).
- The observation of selectively labeled leukocytes within these capillaries (Villringer et al. 1991).
- The continuous assessment of erythrocyte flow within cerebral capillaries under resting and stimulated conditions (this report).

Thus this method seems to be a powerful new approach to assess controversial issues in the cerebral microcirculation such as the existence of capillary recruitment (Weiss 1988; Göbel et al. 1990). However, before CLSM can be applied to the study of the physiology and pathophysiology of the brain microcirculation the potential damage to the tissue has to be considered. In our current experimental paradigm no signs of tissue damage such as extravasation of fluorescein or thrombocyte aggregates have been observed, and the reaction of the blood vessels to stimuli such as hypercapnia and acetazolamide remained intact. Further studies (influence of CLSM on the ultrastructure of brain capillary endothelium, brain protein synthesis, brain tissue ATP levels) on potential damage in our model are underway.

References

Dirnagl U, Villringer A, Haberl RI, Einhäupl KM (1990) In vivo confocal laser scanning microscopy (CLSM): laser light induced alterations of erythrocyte flow in rat brain capillaries sensitized with intravascular fluorescein. Trans R Microsc Soc [New Series] 1:337–340

Dirnagl U, Villringer A, Gebhardt R, Haberl R, Einhäupl KM (1991) Three-dimensional reconstruction of the rat brain cortical microcirculation in vivo. J Cereb Blood Flow Metab 11:353–360

Göbel U, Klein B, Schröck H, Kuschinsky W (1989) Lack of capillary recruitment in the brains of awake rats during hypercapnia. J Cereb Blood Flow Metab 9:491–499

Ivanov KP, Kalinina MK, Levkovich YI (1981) Blood flow velocity in capillaries of brain and muscles and its physiological significance. Microvasc Res 22:143–155

Ma YP, Koo A, Kwan HC, Cheng KK (1974) On-line measurements of the dynamic velocity of erythrocytes in the cerebral microvessels in the rat. Microvasc Res 8:1–13

Morii S, Ngai AC, Winn RH (1986) Reactivity of rat pial arterioles and venules to adenosine and carbon dioxide: with detailed description of the closed cranial window technique in rats. J Cereb Blood Flow Metab 6:34–41

Pawlik G, Rachi A, Bing RJ (1981) Quantitative capillary topography and blood flow in the cerebral cortex of cats: an in vivo microscopic study. Brain Res 208:35–58

Rosenblum WI, Zweifach BW (1963) Cerebral microcirculation in the mouse brain. Arch Neurol 9:414–423

Villringer A, Haberl RL, Dirnagl U, Anneser F, Verst M, Einhäupl KM (1989) Confocal laser microscopy to study microcirculation on the rat brain surface in vivo. Brain Res 504:159–160

Villringer A, Dirnagl U, Gebhardt R, Haberl RL, Einhäupl KM (1990) Non-invasive optical sectioning of structures in the living rat brain. Trans R Microsc Soc [New Series] 1:353–356

Villringer A, Dirnagl U, Them A, Schürer L, Krombach F, Einhäupl KM (1991) Imaging of leukocytes within the rat brain cortex in vivo. Microvasc Res 42:305–315

Weiss HR (1988) Measurement of cerebral capillary perfusion with a fluorescent label. Microvasc Res 36:172–180

Continuous Measurement of Acetazolamide-Stimulated Cerebral Blood Flow by Laser Doppler Flowmetry

R. L. Haberl, M. Boerschel, U. Dirnagl, A. Piepgras, P. Schmiedek, and K. M. Einhäupl

Laser Doppler (LD) flowmetry is a relatively new technique for the measurement of capillary blood flow. It has been used for cerebral blood flow (CBF) measurement in various experimental preparations (Skarphedinsson et al. 1988; Haberl et al. 1989a, b; Dirnagl et al. 1989) and there are preliminary reports on the clinical application of the technique during brain surgery (Rosenblum et al. 1987; Arbit et al. 1989). It has several advantages over alternative methods for CBF evaluation: The LD measurement is continuous, it is noninvasive in that the detection probe does not penetrate the tissue to be analyzed, and it is highly sensitive to small and transient blood flow changes. Disadvantages are that the brain or the dura needs to be exposed through a burr hole or a craniotomy and that the measurement is highly localized.

Methods and Materials

The principle of LC flowmetry has been described in detail previously (Stern et al. 1977). Briefly, low-energy laser light (instrument used; BPM 403, Vasamedics Inc., diode laser; wavelength, ca. 780 nm) in conducted to the tissue by a fiberoptic light guide and penetrates the tissue to a depth of 1–1.5 mm. The light is reflected by stationary tissue cells without frequency shift and by moving particles with a Doppler shift in frequency. Randomly scattered light is guided back to the machine. The frequency-shifted portion of the backscattered light is further processed electronically and digital outputs for the volume and the velocity of the moving particles in the illuminated tissue are produced (arbitrary units). Blood flow corresponds to the arithmetic product of volume times velocity. Due to the principle of the measurement, LD blood flow basically reflects capillary red cell flux in a tissue volume of about 1 mm^3. Unlike ultrasound Doppler sonography, flow information is nondirectional because of random light-scattering events in the tissue.

Changes in LD flow have been shown to correlate well with CBF changes as measured by the hydrogen clearance technique (Skarphedinsson et al. 1988; Haberl 1989a), microspheres (Eyre et al. 1988), and [^{14}C]iodoantipyrine autoradiography (Dirnagl et al. 1989). The LD technique is not appropriate for quantitative CBF measurement. Absolute CBF measurement by autoradiography (in ml/100 g min) did not correlate with arbitrary blood flow units in the LD evaluation (Dirnagl et al. 1989).

Experiments were carried out on anesthetized rabbits equipped with a closed cranial window (Levasseur et al. 1975). The animals were mechanically ventilated, end expiratory CO_2 was continuously measured with a Heyer infrared CO_2 analyzer, and arterial blood samples were periodically evaluated for PCO_2, PO_2, and pH with an AVL 940 blood gas analyzer. Blood pressure was measured through a catheter in the femoral artery. The LD probe (0.84 mm in diameter) was inserted through a port in the steel frame of the cranial window and was positioned over a parietal cortical area free of visible large surface vessels (dura removed). An intracranial pressure of about 5 mmHg was produced by filling the cranial window with artificial CSF (Levasseur et al. 1975) through inlet and outlet openings in the windows and by setting the outflow tube at a fixed height. Diameters of two to three pial arterioles in each rabbit (range, 40–120 μm) were measured with a microscope and videometry. Acetazolamide (Diamox, Lederle FRG) was administered into the femoral vein as bolus injections at concentrations of 1–20 mg/kg body wt. Pial arteriolar diameter responses were measured at 2- to 5-min intervals for 60 min after injection and LD flow was conintuously recorded with a signal averaging time of 5 s.

Results

Figure 1a shows that there was a dose-dependent increase in arterical CO_2 tension and arterial acidosis after i.v. injection of different concentrations of acetazolamide, consistent with red cell carboanhydrase inhibition. Blood gas changes seen in these mechanically ventilated animals were more pronounced than in spontaneously breathing subjects. Within 5 min after acetazolamide injection, LD flow and pial arteriolar diameters increased in a dose-dependent manner (Fig. 1b). Maximum increases were attained at 7 mg/kg body wt. Higher concentrations had similar maximum effects, but vasodilatation and LD flow increase were sustained. Nearly steady-state flow for 10–15 min after acetazolamide injection was produced with concentrations between 10 and 20 mg/kg body wt.

When a further increase in arterial PCO_2 and a decrease in arterial pH were induced by inhalation of 5% CO_2 gas in room air at 5 min following injection of 20 mg/kg body wt. acetazolamide, no vasodilation and flow increase in addition to that seen with acetazolamide was observed. This result may suggest that the mechanism leading to CBF increase is maximally stimulated by 20 mg/kg body wt. acetazolamide and that hypercapnia and acetazolamide share a similar mechanisms to induce the CBF increase. Further studies, however, have to consolidate this assumption.

Discussion

Laser Doppler flowmetry is a valuable technique for instantaneous, continuous measurement of blood flow changes in the brain. It has the potential for clinical use when a burr hole or craniotomy is indicated for other reasons. Stimulated CBF measurement as a bedside follow-up parameter, with the possibility of guiding anti-ischemic therapy or intracranial pressure therapy in critically ill patients, may be possible with the laser Doppler technique.

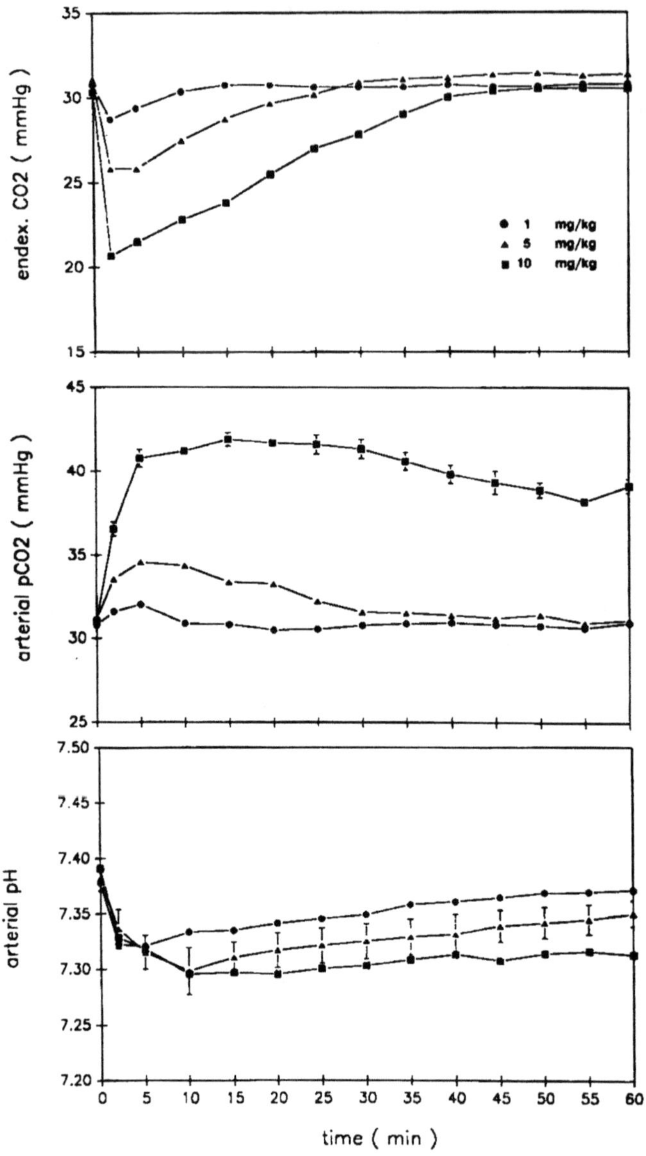

Fig. 1a. Effect of different acetazolamide concentrations on end expiratory CO_2, arterial PCO_2, arterial PO_2, arterial pH

Fig. 1b. Response of pial arteriolar diameters and LD flow to acetazolamide. Each acetazolamide concentration was tested in a separate group of four rabbits. The baseline diameter of all vessels was 73±2.2 μm (mean ± SEM, n=62). Note that arterial blood gas and arterial pH changes were not likely to be causally related to the blood flow changes seen. Rather, *perivascular* acidosis due to reduced transport of CO_2 from the brain to the blood may induce the diameter and blood flow response.

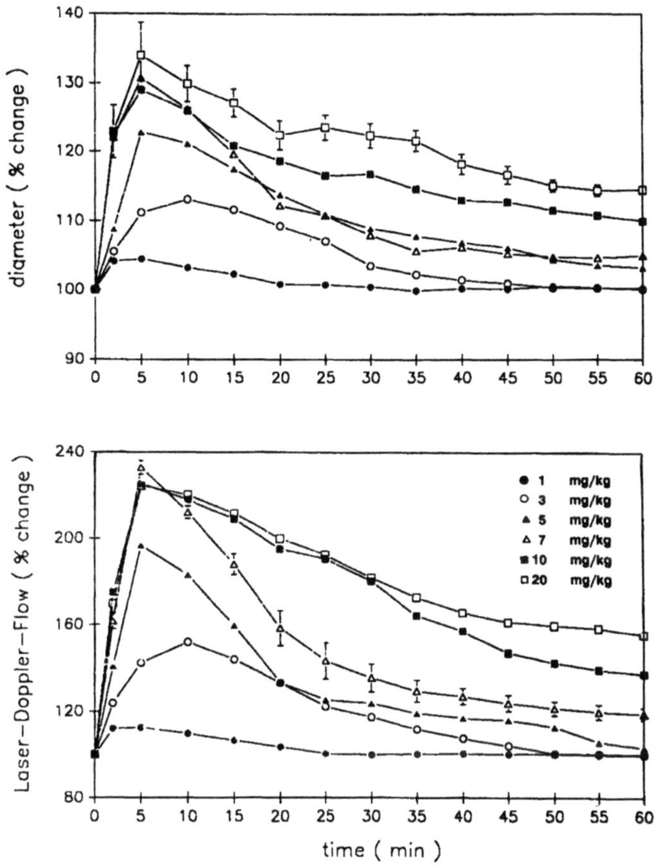

References

Arbit E, DiResta GR, Bedford RF, Shah NK, Galicich JH (1989) Intraoperative measurement of cerebral and tumor blood flow with laser Doppler flowmetry. Neurosurgery 24:166–170

Dirnagl U, Kaplan B, Jacewicz M, Pulsinelli W (1989) Continuous measurement of cerebral cortical blood flow by laser Doppler flowmetry in a rat stroke model. J Cereb Blood Flow Metab 9:589–596

Eyre JA, Essex TJ, Flecknell PA, Bartholomew PH, Sinclair JI (1988) A comparison of measurements of cerebral blood flow in the rabbit using laser Doppler spectroscopy and radionuclide labelled microspheres. Clin Phys Physiol Meas 9:65–74

Haberl RL, Heizer ML, Marmarou A, Ellis EF (1989a) Laser Doppler assessment of brain microcirculation: effect of systemic alterations. Am J Physiol 256:H1246–H1254

Haberl RL, Heizer ML, Ellis EF (1989b) Laser Doppler assessment of brain microcirculation: effect of local alterations. Am J Physiol 256:H1255–H1260

Levasseur JE, Wei EP, Raper AJ, Kontos HA, Patterson JL (1975) Detailed description of a cranial window technique for actue and chronic experiments. Stroke 6:308–317

Rosenblum BR, Bonner RF, Oldfield EH (1987) Intraoperative measurement of cortical blood flow adjacent to cerebral AVM using laser Doppler velocimetry. J Neurosurg 66:396–399

Skarphedinsson JO, Harding H, Thoren P (1988) Repeated measurement of cerebral blood flow in rats. Comparisons between the hydrogen clearance method and laser Doppler flowmetry. Acta Physiol Scand 124:133–142

Stern MD, Lappe DL, Bowen PD, Chimosky JE, Holloway GA Jr, Keiser HR, Bowman RL (1977) Continuous measurement of tissue blood flow by laser Doppler spectroscopy. Am J Physiol 232:H441–H448

Transcranial Doppler Ultrasound and Regional Cerebral Blood Flow Assessment of Cerebral Hemodynamics: The Acetazolamide Test

A. Dahl, R. Nyberg-Hansen, D. Russell, and K. Rootwelt

Introduction

Evaluation of the cerebral perfusion reserve is important in one way or another in patients with impaired circulation of the brain. Cerebral hemodynamics can be assessed noninvasively by both single photon emission computed tomography (SPECT) and transcranial Doppler ultrasound (TCD). SPECT measures global and regional cerebral blood flow (rCBF) (Lassen 1985), while TCD enables blood flow velocities to be measured in basal intracranial inflow arteries (Aaslid et al. 1982). Although TCD does not directly measure flow, there is a linear relationship between flow and velocity in a particular artery if the diameter of the vessel remains constant. The relationship between velocity and flow in a defined cerebral artery system is, however, complex. Velocity depends not only on the diameter of the vessel, but also upon rCBF in its perfusion territory and the size of the territory in question (Sorteberg et al. 1989).

The capacity of the cerebral perfusion reserve may be determined by assessing vasoreactivity using a potent vasodilator stimulus such as CO_2 or acetazolamide (Gibbs et al. 1984; Brown et al. 1986; Bullock et al. 1985; Schroeder et al. 1987; Vorstrup et al. 1986; Herold et al. 1988; Russell et al. 1990, Piepgras et al. 1990). The response provides a measure of the capacity of the cerebral circulation for further vasodilation. The present paper discusses some aspects of cerebral hemodynamics obtained by SPECT and TCD studies in healthy subjects and in patients with carotid occlusive disease. Particular emphasis is paid to the use of the *acetazolamide test* in the assessment of cerebral vasoreactivity.

Material and Methods

We studied the relationship between velocity in the middle cerebral artery (MCA) and rCBF in its perfusion territory by TCD and SPECT recordings in *healthy volunteers*. rCBF was studied in 33 subjects (Dahl et al. 1989; Nyberg-Hansen et al. 1990). Measurements were made before and approximately 20 min after the i.v. administration of 1 g acetazolamide. TCD recordings were performed *simultaneously* with SPECT in 20 of the control subjects using probes which were permanently fixed throughout the examination. Cerebral vasoreactivity was calculated as the difference between the two rCBF and velocity values.

Two groups of *patients* with carotid occlusive disease have been studied (Dahl et al. 1990a, b): (a) unilateral internal carotid artery (ICA) stenosis with a greater than 50%

diameter reduction (n=11) and (b) occlusion of one ICA and a normal vessel or a stenosis less than 50% on the contralateral side (n=9). rCBF measurements were made before and approximately 20 min after acetazolamide administration, while blood velocity was measured before the first and immediately after the second SPECT study.

Regional Cerebral Blood Flow Examination

Regional cerebral blood flow was studied by xenon-133 inhalation and a SPECT machine with rapidly rotating detectors (Tomomatic 64, Medimatic Inc., Copenhagen, Denmark). Using high-sensitivity collimators, three slices of the brain were studied simultaneously (Stokely et al. 1980; Lassen 1985; Rootwelt et al. 1986). The slices were 2 cm thick and routinely positioned 2, 6, and 10 cm above the orbitomeatal (OM) plane. The resolution in the plane of each slice was 1.7 cm (full width, half maximum, FWHM). rCBF was calculated in milliliters per 100 g per minute from slice 2 (OM + 6 cm) in a standardized region of interest in each hemisphere corresponding approximately to the estimated perfusion territory of the MCA at that slice level. This was obtained using a software package for automatic calculation of flow values in regions of interest (Rootwelt et al. 1986).

Transcranial Doppler Ultrasound Examination

Blood velocity was measured with a 2-MHz range-gated pulsed wave Doppler instrument with on line spectrum analysis (TCD 2-64 EME, Überlingen, FRG). Peak systolic velocity, diastolic velocity, and mean velocity (the time mean from spectrum outline) were measured in the proximal segment of the MCA on both sides from at least ten cardiac cycles for comparison with the rCBF findings. The pulsatility index (PI = max. systolic – max. diastolic velocity/mean velocity) (Gosling and King 1974) and the pulsatility transmission index (PTI) (Lindegaard et al. 1985) were calculated. The PTI was obtained by dividing the PI on the side of the lesion by the PI of the contralateral MCA. No correction of either rCBF or velocity values for PCO_2 was carried out in this study.

Results

Healthy Subjects

In healthy subjects both rCBF and velocity increased after administration of acetazolamide (Dahl et al. 1989; Nyberg-Hansen et al. 1990). There was an uniform increase in hemispheric CBF without changing the regional flow pattern. Since the two sides of the brain cannot be considered independent of each other, flow and velocity were compared on each side separately. The increase in rCBF in the MCA perfusion territory after administration of acetazolamide was 16.2±0.9 (SEM) and 16.4±0.8 ml/100 g per minute on the right and left side, respectively. The corresponding increase in mean MCA blood velocity was 23.2±1.8 (SEM) and 24.7±1.9 cm/s on the right and left side, respectively. There was no significant side-to-side asymmetry of the increase after acetazolamide in either rCBF or blood velocity.

Fig. 1 A, B. Relationship between mean blood velocity in the MCA and rCBF in the corresponding perfusion territory on the right side under baseline conditions **(A)**, and on the left side after acetazolamide administration **(B)** in 20 healthy volunteers

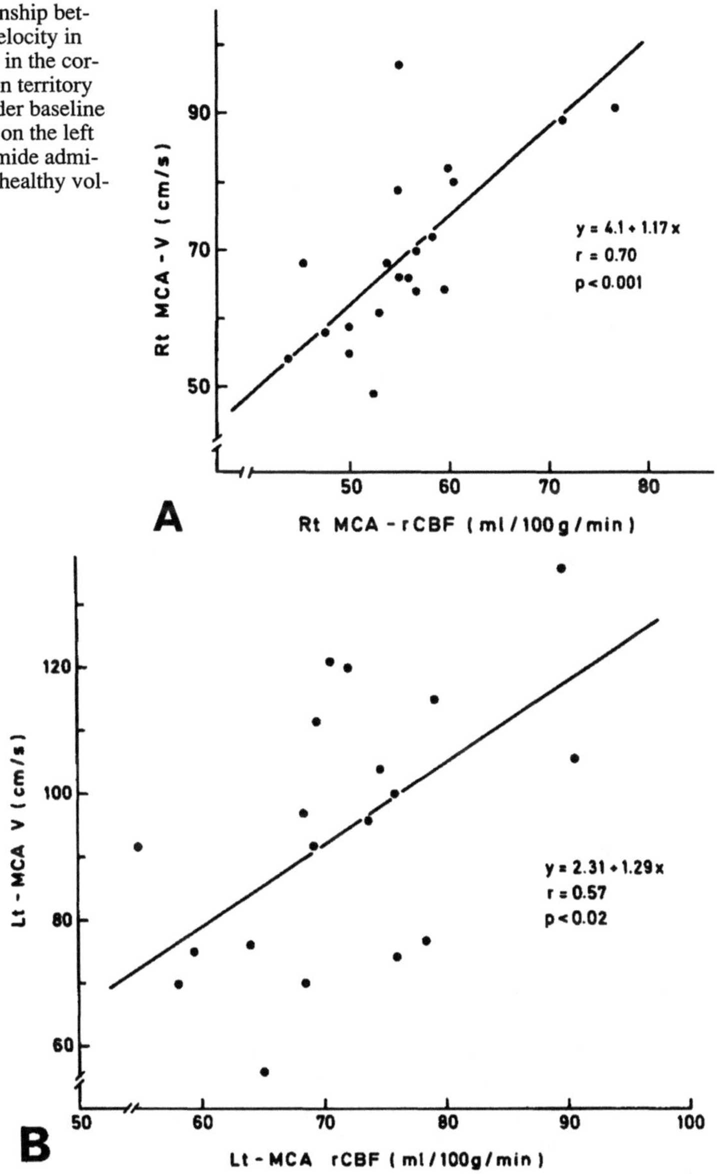

There was a good correlation between rCBF and mean velocity both under baseline conditions (right side: r=0.70, p<0.001; left side: r=0.64, p<0.005) and after acetazolamide administration (right side: r=0.64, p<0.005; left side: r=0.57, p<0.02) in the 20 subjects studied simultaneously by SPECT and TCD. The correlation was best under baseline conditions (Fig. 1).

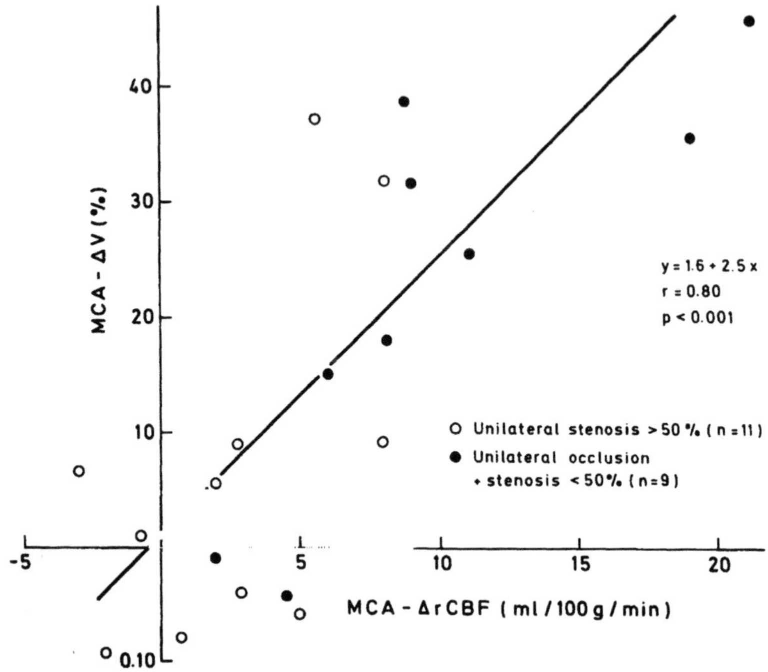

Fig. 2. Relationship between the side-to-side asymmetry of the increase in mean MCA velocity and the increase in rCBF in the MCA perfusion territory after acetazolamide administration in 20 patients with carotid occlusive disease

Patients with Carotid Occlusive Disease

The SPECT and TCD findings were compared on the right and left side in order to assess side-to-side asymmetry of the response to acetazolamide in the two groups of patients with carotid occlusive disease (Dahl et al. 1990a, b). Reduced vasoreactivity was demonstrated on the side of the lesion (occlusion, stenosis) with both techniques. The asymmetry was much greater in patients with occlusion than in those with stenoses with regard to both flow and velocity. The asymmetry of the increase in rCBF was significantly higher than in the controls both in the group with occlusion ($p<0.01$) and in the group with stenosis ($p<0.05$). Due to the restricted number of patients and the considerable spread in velocity values, the asymmetry of the increase in mean velocity reached statistical significance only in the former ($p<0.01$), but not in the latter group. There was a good correlation between the asymmetry of the increase in mean velocity and the increase in rCBF after acetazolamide administration in the two groups of patients with carotid occlusive disease taken together ($r=0.80$, $p<0.001$) (Fig. 2).

The asymmetry of vasoreactivity found in the SPECT studies was compared with the PTI recorded on baseline TCD examination. A good correlation was also observed between these two parameters ($r=0.64$, $p<0.01$). We also found that the estimated PTI giving asymmetry in rCBF acetazolamide response = 0 was not significantly different from 1 (Fig. 3).

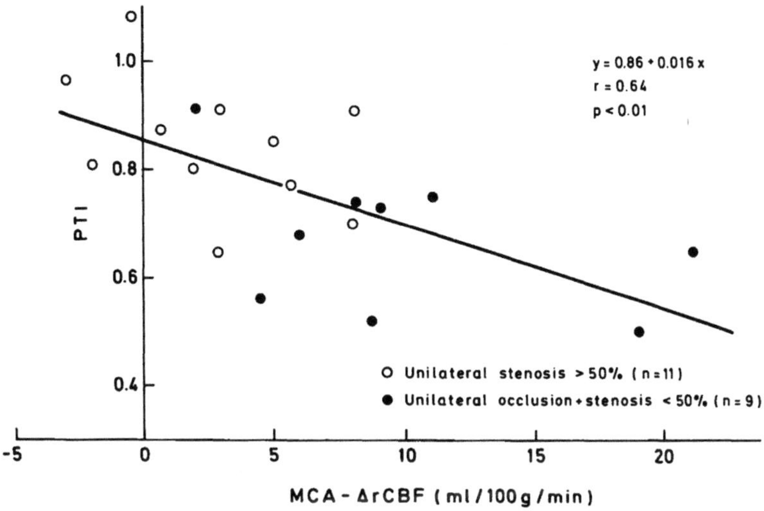

Fig. 3. Relationship between PTI recorded on baseline TCD examination and the asymmetry of the increase in rCBF after acetazolamide administration in 20 patients with carotid occlusive disease

Discussion

Evaluation of cerebral vasoreactivity and the perfusion reserve of the brain may prove to be important in the assessment of patients with cerebrovascular disease. We have found the acetazolamide test a useful tool for this purpose both in SPECT and TCD studies (Dahl et al. 1990a, b; Nyberg-Hansen et al. 1990). SPECT measures rCBF in brain parenchyma and TCD measures blood velocities in cerebral inflow arteries. However, by simultaneous recordings in healthy volunteers, we have found a relatively good correlation between the results obtained by these two techniques, both under baseline conditions and when testing cerebral vasoreactivity with acetazolamide (Dahl et al. 1989, Nyberg-Hansen et al. 1990). When direct comparison is made, it is essential that the measurements are performed under conditions identical with regard to PCO_2, preferably with simultaneous recordings.

A relatively good correlation between SPECT and TCD has been found when cerebral vasoreactivity is assessed by the acetazolamide test in patients with carotid occlusive disease (Dahl et al. 1990a, b; Nyberg-Hansen et al. 1990; Piepgras et al. 1990). We have observed a good correlation between the asymmetry of the increase in mean velocity and the increase in rCBF in the MCA territory, and between PTI recorded on baseline TCD examination and the asymmetry of the increase in rCBF after acetazolamide administration. The PTI was obtained by dividing the PI on the side of the lesion by the PI of the contralateral MCA. The PI is an indicator of cerebral vascular resistance (Gosling and King 1974), and asymmetry in baseline values may predict asymmetry in vasoreactivity. This suggestion is confirmed in the present SPECT study when using the acetazolamide test to assess vasoreactivity.

By simultaneous SPECT and TCD recordings in healthy volunteers, we have previously shown that acetazolamide leads to an increase in mean MCA velocity proportional to the baseline value, while this is not the case with regard to rCBF (Dahl et al. 1989; Nyberg-Hansen et al. 1990). There is a positive correlation between the increase in velocity and baseline velocity. However, the increase in flow is not dependent on baseline flow values. Approximately the same increase occurs irrespectively of baseline rCBF (Rootwelt et al. 1986; Dahl et al. 1989; Nyberg-Hansen et al. 1990). When assessing cerebral vasoreactivity with the acetazolamide test, it is therefore probably correct to report the response as an absolute increase in flow with regard to rCBF, and a percentage increase when blood velocity is recorded in TCD studies.

Acetazolamide is known to cause a uniform increase in CBF, which is considered to be caused by vasodilation of resistance vessels (Posner and Plum 1960; Ehrenreich et al. 1961). The exact mechanism is not known, but a decrease in cerebral pH due to inhibition of carbonic anhydrase in the brain, causing carbonic acidosis, has been suggested (Severinghaus et al. 1969). A recent study indicates that the increase in CBF after short-term administration of acetazolamide is caused by a transient extracellular acidosis (Friberg et al. 1990). However, during prolonged oral treatment with the drug, CBF returns to normal values within 2 days, indicating that an adaptation has taken place returning the pH around the brain arterioles to normal values. At this time a delayed intracellular acidosis probably occurs.

The acetazolamide test has proved very useful in identifying patients with a limited perfusion reserve (Vorstrup et al. 1986; Schroeder et al. 1987; Russell et al. 1990; Piepgras et al. 1990). A significant change in flow pattern after acetazolamide administration indicates that some regions of the brain have less perfusion reserve than others. This test may be used as an alternative to CO_2 inhalation when testing vasoreactivity. The vasodilatory effect has been found to be at least as effective as 5% CO_2 inhalation (Ehrenreich et al. 1961). Acetazolamide offers several practical advantages and causes no or little discomfort to the patients. No side effects were observed in the present study. The cerebral metabolic rate for oxygen is reported to remain unchanged after short-term acetazolamide administration, and there is no significant change in systemic arterial blood pressure or arterial PCO_2 (Posner and Plum 1960; Vorstrup et al. 1984). The end-expiratory PCO_2 usually decreases 3–4 mmHg (Rootwelt et al. 1986) since inhibition of carbonic anhydrase in the erythrocytes impedes unloading of CO_2 in the lungs (Rootwelt et al. 1986). End-tidal PCO_2 therefore does not reflect the CO_2 tension in brain parenchyma.

Conclusions

There is a positive correlation between mean blood velocity in the MCA obtained by TCD examination and rCBF in the corresponding perfusion territory measured in SPECT studies under baseline conditions in healthy volunteers. When using the acetazolamide test to assess the capacity of the cerebral perfusion reserve, there is a relatively good correlation between the results obtained by TCD and SPECT in the MCA perfusion system, both in healthy subjects and in patients with carotid occlusive disease. The acetazolamide test has proved to be very useful for assessing the capacity of the perfusion reserve in patients with cerebrovascular disease.

References

Aaslid R, Markwalder TM, Nornes H (1982) Noninvasive transcranial Doppler ultrasound recording of flow velocity in basal cerebral arteries. J Neurosurg 57:769–774

Brown MM, Wade JPH, Bishop CCR, Russell RWR (1986) Reactivity of the cerebral circulation in patients with carotid occlusion. J Neurol Neurosurg Psychiatry 49:899–904

Bullock R, Mendelow AD, Bone I, Patterson J, Macleod WN, Allardice G (1985) Cerebral blood flow and CO_2 responsiveness as an indicator of collateral reserve capacity in patients with carotid arterial disease. Br J Surg 72:348–351

Dahl A, Russell D, Nyberg-Hansen R, Rootwelt K (1989) Cerebral vasoreactivity: simultaneous assessment by transcranial Doppler and rCBF studies. J Cereb Blood Flow Metab [Suppl 1] 9:364

Dahl A, Russell D, Nyberg-Hansen R, Lindegaard K-F, Rootwelt K (1990a) Assessment of cerebral vasoreactivity by blood velocity and rCBF measurements in unilateral carotid occlusive disease. J Neurol 237:157

Dahl A, Russell D, Nyberg-Hansen R, Lindegaard K-F, Rootwelt K (1990b) Vasoreactivity in carotid occlusive disease: a comparison of transcranial Doppler (TCD) and rCBF. Neurology [Suppl 1] 40:191

Ehrenreich DL, Burns RA, Alman FN, Fazekas J (1961) Influence of acetazolamide on cerebral blood flow. Arch Neurol 5:227–232

Friberg L, Kastrup J, Rizzi D, Jensen JB, Lassen NA (1990) Cerebral blood flow and end-tidal PCO_2 during prolonged acetazolamide treatment in humans. Am J Physiol 258:H954–H959

Gibbs JM, Wise RJS, Leenders KL, Jones T (1984) Evaluation of cerebral perfusion reserve in patients with carotid-artery occlusion. Lancet 1:310–314

Gosling RG, King DH (1974) Arterial assessment by Doppler-shift ultrasound. Proc R Soc Med 67:447–449

Herold S, Brown MM, Frackowiak RSJ, Mansfield AO, Thomas DJ, Marshall J (1988) Assessment of cerebral haemodynamic reserve: correlation between PET parameters and CO_2 reactivity measured by the intravenous ^{133}Xenon injection technique. J Neurol Neurosurg Psychiatry 51:1045–1050

Lassen NA (1985) Cerebral blood flow tomography with Xenon 133 inhalation – methodological considerations. In: Hartmann A, Hoyer S (eds) Cerebral blood flow and metabolism measurement. Springer, Berlin Heidelberg New York, pp 224–233

Lindegaard K-F, Bakke SJ, Gromilund P, Aaslid R, Huber P, Nornes H (1985) Assessment of intracranial hemodynamics in carotid artery disease by transcranial Doppler ultrasound. J Neurosurg 6:890–898

Nyberg-Hansen R, Dahl A, Russell D, Rootwelt K (1990) Simultaneous assessment of blood velocity and rCBF in the middle cerebral artery system. J Neurol 237:159

Piepgras A, Schmiedek P, Leinsinger G, Haberl RL, Kirsch CM, Einhäupl KM (1990) A simple test to assess cerebrovascular reserve capacity using transcranial Doppler sonography and acetazolamide. Stroke 21:1306–1311

Posner JB, Plum F (1960) The toxic effects of carbon dioxide and acetazolamide in hepatic encephalopathy. J Clin Invest 39:1246–1258

Rootwelt K, Dybevold S, Nyberg-Hansen R, Russell D (1986) Measurement of cerebral blood flow with ^{133}XE inhalation and dynamic single photon emission computer tomography. Normal values. Scand J Clin Lab Invest [Suppl 184] 46:97–105

Russell D, Dybevold S, Kjartansson O, Nyberg-Hansen R, Rootwelt K, Wiberg J (1990) Cerebral vasoreactivity and blood flow before and 3 months after carotid endarterectomy. Stroke 21:1029–1032

Schroeder T, Sillesen H, Engell HC (1987) Hemodynamic effect of carotid endarterectomy. Stroke 18:294–309

Severinghaus JW, Hamilton FN, Cotev S (1969) Carbonic acid production and the role of carbonic anhydrase in decarboxylation in brain. Biochem J 114:703–705

Sorteberg W, Lindegaard K-F, Rootwelt K, Dahl A, Russell D, Nyberg-Hansen R, Nornes H (1989) Blood velocity and regional blood flow in defined cerebral artery systems. Acta Neurochir (Wien) 97:47–52

Stokely EM, Sveinsdottir E, Lassen NA, Rommer P (1980) A single photon dynamic computer assisted tomography (DCAT) for imaging brain function in multiple cross sections. J Comput Assist Tomogr 4:230–240
Vorstrup S, Henriksen L, Paulson OB (1984) Effect of acetazolamide on cerebral blood flow and cerebral metabolic rate for oxygen. J Clin Invest 74:1634–1639
Vorstrup S, Brun B, Lassen NA (1986) Evaluation of the cerebral vasodilatory capacity by the acetazolamide test before EC-IC bypass surgery in patients with occlusion of the internal carotid artery. Stroke 17:1291–1298

Continuous Monitoring of Cortical Blood Flow and Intracranial Pressure in Severe Cerebral Trauma

L. CARTER AND C. A. DICKMAN

Introduction

It is commonly accepted practice to monitor intracranial pressure (ICP) in patients with severe head injury. Elevation of ICP is treated with appropriate measures to normalize ICP such as hyperventilation, diuretics, mannitol, drainage of CSF, and barbiturates. The various treatment modalities affect cerebral blood flow (CBF) flow differently. Therefore, knowing the CBF may help in selecting the proper treatment modality. Jaggi et al. (1990) demonstrated that patients who do poorly may either have markedly elevated CBF (hyperemia) or very low blood flows (ischemia). It may be that these two groups need to be treated in a different fashion. A continuous monitor of CBF may allow more appropriate treatment and hopefully decrease the risk of secondary neurological deficit.

Methods

Continuous monitoring of CBF may be obtained with either laser Doppler or thermal diffusion flow techniques. Because of the ease of use of the thermal system, we have chosen this to incorporate into a subdural ICP monitor so that CBF and ICP can be recorded simultaneously. Most other forms of monitoring CBF are intermittent such as stable xenon or radioactive clearance. We have incorporated a Flowtronics cerebral flow sensor (Flowtronics Inc., 10250 North 19th Avenue, Phoenix, Arizona, United States). The CBF sensor consists of two gold plates which rest on the cortex; one gold plate is heated and the other is neutral. The difference between these gold plates is recorded with thermistors; as the blood flow increases, the delta-T (temperature difference) decreases. This change in delta-T has been correlated with other methods of measuring CBF and is quantitative as described by Carter et al. (1981). In the same probe a fluid column can be connected to a transducer to monitor subdural ICP. Continuous monitoring of ICP and CBF can be carried out with this sensor, which is connected to a microprocessor, allowing immediate results and changes in ICP to be correlated with changes in CBF. This equipment has been used in patients with cerebral vascular disease, brain tumors, and cranial trauma.

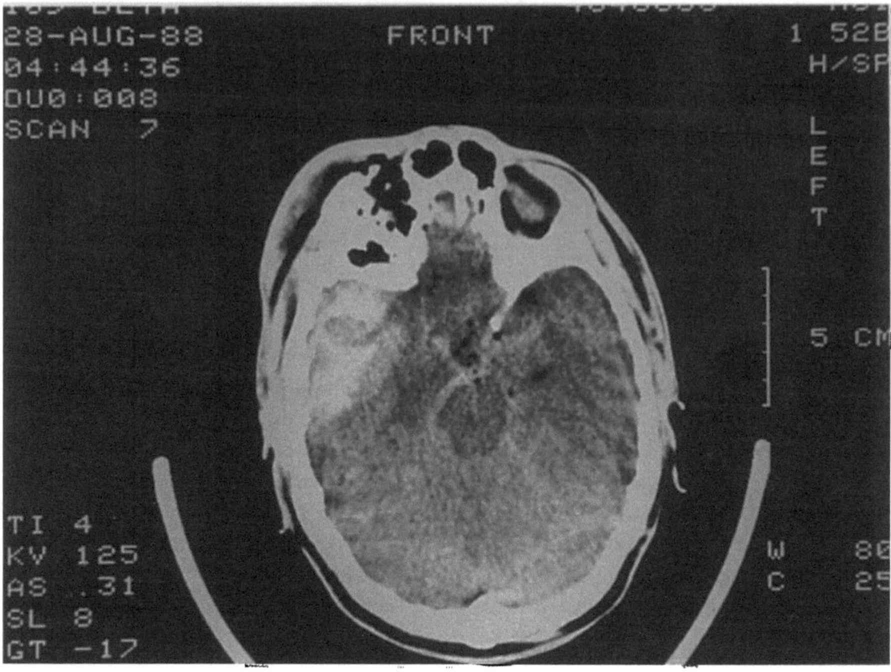

Fig. 1. A CT scan demonstrating a right temporal epidural hematoma, in case No. 1

Cases

We monitored ICP and CBF in 12 patients with severe cranial cerebral trauma. There were eight males and four females with a mean age of 31 years and an age range of 7–65 years. The probe was placed following operation 11 times and on one occasion was placed through a burr hole which was placed in the intensive care unit. The lesions monitored were seven subdural hematomas, four cerebral contusions, and one epidural hematoma. In two patients, increases in CBF preceded elevation of ICP and allerted the physicians to impending secondary elevations of ICP due to malignant cerebral edema. One patient did develop traumatic vasospasm and demonstrated a reduced CBF. Six of these patients proceeded to brain death, which was confirmed with clinical and electrographic findings. An example of two recordings of ICP and CBF follows.

Case No. 1 was on 22-year-old white male who was involved in a vehicular accident. The patient was obtunded with a left hemiparesis and on computerized tomography (CT) scan (Fig. 1) a right epidural hematoma was identified. Following surgical evacuation of the hematoma, a subdural monitor was placed. The patient's ICP and CBF were recorded in Fig. 2 and demonstrated ICPs in the normal range of 5–10 Torr and a CBF in the range of 35–40 ml/100 g per minute initially, subsequently up to 55–60 ml/100 g per minute when the monitor was removed. This patient had an uneventful recovery and an essentially normal ICP and improved CBF following the injury.

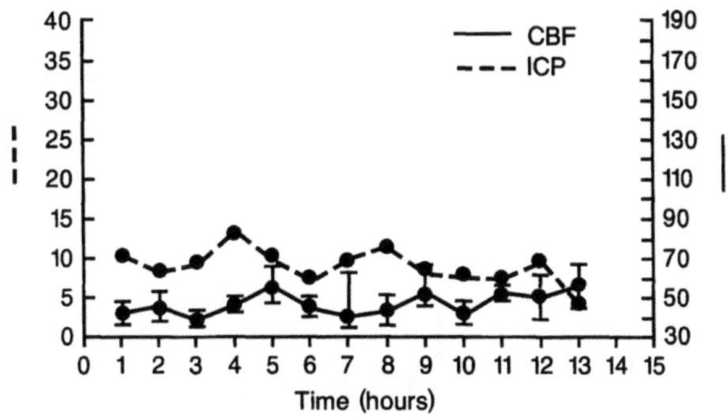

Fig. 2. Intracranial pressure and CBF monitoring of patient No. 1 with epidural hematoma. *Dashed line*, ICP; *solid line*, CBF

Case No. 2 was a middle-aged woman who was also involved in a vehicular accident and presented with severe head injury. Her initial Glasgow coma scale was 5 with a right third nerve palsy. She had severe right temporal contusions and was taken to surgery for evacuation of the contusions and a small subdural hematoma. The CT scan is shown in Fig. 3. Postoperatively, the patient was monitored and was found to have an initially high ICP with an ischemic CBF. The ICP subsequently fell to 0 and she was declared brain dead. This is illustrated in Fig. 4.

These two cases illustrate normal and abnormal CBF responses.

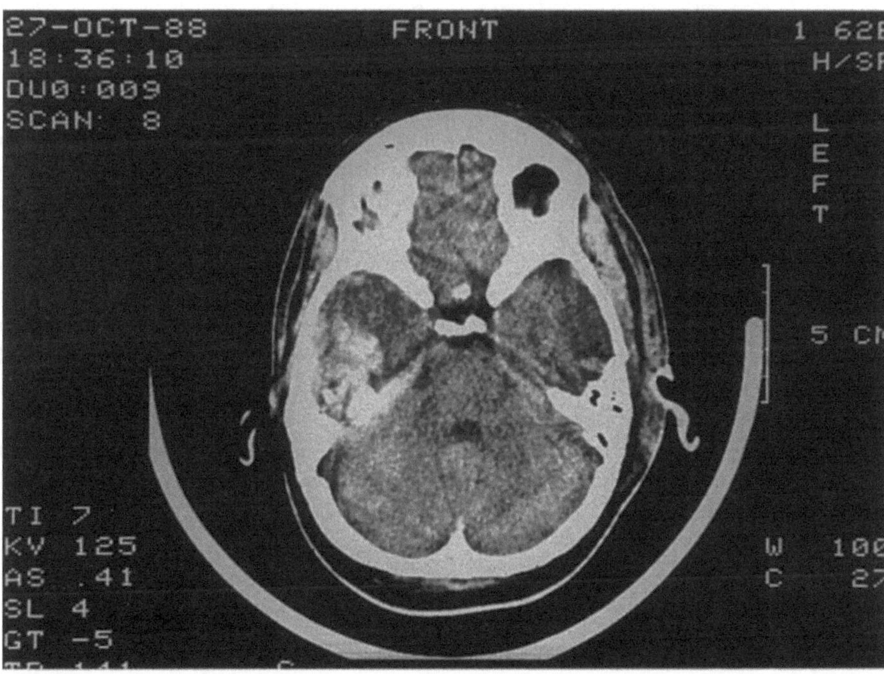

Fig. 3. Computerized tomography scan demonstrating a right temporal contusion in patient No. 2 with severe cranial cerebral trauma

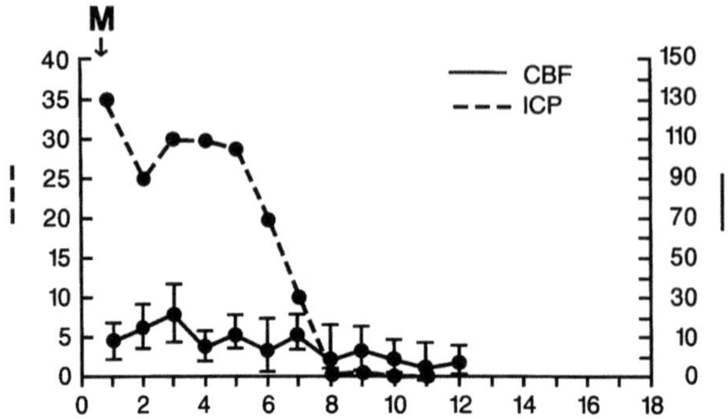

Fig. 4. Patient No. 2 with continuous monitoring of ICP and CBF. *Hatched line,* ICP; *solid line,* CBF. This demonstrates a significant elevation of ICP under conditions of cerebral ischemia. This condition of ischemia proceeded to brain death

Discussion

Thermal diffusion measured CBF is an additional parameter that can readily be monitored in trauma patients. The thermal diffusion blood flow probe has the advantage of providing a continuous real-time recording. The probe must be placed over normal cortex in areas away from contusion or surface vessels. The main disadvantage of the probe is that it monitors only a small area of cortex which one must assume is representative of the majority of the cortex. Artifact occurs if the probe loses contact with the cortex. This can be detected by a confidence factor which is identified by the microprocessor. The microprocessor turns off the heat and measures the temperature of the two plates. If they are in contact with the same tissue then the temperature is identical. This gives a confidence factor. The recording appears to be accurate if the confidence factor is 0.85 or greater.

No complications such as infection, hematomas, or brain injury occurred from the use of the ICP/CBF sensor. Sustained ischemic responses were associated with very poor prognosis while marked hyperemia frequently also had a poor prognosis. Hyperemia frequently preceded or was coincident with elevations of ICP.

Thermal CBF monitoring offers the opportunity to assess cerebral circulation and may potentially influence therapy. For example, if ICP is elevated with a low CBF, hyperventilation and barbiturates are not indicated. However, mannitol and elevation of blood pressure may help in improving cerebral perfusion. On the other hand, if ICP is elevated with a high CBF, then reduction of CBF may be achieved by hyperventilation and institution of barbiturate therapy.

The thermal diffusion flow probe has been tested extensively in the laboratory and in surgery (Carter et al. 1978, 1981, 1982). It now appears to be an excellent tool for postoperative monitoring.

Conclusion

Continuous monitoring of ICP and CBF in severe cerebral trauma is safe and feasible. It offers an innovative ability to study an additional parameter in the neurologically compromised head injury patient. Poor prognosis occurs in patients with severe ischemia and hyperemia. It may be that therapy should be directed toward improving cerebral circulation under these circumstances. A continuous CBF monitor may allow such therapeutic endeavors.

References

Carter LP, White WL, Atkinson JR (1978) Regional cortical blood flow at craniotomy. Neurosurgery 2:223–229

Carter LP, Erspamer R, Bro WF (1981) Cortical blood flow: thermal diffusion vs. isotope clearance. Stroke 12:513–518

Carter LP, Erspamer R, White WL, Yamagata S (1982) Cortical blood flow during craniotomy for aneurysm. Surg Neurol 17:204–208

Carter LP, Raudzens RA, Gaines C, Crowell RM (1984) Somatosensory evoked potentials and cortical blood flow during craniotomy for vascular disease. Neurosurgery 15:22–28

Jaggi JL, Obrist WD, Gennarelli TA, Langfitt TW (1990) Relationship of early cerebral blood flow and metabolism to outcome in acute head injury. J Neurosurg 72:176–182

Role of Cerebral Blood Flow Imaging in the Evaluation of Subarachnoid Hemorrhage and Intracranial Arteriovenous Malformations

H. H. Batjer

In 1984, Ackerman stated that "despite a considerable output of time, effort, and money, techniques for measuring CBF produced relatively little information that proved to be of clinical value in ischemic stroke disease". While this pessimism concerning the value of cerebral blood flow (CBF) measurement may be challenged in individual circumstances and certainly in management failures, subsequent studies with positron emission tomography (PET) scanning as well as large cooperative studies on the issue of cerebral revascularization have confirmed this somewhat nihilistic viewpoint for the larger group of patients presenting with complaints related to occlusive disease. Nevertheless, certain subgroups of patients definitely do become candidates for clinical CBF studies which can contribute to the decision-making process. In addition, the judicious acquisition of these data can lead to significant insight into pathopyhsiology both in the clinic and in the laboratory.

It is my belief, however, that we will never see such a negative conclusion about the use of CBF measurement in patients suffering from hemorrhagic stroke. The unique problems associated with the diagnosis of intracranial vascular malformations as well as the impact on the surrounding brain tissue of sequential arteriovenous malfunction (AVM) obliteration render this condition ideal for the acquisition of hemodynamic information of great clinical utility not obtainable through monitoring of clinical, radiographic, or systemic physiological parameters. The same points can be made concerning the management of aneurysmal disease both in the context of planned sacrifice of intracranial vessels (either temporary of permanent) and for the monitoring and therapeutic reversal of the myriad of hemodynamic derangements that accompany subarachnoid hemorrhage (SAH). This presentation will focus on information acquired from our center as well as others in the systematic evaluation and treatment of these disease states. Particular attention will be directed toward the major clinical problems encountered in the treatment of hemorrhagic stroke patients and on the potential roles that CBF measurement may play in the elucidation of pathophysiolocial mechanisms as well as in the very practical therapeutic decisions required in managing these patients.

Intracranial Arteriovenous Malformation

Intracranial AVMs remain a difficult and controversial disease entity associated with persistent management problems. While the best natural history data available to date stems from the experience of Ondra et al. (1990) in Finland, where an annual risk of rehemorrhage of 4% has been documented regardless of whether prior bleeding episodes have occurred, it is very likely that subgroups exist within the AVM population at large. All clinicians have seen patients whose AVMs repetitively bled or in whom neurological deficits relentlessly progressed to death or disability. We currently have little means of prospectively identifying these subgroups. Due to the current availability of multiple therapeutic modalities including primary embolization, stereotactic radiation therapy, and traditional microsurgery, it is becoming increasingly important to tailor therapy to the individual patient. For this reason an accurate determination of the etiology of the patient's symptoms becomes important. Currently it is extremely difficult to know whether a patient with a progressive neurological decline is sustaining repeated small hemorrhages or suffering from ischemic complications of his or her malformation. Magnetic resonance imaging (MRI) has certainly helped in this regard but the presence of hemosiderin around a malformation by MRI criteria is of limited value as many presumed unruptured AVMs are found at surgery to have definite areas of prior hemorrhage. Perhaps the most important single factor in the initial evaluation of the AVM patient concerns identification of risk factors for the various therapeutic modalities. We currently have little to go on in this regard except the surgeon's consideration of the size and eloquence of the malformation, the patient's general medical condition, and an awareness of the surgeon's own unique microsurgical skill and experience. Attempts at classification of AVMs have proven helpful, but to date concern largely radiographic criteria (Spetzler and Martin 1986). The risk of embolization therapy as a primary mode of treatment is difficult to assess but in our own experience involves approximately a 5% risk of hemorrhagic complication for each endovascular procedure performed (Purdy et al. 1990). The risk of stereotactic radiation therapy (brain necrosis, cranial neuropathy, ischemia) will become increasingly obvious as this modality becomes offered to wider aspects of the AVM population. As will be discussed below, a variety of hemodynamic disturbances are possible during and following treatment for AVM and have been associated with substantial morbidity and mortality. We currently have very limited means of diagnosing these complications in their precatastrophic period as well as limited means of monitoring therapeutic intervention in their management.

A number of physiological observations have been made regarding flow dynamics in AVMs. Nornes and Grip (1980) have detected flow values of up to 550 ml/min in individual AVM feeding vessels as well as increased venous pressures leading to poor metabolite delivery. In addition, cortical blood flow measured at sites remote from the actual AVM have been shown to increase significantly following removal of the AVM (Barnett et al. 1987). The high-flow low-resistance nature of the intracranial shunt has been felt to contribute to hypoperfusion in adjacent cerebral tissue and it is well known that progressive neurological deficits are common in patients with AVMs (Spetzler and Selman 1984). As early as 1949, Norlen observed improvement in hemiparesis following resection of an AVM. The concept of cerebral "steal" was described by Feindel and Perot in 1965. Pathological documentation of this phenomenon was noted by Constantino and Vintners in 1966 when neuronal dropout in an ipsilateral hippocampus was noted in an AVM patient. Spetzler et al. in 1978 performed unique physiological experiments in the feline in which an anastomosis was performed between the rostral carotid and the caudal jugular vein extracranially. The resultant extracranial fistula produced retrograde flow down the ipsilateral carotid artery resulting in a steal phenomenon of the ipsilateral hemisphere. In five cats, marked vasodilation of the afferent and efferent vessels occurred. When the fistula was temporarily occluded, autoregulation and PCO_2 control recovered immediately in all animals studied except the five cats in which vasodilation had occurred. Two of these cats became hemiparetic. These investigators concluded that CO_2 reactivity and autoregulation were lost in the presence of large arteriovenous shunts and that there was low resistance to flow in the AVM and high resistance in the surrounding vasculature. They postulated that small vessels maximally dilated to divert flow competitively from the AVM ultimately resulting in dysautoregulation, not unlike vessels in ischemic brain regions from any cause. At the time of sudden fistula occlusion, flow is redirected to the adjacent vessels whose arterioles cannot constrict to protect the capillaries, resulting in edema and hemorrhage. This phenomenon was termed the normal perfusion pressure breakthrough theory and explained occasionally dramatic clinical complications (Spetzler et al. 1978). Anecdotal evidence from clinical studies suggested that certain risk factors for hyperemic postoperative complications included large size, high flow, clinically obvious ischemia, radiographic evidence of hypoperfusion, and the presence of long tortuous feeding arteries.

We hoped that it might be possible to identify preoperative risk factors for the development of perioperative hemodynamic disturbances as well as poor clinical outcome by measuring regional CBF. We studied 62 patients referred to our center who ultimately underwent microsurgical resection of their AVM (Batjer et al. 1988b, 1989a–c). Clinical characteristics of the patient group including sex, age, and presenting symptoms were recorded as were radiographic characteristics including size, location, the presence or absence of intracerebral hematoma, the number of major feeding vessels, the presence of perforator recruitment, patterns of venous drainage (superficial, deep, or both), the sum of diameter of feeding vessels, and angiographic steal phenomena. CBF was performed with single photon emission computed tomography (SPECT) using xenon-133 inhalation. rCBF characteristics evaluated included total brain flow (average of right and left hemispheric flow) and steal regions (hand-drawn regions of ipsilateral and contralateral hypoperfusion). From these data, a "steal index" was calculated for ipsilateral and contralateral regions in which the "steal index" was defined as rCBF (steal area) divided by total brain flow. Hyperemic complications were liberally defined as unexpected intraoperative brain swelling or hemorrhage unrelated to technical error, postoperative CT evidence of edema unrelated to inadvertent proximal occlusion, or postoperative hemorrhage following angiographically proven AVM resection. These criteria for hyperemic complications were relatively liberal and based on the assumption that the full-blown catastrophic manifestations of "breakthrough" occurred relatively rarely, but that the same pathophysiological mechanisms were operant in many milder manifestations of the same syndrome. Outcome was defined as good (capable of independent life), poor (not capable of independent life), or dead. This patient series proved to be relatively representative of most large series of patients; nearly 50% presented with intracranial hemorrhage, 34% presented with progressive neurological deficit, 44% had a history of seizures, and 18% of patients had a serious headache history. Intracranial hematomas were detected in 13%, angiographic steal phenomena were documented in 37%, and perforating arteries were recruited into the feeding system in 31% of patients. As defined, hyperemic complications occurred in 21% of these patients. Analysis of the purely clinical and radiographic data demonstrated a number of interesting relationships (Batjer et al. 1989c). Older patients were found more frequently to present with progressive deficits; 44% of patients greater than 50 years old had ischemic symptoms while only 16% of patients younger than 30 years had similar complaints ($p<0.05$). The presence of perforator recruitment into the feeding system was associated with progressive neurological deficits; 53% of patients with perforator recruitment had ischemic deficits while only 26% of those without perforator recruitment had similar findings ($p<0.05$). Interestingly, the presence or absence of angiographically documented steal phenomena was not predictive of patients found to have progressive neurological deficits. Clinical and radiographic factors were analyzed to determine which of these characteristics were associated with the development of hyperemic complications. We found that the presence of angiographic steal was associated with hyperemic events; 35% of those patients with angiographic steal ultimately developed hyperemia while only 13% of those patients without angiographic steal developed similar complications ($p<0.05$). A striking relationship was noted in patients with perforator recruitment: while only 7% of patients without perforators recruited developed hyperemia, 53% of those with perforator recruitment developed these complications ($p<0.001$). Clinical outcome was surprisingly independent of most clinical and radiographic findings except the recruitment of perforating vessels. Eighty-eight percent of patients without perforating vessels recruited ultimately had a good outcome while only 68% of those with perforator recruitment had a good outcome ($p<0.07$). Hyperemic complications had a profound influence on outcome such that 92% of the patients who did not develop hyperemic complications ultimately recovered well while less than half of those patients developing hyperemic complications had similar favorable recoveries ($p<0.001$).

While all patients were found to have some visually identifiable brain region which was hypoperfused on rCBF imaging, these areas of steal were categorized as severe, moderate, or mild. (These categories were defined such that approximately one-third of patients fell into each group) (Batjer et al. 1988b, 1989a, b). Interestingly, the severity of steal was clearly predictive of patients presenting with progressive neurological deficits whereas angiographic phenomena had not been. Ninety percent of patients presenting with progressive deficits had steal indices of a severe or moderate degree while 41% of patients without progressive deficits were found to have steal indices in the mild category ($p<0.05$). A converse relationship was noted in patients who had presented with intracranial hemorrhage. Forty-three percent of those patients who had initially bled had a steal index in the mild category, while of the patients who had not suffered hemorrhage 47% where found to have severe steal, 34% had intermediate severity steal, and only 19% were noted to have a steal index in the mild range ($p<0.08$). A substantially larger patient series and perhaps prospective study would be required to determine whether two independent subgroups of patients exist: (a) those with depressed CBF around their malformation who may be at low risk of subsequent hemorrhage but at high risk of ischemic sequelae and (b) a group with higher flow around the AVM (less severe steal) who may be at higher risk of hemorrhage. No relationship was noted between the severity of ipsilateral steal (as calculated by steal index) and the size of the malformation, the number of feeding vessels involved, the presence of a hematoma, perforator involvement, angiographic steal, or the pattern of venous drainage. An interesting paradoxial relationship was frequently observed between angiographic criteria of hypoperfusion and rCBF evidence of steal. A number of patients with apparent angiographic steal phenomena were found to have surprisingly normal rCBF images while some patients with very early angiographic opacification of adjacent brain parenchyma were found to have severely depressed adjacent rCBF.

Early in our experience, we were performing routine acetazolamide (Diamox)-activated rCBF studies in patients with occlusive cerebral vascular disease in hopes of identifying patients with threatened perfusion reserve. The same provocative maneuver seemed to be an ideal mechanism to identify patients who could be at risk for hyperemic therapeutic complications. If the adjacent brain parenchyma of AVM patients behaved as tissue rendered chronically ischemic from occlusive disease, one would predict two possible responses to the administration of a vasodilator (acetazolamide). In the circumstance of intact vasoreactivity, one would expect to see flow augmentation in normal brain regions as well as in ischemic (steal) regions surrounding the AVM. In cases with failed vasoreactivity one would expect to see normal flow augmentation in normal brain tissue but to see no further vasodilation in the maximally dilated steal region. This maximally vasodilated tissue would logically be presumed to be at acute risk at the time of sudden flow redistribution during shunt obliteration (AVM resection). At the time of preparation of this manuscript, further data analysis is being performed on a large number of patients who were preoperatively challenged with acetazolamide but our preliminary experience suggests that our original hypothesis may have been incorrect. A patient that we have previously reported (Batjer et al. 1988a) was studied both with and without acetazolamide activation preoperatively. This patient ultimately developed fatal intraoperative and postoperative hyperemic complications resulting in severe hemorrhage and brain edema. The results of his pre- and postembolization rCBF studies were compared with four other patients with similar supratentorial malformations treated in similar fashion with aggressive preoperative embolization in whom baseline and acetazolamide rCBF studies were performed preoperatively and after embolization. These four control patients had uneventful perioperative courses and made normal recoveries. Several interesting features were noted from analysis of these rCBF studies (a). The patient with fatal outcome had a significantly depressed rCBF before treatment in both ipsilateral and contralateral hemispheres compared with the controlled group. (b) Therapeutic embolization resulted in a dramatic increase in rCBF in both hemispheres in this patient while changes in the control group were slight. (c) Acetazolamide augmented rCBF in the patient with fatal outcome both before and after embolization significantly more than in the control patients in the ipsilateral hemisphere. This pathological and paradoxical augmentation of flow to acetazolamide was a significant surprise. One would expect vessels in the surrounding brain regions to have been maximally dilated and totally unable to respond further to a vasodilating agent. This finding led us to postulate that there might be a potential dissociation in vasoreactive properties in vessels surrounding an AVM such that pharmacological or metabolic stimuli (or a sudden volume challenge) may induce further vasodilation, but that protective vasoconstriction may not be prompted by acute hemodynamic redistribution during shunt obliteration. If this theory is valid, one could postulate that similar untoward events (although perhaps somewhat milder in severity) might occur during endovascular embolization procedures in which modest flow redistribution occurs into surrounding tissue (Batjer et al. 1988a, 1989d).

Analysis of all clinical, radiographic, and rCBF data in our series led us to conclude that certain characteristics were associated with hyperemic complications and unfavorable outcome. The occurence of hyperemic complications was associated with the following variables: (a) recruitment of perforating vessels, (b) angiographic steal, (c) large AVM size, (d) larger sum of diameter of feeding vessels, (e) intermediate contralateral steal severity, (f) dramatic increase in hemispheric rCBF after therapeutic embolization, and (g) abnormal vasoreactivity. Enhanced vasodilation to acetazolamide may be a marker. Unfavorable outcome appeared to be associated with: (a) older patients, (b) recruitment of perforating vessels, (c) right hemispheric AVMs, (d) large AVM size, (e) depressed total brain blood flow, (f) mild ipsilateral steal severity, (g) mild contralateral steal severity, and (h) hyperemic complications. (f and g above imply relatively higher flow in areas around the AVM).

From this preliminary experience with the measurement of CBF in AVM patients, a number of potential roles for this modality to assist the clinician in evaluating and managing these patients becomes apparent. The evidence of and location of hypoperfused regions in patients presenting with ischemic symptoms can be accurately quantitated with accurate rCBF studies. This finding may assume great importance in the elderly patient with medical contraindications to a major surgical procedure who has a limited life expectancy in whom endovascular therapy may be able to selectively redistribute flow into ischemic regions to temporarily improve neurological function. Regional CBF determination offers some hope for the identification of subgroups of AVM patients whose natural history may be more malignant or more benign than the group of patients as a whole. With the availability of modern endovascular techniques myriads of new questions arise regarding which patients should be embolized, how many times they should be embolized, and what intervals should be used to separate these embolization attempts. Substantial controversy continues to exist regarding the timing of surgery after intracranial hemorrhage and after a final embolization procedure. This issue may be accurately resolved with the prospective use of MRI and rCBF measurement to maximize the brain's accommodation to new flow dynamics and minimize the risk of recruitment of collateral circulation to the AVM. Patients with postoperative deficits continue to pose a very difficult problem for the treating clinician. While postoperative angiography and sequential CT scanning provide some insight, it remains quite difficult in many circumstances to determine whether a given deficit and structural abnormality on CT scanning is related to an ischemic complication or brain edema that may be associated with poor tolerance of redistribution phenomena. The treatment for these alternate diagnoses may be quite different in selected cases. For the patient who develops a hyperemic state postoperatively, we have no standardized clinical or radiographic means to monitor our therapy for this condition. Regional CBF imaging holds major promise for assisting the clinician to optimize the patient's hemodynamic state. And finally perhaps the most important contribution that rCBF measurement could provide to this patient group involves the determination of markers for morbidity. Identification of an rCBF "fingerprint" that is associated with strikingly high therapeutic risk would be an invaluable contribution to clinical care of the patient.

Intracranial Aneurysm

Subarachnoid hemorrhage with the numerous structural and hemodynamic sequelae which occur over the ensuing days and weeks comprises a complex clinical laboratory in which we currently have limited ability for pathophysiological monitoring and intervention. Current clinical problems which contribute to the dismal prognosis for subarachnoid hemorrhage patients include structural tissue damage from the initial hemorrhage, delayed cerebral ischemia (vasospasm), rehemorrhage prior to surgery, and morbidity encountered as a result of errors in timing or execution of surgical therapy.

Management of the poor-grade patient remains difficult and controversial. All aneurysm surgeons have treated comatose patients with focal intraparenchymal or extraaxial hematomas from aneurysmal rupture who ultimately made excellent recoveries following emergent surgery. These same surgeons have also treated patients with identical clinical presentations who remained comatose postoperatively and ultimately died. There may be rCBF characteristics which could predict those patients in whom salvage was possible.

Cerebral vasospasm and resultant ischemia remains the major cause of death and disability following subarachnoid hemorrhage (Kassell and Torner 1983, 1984). Patients who tolerate their aneurysm clipping well and remain in good condition for several days may quickly develop dense and irreversible ischemic deficits refractory to all management modalities toward the end of the first posthemorrhage week. Meticulous and sequential neurological examinations can pinpoint the moment at which focal cerebral perfusion is diminished beyond the ischemic threshold, but the bedside clinician has little insight into the dynamics occurring over the hours and days previous to that event. Angiography can certainly diagnose angiographic vascular narrowing of variable degrees but this finding is notoriously unreliable in predicting the patients who are going to develop ischemic symptoms. CT scanning may document the establishment of cerebral infarction but yields little insight into the events prior to its occurrence. MRI may be more sensitive at documentation of early signs of infarction but this modality also provides little help to the clinician in predicting which patients should be treated aggressively early. Transcranial Doppler is emerging as a very helpful bedside technique from which important information may develop regarding the rapidity of the increase in flow velocity occurring over time. The slope of this curve may help predict which patients will develop symptoms and which will not. Nevertheless, the actual information acquired from this modality consists of blood velocity and not tissue blood flow. It is possible that sequential CBF imaging may provide insight into the patients who should be treated prophylactically by endovascular angioplasty or the administration of pressors (Yonas et al. 1989).

While Hunterian ligation may seem to be a historical methodology in the treatment of aneurysm patients, employment of this technique continues to play some role in the management of giant and thrombotic subarachnoid aneurysms and as well as skull base giant aneurysms not amenable to direct clipping. In these patients, we have found it extremely helpful to perform a diagnostic trial of parent vessel occlusion in the angiography suite with the patient awake. This type of physiological monitoring provides substantial insight into the patient's collateral potential and the ultimate safety of subsequent vessel sacrifice. We have found that between 80% and 85% of patients will tolerate a 45-min period of carotid occlusion when it is performed in this manner. When possible, it is our routine to perform CBF studies prior to and at the time of balloon inflation as has been previously described (de Vries et al. 1990; Erba et al. 1988; Steed et al. 1990). We have not had a patient develop subsequent ischemic neurological deficit at the time of vessel sacrifice who retained a normal rCBF distribution during temporary occlusion. Our sole ischemic complication involving carotid occlusion in a patient who had previously tolerated a 45-min provocative trial occurred in a woman on whom we were unable to obtain preoperative cerebral blood studies. This patient developed a progressive middle cerebral ischemic syndrome with minor CT evidence of infarction and ultimately stabilized after extracranial-intracranial arterial bypass. SPECT studies obtained during the progression of her neurological symptoms confirmed diffuse middle cerebral hypoperfusion with evidence of poor perfusion reserve on acetazolamide challenge and this state was improved following the bypass procedure.

From our preliminary experience in studying patients with a variety of disease states related to intracranial aneurysms, a number of potential roles for the widespread application of clinical rCBF measurement become apparent. There may be apparent rCBF correlates to explain why patients are initially poor clinical grade. A finding that hemodynamic disturbances may be operant in the very early posthemorrhage patient may provide avenues for therapy that would be ineffective in patients who simply suffered irreversible destructive structural damage. The timing of surgical intervention remains a major challenge and it is possible that rCBF imaging together with clinical variables may provide immeasurable assistance to the clinician in maximizing the patient's chances of undergoing successful aneurysm surgery. In this context, it may be possible to define a given patient's optimal preoperative hemodynamic state regarding crystalloid and colloid fluid administration as well as the administration of vasoactive agents. The hemodynamic affect of our various therapies for delayed cerebral ischemia are clinically assessable only by neurological parameters. Regional CBF measurement could conceivably provide insight into the degree of hemodilution necessary to maximize cerebral perfusion, the degree of volume expansion which optimizes perfusion, and the degree of induced hypertension necessary to augment flow. In this context, a number of patients are injured by the injudicious administration of these hemodynamic therapies (Adam and Batjer 1988; Batjer and Samson 1989). A number of patients develop substantial brain edema that likely results from the persistence of hyperdynamic therapy in the setting of established infarction. This clinical misadventure can convert a patient with a middle cerebral infarction who would ultimately make an acceptable neurological recovery into a patient with a life-threatening intracranial mass. CBF measurement may potentially provide insight into the question of when to convert hyperdynamic therapy to an alternate modality using aggressive diuresis and perhaps hypotension. The presence or absence of autoregulatory disturbances after subarachnoid hemorrhage could be feasibly documented with stimulated rCBF studies. The implications of these findings may have a profound influence on pertinent clinical questions concerning the selection of intraoperative blood pressure parameters as well as the surgeon's willingness to apply temporary arterial occlusion and how long such occlusion may be tolerated. In addition, as previously mentioned, it is our initial impression that rCBF measurement may provide further safety to parent vessel sacrifice in the treatment of giant aneurysm.

Clinical CBF Imaging

In my opinion, the sluggish application of rCBF measurement into routine clinical practice has resulted from several easily definable problems. The principle focus of most studies reported to date concerns the confirmation of information otherwise available on physical examination, CT, cerebral angiography, MRI, or transcranial Doppler. In many centers, the location of the CBF laboratory is at some distance from the inpatient setting. While there may substantial capability for the routine study of outpatients, in general the hemorrhagic stroke population will be in acute care centers and often in the intensive care unit environment. While convenience is a priority, patient safety is the critical factor. Patients in the acute phase following subarachnoid hemorrhage or following craniotomy for AVM simply cannot be moved routinely from their critical care environment. A very useful analogy may be invoked for the determination of prospective locations of CBF-measuring instruments. If a planned location is more difficult to access than the CT scanning suite, the results more difficult for the clinician to acquire than standard CT results, one may presume that the instrument will not be routinely available to the critically ill patient. In fact, the ideal location for such an instrument would be immediately adjacent to the CT scanner so that patients would ideally undergo both studies on the same trip from the intensive care unit, thus minimizing transit time and the period of least effective patient monitoring. The cost of rCBF studies (not including PET) should prove to be a trivial obstacle to the routine application of the studies in clinical practice if clear utility and safety are documented in the various disease states. As a clinician actively involved in the care of a large number of subarachnoid hemorrhage and AVM patients, it is clear to met that rCBF imaging is potentially an extremely powerful clinical tool. There can be little doubt that this technology has tremendous potential benefit in the elucidation of various pathophysiological states but it is my belief that direct and practical patient care can be substantially impacted and improved by the availability of these studies. Widespread adoption of these techniques to the care of hemorrhagic stroke victims in the academic as well as private setting is critically dependent on careful planning by the radiologist so that the rCBF laboratory is no more difficult to use than the CT scanner in a critical care setting. In addition, at this early time, it is critical to establish protocols on identifiable clinical problems and prospectively accumulate data that will yield insight into solving these problems.

References

Ackerman RH (1984) Of cerebral blood flow, stroke, and SPECT. Stroke 15:1–4

Adamson T, Batjer H (1988) Aneurysm recurrence associated with induced hypertension and hypervolemia. Surg Neurol 29:57–61

Barnett GH, Little JR, Ebrahim ZY, Jones SC, Friel HT (1987) Cerebral circulation during arteriovenous malformation resection. Neurosurgery 20:836–842

Batjer HH, Samson DS (1989) Causes of morbidity and mortality from surgery of aneurysms of the distal basilar artery. Neurosurgery 25:904–916

Batjer HH, Devous MD, Meyer YS, Purdy PD, Samson DS (1988a) Cerebrovascular hemodynamics in arteriovenous malformation complicated by normal perfusion pressure breakthrough. Neurosurgery 22:503–509

Batjer HH, Devous MD Sr, Seibert GB, Purdy PD, Ajmani AK, Delarosa M, Bonte FJ (1988b) Intracranial arteriovenous malformation: relationship between clinical and radiographic factors and ipsilateral steal severity. Neurosurgery 23:322–328

Batjer HH, Devous MD, Seibert GB, Purdy PD, Ajmani AK, Delarosa M, Bonte FJ (1989a) Intracranial arteriovenous malformation: relationship between clinical factors and cerebral blood flow. Neurol Med Chir (Tokyo) 29:395–400

Batjer HH, Devous MD, Seibert GB, Purdy PD, Ajmani AK, Delarosa M, Bonte FJ (1989b) Intracranial arteriovenous malformation: contralateral steal phenomena. Neurol Med Chir (Tokyo) 29:401–406

Batjer HH, Devous MD, Seibert GB, Purdy PD, Bonte FJ (1989c) Intracranial arteriovenous malformation: relationship between clinical factors and surgical complications. Neurosurgery 24:75–79

Batjer HH, Purdy PD, Giller CA, Samson DS (1989d) Evidence of blood flow redistribution during treatment for intracranial arteriovenous malformation. Neurosurgery 25:599–605

Constantino A, Vintners HV (1986) A pathogenic correlate of the "steal" phenomena in a patient with cerebral arteriovenous malformation. Stroke 17:103–106

De Vries EJ, Sekhar LN, Horton JA, Eibling DE, Janecka IP, Schramm VL, Yonas H (1990) A new method to predict safe resection of the internal carotid artery. Laryngoscope 100:85–88

Erba SM, Horton JA, Latchaw RE, Yonas H, Sekhar L, Schramm V (1988) Balloon test occlusion of the internal carotid artery with stable Xenon/CT cerebral blood flow imaging. Am J Neuroradiol 9:533–538

Feindel W, Perot P (1965) Red cerebral veins: a report on arteriovenous shunts in tumors and cerebral scars. J Neurosurg 22:315–325

Kassell NF, Torner JC (1983) Aneurysmal rebleeding: a preliminary report from the Cooperative Aneurysm Study. Neurosurgery 13:479–481

Kassell NF, Torner JC (1984) The International Cooperative Study on Timing of Aneurysm Surgery: an update. Stroke 15:566-570

Norlen G (1949) Arteriovenous aneurysms of the brain: report of 10 cases of total removal of the lesion. J Neurosurg 6:475–494

Nornes H, Grip A (1980) Hemodynamic aspects of cerebral arteriovenous malformations. J Neurosurg 53:456–464

Ondra SL, Troupp H, George ED, Schwab K (1990) The natural history of symptomatic arteriovenous malformations of the brain: a 24-years followup assessment. J Neurosurg 73:387–391

Purdy PD, Samson D, Batjer HH, Risser RC (1990) Preoperative embolization of cerebral arteriovenous malformation with polyvinyl alcohol particles: experience in 51 adults. Am J Neuroradiol 11:501–510

Spetzler R, Martin N (1986) A proposed grading system for arteriovenous malformations. J Neurosurg 65:476–483

Spetzler RF, Selman WR (1984) Pathophysiology of cerebral ischemia accompanying arteriovenous malformation. In: Wilson CB, Stein BM (eds) Intracranial arteriovenous malformations. Williams and Wilkins, Baltimore, pp 24–31

Spetzler RF, Wilson CB, Weinstein P, Mehdorn M, Townsend J, Telles D (1978) Normal perfusion pressure breakthrough theory. Clin Neurosurg 25:651–672

Steed DL, Webster MW, de Vries EJ, Jungreis CA, Horton JA, Sekhar L, Yonas H (1990) Clinical observations of the effect of carotid artery occlusion on cerebral blood flow mapped by xenon computed tomography and its correlation with carotid artery back pressure. J Vasc Surg 11:38–43

Yonas H, Sekhar L, Johnson DW, Gur D (1989) Determination of irreversible ischemia by xenon-enhanced computed tomographic monitoring of cerebral blood flow in patients with symptomatic vasospasm. Neurosurgery 24:368–372

Hemodynamic Assessment of Carotid Artery Obstructive Lesions: Comparison of PET and SPECT

J. M. DERLON, G. BOUVARD, M. C. PETIT, F. VIADER, B. LECHEVALIER, P. MORIN, and J. P. HOUTTEVILLE

Introduction

Internal carotid artery (ICA) obstructive lesions (stenoses and occlusions) can cause brain ischemic disorders in two ways: by embolism of the proximal stump to a distal intracranial arterial branch, or by an acute decrease in cerebral perfusion pressure (CPP) downstream to the reduction in lumen size. There is no means by which the occurence of the former mechanism can be predicted. There is some evidence, gathered by previous studies, that the latter mechanism could occur only in patients in whom there was already a permanent (chronic) impairment of the CPP, even if it was previously asymptomatic. Over the past 10 years, several studies have tried to assess as accurately as possible the cerebral perfusion reserve (CPR) in such patients, with isotopic methods. The theoretical aims of such assessments are:

– Prediction of neurological outcome of patients with symptomatic or asymptomatic ICA lesions.
– Supply of helpful information for the perioperative management of patients with a decreased CPR, who are threatened both by low-flow ischemia [during systemic arterial pressure (SAP) lowering, or arterial clamping] and by reperfusion disaster (edema or hemorrhage).
– Assessment of the pyhsiological hemodynamic benefit of revascularization procedures, surgical or pharmacological.

There has been no scepticism regarding the reliability and accuracy of position emission tomography (PET) methods for such assessments, even if many questions remain unanswered, for instance, the prognostic significance of a long-term reduction in CPR. More questions have been raised about the reliability of single photon emission computed tomography (SPECT) methods, noticeably because quantification has remained poor with most devices, tracers, and models. We present here data which provide both a theoretical and methodological picture of the reliability of SPECT methods in the assessment of brain hemodynamics in ICA obstructive lesions, in order to define their limits and the means by which they could be improved in daily clinical practice.

Methods

All patients were assessed clinically, were given a computed tomography (CT)-scan, and a combined study of rCBF (regional cerebral blood flow) and rCBV (regional cerebral blood volume) was performed. rCBF was measured after inhalation of ^{133}Xe using a Novo-Cerebrograph (Novo Diagnostic Systems, Denmark) with 16 probes over each hemisphere. The parameter used in this study was the initial slope index (ISI). We assessed interhemispheric asymmetries by considering those lying outside ± SDs as significant in a group of 23 normal subjects. Normal asymmetries of 9% for hemispheric CBF and 16% for rCBF were recorded. In most patients, the rCBF study was performed with the patient at rest and after intravenous injection of 1 g acetazolamide. In a series of ten subjects without carotid artery disease or CT scanner lesions, we have previously observed, as have others (Schroeder 1986; Schroeder et al. 1986), an increase in CBF of 15%–45% (mean = 30%) symmetrically and simultaneously in all areas of each hemisphere.

Relative measurement of rCBV was performed by SPECT. 15 min after infusion of autologous erythrocytes labeled with 740 MBq [^{99m}Tc] pertechnetate. Erythrocyte labeling was stable: measurements performed on blood samples 45 min after injection showed an erythrocyte/whole blood activity ratio of 97.1%±1.1% (n=26). Tomographic date were acquired with a digital gamma camera (Elscint Apex 415 ECT) (Elscint Ltd., Haifa, Israel), using a low-energy, high-resolution collimator and rotating around the patient's head with angular sampling every 4°. Each slice was reconstructed parallel to the canthomeatal line, by filtered backprojection in a 64x64 matrix, with a mean of 200000 events for each image. Right and left count rates were compared for whole hemispheres or for regions of interest (ROIs) (of about 8 cm^3). The interhemispheric or interregional ratio in each slice was expressed by the index I:

$$I = \frac{\text{(higher activity)} - \text{(lower activity)}}{\text{(lower activity)}}$$

A hemispheric asymmetry index of 4.2%±2.6% was calculated for nine normal subjects and a value of 6.9%±3.2% was obtained for the ROIs. Confidence intervals ($p<0.05$) of 10% for the interhemispheric ratio and 14% for the interregional ratio were used. Hemodynamic studies (rCBF and rCBV) were performed within 24 h of each other. In those patients in whom rCBF was measured before and after IV acetazolamide injection, the rCBV asymmetry index was also measured under the same conditions. Four types of hemodynamic pattern were demonstrated (Table 1) in patients with unilateral lesions.

Type I ("normal"): No asymmetriy of rCBF or rCBV in resting conditions; symmetrical normal increase in rCBF after IV acetazolamide injection, with symmetrical rCBV.

Type II: A relative decrease of both resting rCBF and rCBV on the side of the ICA lesion; after IV acetazolamide injection the asymmetry persisted or was accentuated.

Type III: Moderate decrease of resting rCBF distal to the ICA lesion with symmetrical rCBV; bilateral increase of rCBF after IV acetazolamide injection, with persistant asymmetry of rCBF in the face of a symmetrical rCBV.

Table 1. Hemodynamic patterns ■, side of ICA occlusion; □, normal side

Type \ Parameter		rCBF	rCBV
I	Resting Acetazolamide	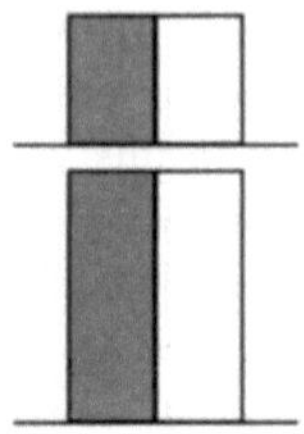	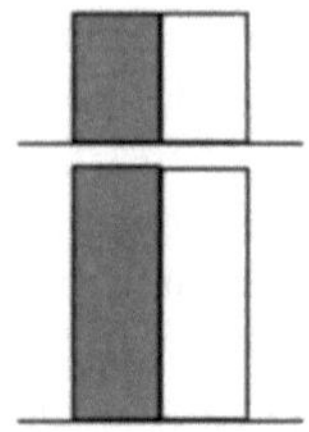
II	Resting Acetazolamide	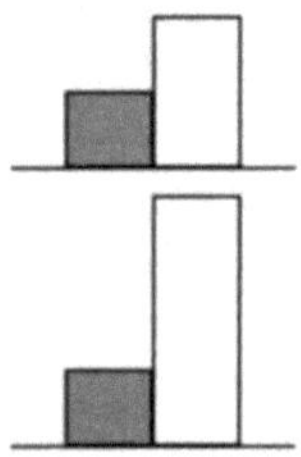	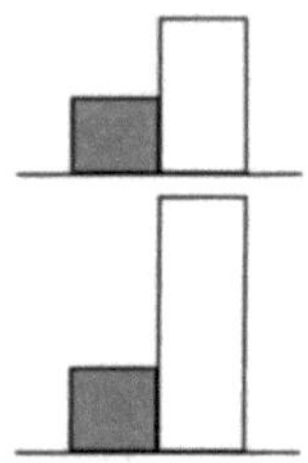
III	Resting Acetazolamide	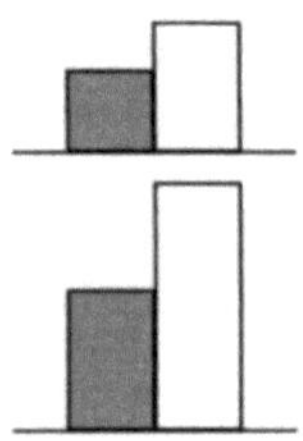	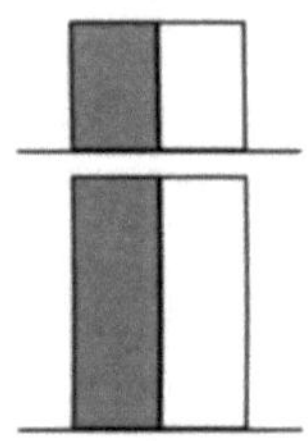
IV	Resting Acetazolamide	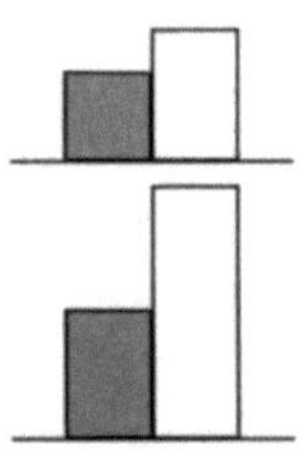	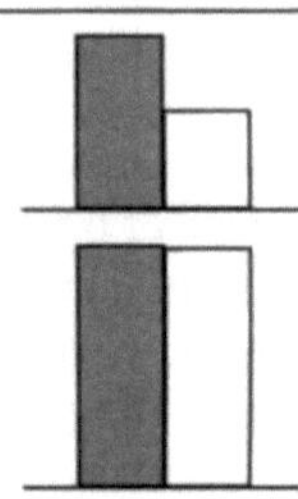

Type IV ("impaired hemodynamic reserve") (Fig. 1): Resting rCBF was normal or decreased on the occluded side, while rCBV was increased; after IV acetazolamide injection rCBF increased mainly or exclusively on the patent side (with consequent accentuation of the rCBF asymmetry); this was associated with a disappearance of the rCBV asymmetry.

We shall present and discuss below the results obtained in patients with bilateral lesions.

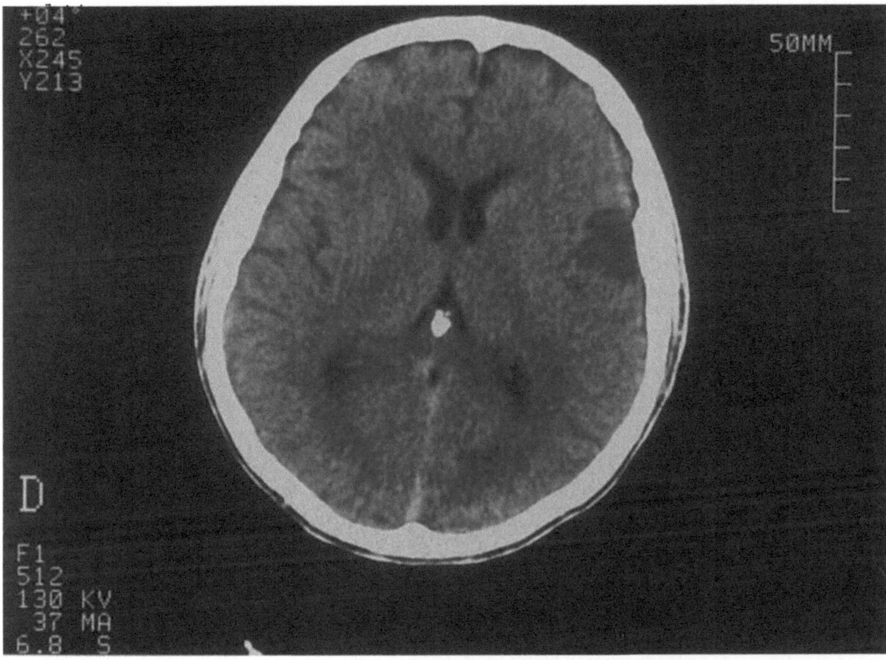

Fig. 1A–F. A case with CPR impairment (type IV pattern). **A** CT scanner: mild left hemispheric infarction;

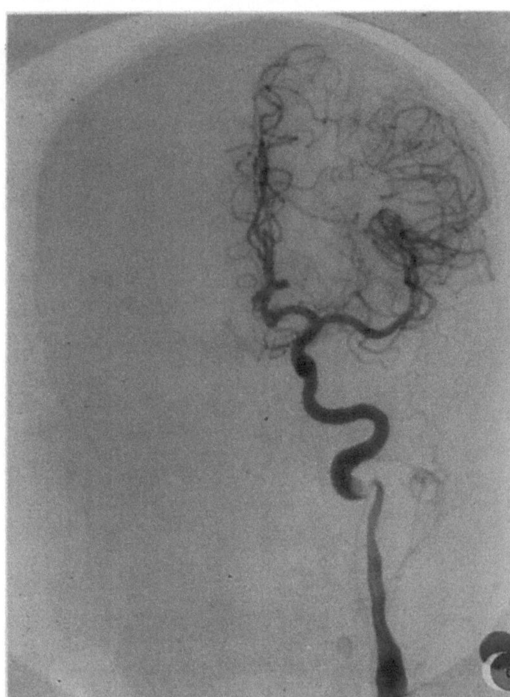

B arteriography: left ICA spontaneous dissection with only a slight residual lumen;

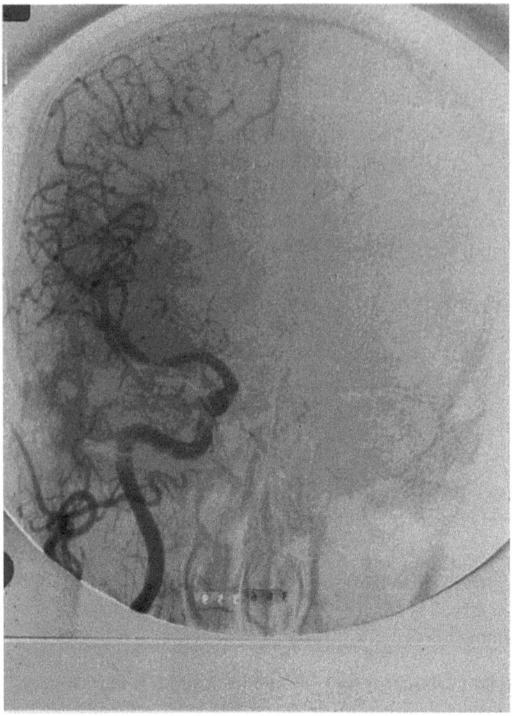

C arteriography: right ICA angiogram showing no cross-filling through the arterior communicating artery (ACOA);

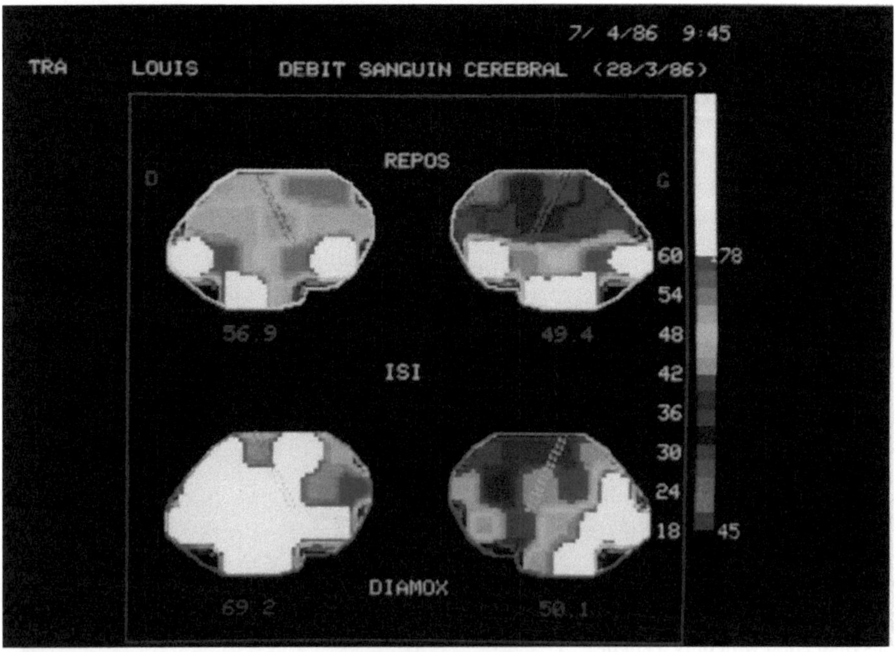

D CBF before and after IV acetazolamide injection;

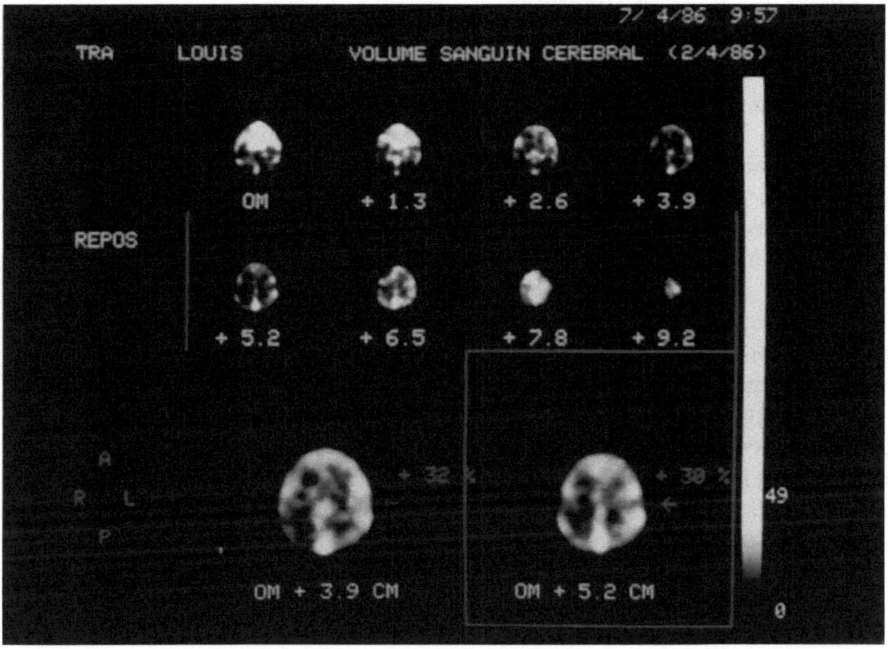

E resting CBV measurement: significant relative increase on the obliterated ICA side (left);

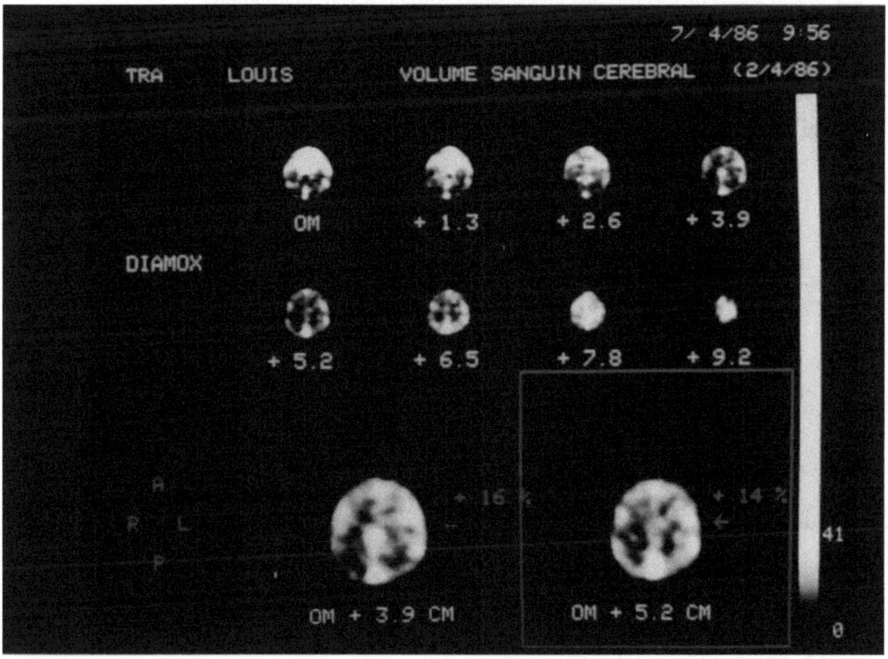

F activated CBV measurement (after 1 g IV acetazolamide injection): reduction of the asymmetry

Theoretical Analysis of SPECT Data

Patients with No or Mild Infarction

For such patients, data gathered from PET investigations should predict that a CBV asymmetry is not due to a reduction of the intravascular space on the side of the lesion – since there is no major parenchymal damage and decreased metabolic demand – but is due solely to a CBV increase on the side of the ICA obstruction, when it induces an autoregulatory response with distal vasodilation (Gibbs et al. 1984).

We initially investigated 130 patients (Derlon et al. 1987) with various clinical (Table 2). CT scan (Table 3), and angiographic patterns (Table 4). In each clinical or CT group we found some cases with rCBF and/or rCBV asymmetry. But only patients with a severe unilateral or bilateral ICA obstruction (stenosis or occlusion) sometimes had CBV asymmetry. In patients with unilateral lesions, this asymmetry was always due to a relative CBV increase on the side of the lesion. In patients with bilateral lesions, it was observed on the symptomatic side. As a whole, 24 out of 78 patients with such severe ICA lesions (of the complete series of 130 patients) exhibited an impaired hemodynamic pattern (type IV). In the others, either a normal (type I) or a type III pattern was demonstrated, with none having a type II pattern. The occurrence of a decreased CPR therefore accounted for only 30% of all patients with severe obstructive lesions.

Table 2. Clinical status of 130 patients investigated with no severe brain infarct

	rCBF		rCBV	
Clinical status	Symptomatic	Asymptomatic	Symptomatic	Asymptomatic
Asymptomatic ($n = 37$)	33	4	35	2
TIA ($n = 44$)	36	8	37	7
CS ($n = 49$)	26	23	34	15

TIA, transient ischemic attack; CS, completed stroke

Table 3. Computed tomography classification of 130 patients investigated with no severe brain infarct

	rCBF		rCBV	
CT classification	Symmetrical	Asymmetrical	Symmetrical	Asymmetrical
N ($n = 33$)	26	7	31	2
A ($n = 15$)	13	2	12	3
I ($n = 32$)	14	18	20	12

N, normal; A, atrophy; I, mild infarct

Table 4. Arteriographic classifications of 130 patients investigated with no severe brain infarct

Arteriographic classification	rCBF		rCBV	
	Symmetrical	Asymmetrical	Symmetrical	Asymmetrical
G1 ($n = 12$)	11	1	12	0
G2 ($n = 40$)	35	5	40	0
G3 ($n = 65$)	37	28	45	20
G4 ($n = 13$)	10	3	9	4
Total = 130				

G1, normal ICAs; G2, mild uni-or bilateral ICA stenosis; G3, severe unilateral ICA stenosis (> 80% reduction in lumen diameter) or occlusion; G4, severe bilateral ICA stenosis or occlusion

Since this early series, a larger number of patients have been assessed with resting and activated rCBF and rCBV parameters. For most, the CBF increase after IV acetazolamide injection was significantly impaired or absent on the side with a resting CBV incrase. In all, the CBV asymmetry resumed after IV acetazolamide injection, which can be explained by a CBV increase only on the side which still had a normal autoregulatory capacity (the so-called "healthy" side, see Table 1, Fig. 1). Cases with discrepancies between resting and activated results will be discussed further.

Pre- and Postoperative Results

Positron emission tomography results and related physiological theory should predict that, after reestablishment of a normal arterial lumen and downstream intravascular pressure, autoregulation is no longer present, with the disappearance of any preoperative type IV pattern. In the series of 130 patients previously analyzed, 44 underwent a surgical revascularization procedure, by either endarterectomy or extracranial – intracranial (ECIC) bypass (Table 5). Of 39 patients submitted for unilateral endarterectomy, 8 had a preoperative relative CBV increase on the operated side, which disappeared within 1 week postoperatively in 7. It is notable that, in three patients in whom an early postoperative assessment was also performed (within 3 days), the CBV asymmetry was still present, indicating that the autoregulatory vasodilation can be delayed in some patients in whom intravascular pressure has nevertheless been restored. This transient state of "lack of autoregulation" – distinct from the preoperative "saturated autoregulation" – could explain postoperative hyperemic syndromes described by some Doppler and clinical studies. In particular, it could be responsible for the reperfusion edema and hemorrhage reported by some authors. No patient in this early series had such a problem. But, in more recent cases, we had two patients with a preoperative type IV pattern who had a severe immediate neurological deficit with coma in the

Table 5. Postoperative modifications of resting CBV

	rCBV			
Preoperative	Symmetrical (33)		Asymmetrical (11)	
	Symmetrical	Asymmetrical	Symmetrical	Asymmetrical
Postoperative endarterectomy (39)	29	2	7	1
Postoperative ECIC bypass (5)	2	0	3	0

recovery room: one had a massive infarction (probably due to a perianesthetic systemic arterial pressure decrease in a patient operated on without a shunt), and the second had a hemorrhage – not explained by excessive anticoagulation or a previous infarction.

In the previous group of 39 endarterectomized patients, 31 showed no preoperative CBV asymmetry, and the postoperative situation remained unchanged except in 2, who showed a relative CBV increase on the contralateral nonoperated side, which in both had an ICA occlusion. It is therefore likely that there was initially a bilateral CBV increase, which resumed only on the operated side. In the small series of patients undergoing an ECIC bypass, the CBV asymmetry disappeared in all three patients who initially had this pattern.

In all patients investigated since the introduction of activated measurements after IV acetazolamide injection, the postoperative results were consistent with these early data. Patients who had both a resting relative CBV increase and a poor CBF response to IV acetazolamide injection on the side of the ICA lesion resumed a normal pattern simultaneously for both parameters in the postoperative course.

Assessment and Follow-up of Patients with Chronic ICA Occlusion

From the clinical experience gathered in previous series of patients, we could therefore confirm that:

– Resting CBF was of little value for the assessment of the CPR, since it could be reduced in patients with no hemodynamic deficit, or normal in patients with a clearly decreased CPR (assessed with CBV measurements and activation studies).

– Resting CBV was highly correlated with the expected hemodynamic status, as clearly demonstrated by postoperative studies.

– Resting and IV acetazolamide activated CBVs, and the CBF data showed a fair consistency with the previous theoretical approach.

We later used this tool for the assessment and follow-up of patients with ICA chronic occlusion, who showed a large variety of both clinical and anatomical patterns. The retrospective study of 75 patients (Table 6) with unilateral or bilateral ICA occlusion demonstrated a type IV hemodynamic pattern (Table 1, 7) in only 27% of the whole series of patients, and in 35% of those who would have been "eligible," from a clinical and radiological point of view, for inclusion in the ECIC Bypass Cooperative Study

(Table 8). In other words, an actual hemodynamic deficit was seen in one-third of the population who would have been considered as showing good indication for reperfusion surgery some years ago. Of the other hemodynamic patterns (Table 1, 7), type II should be considered, which was seen only in patients with a severe stroke and CT scan massive infarction, and therefore not suitable for surgery. This pattern is the opposite of type IV. and again is consistent with the theoretical expectations: under

Table 6. Results of the angiographic study in 75 patients with chronic ICA occlusion

Extent of the disease	
Unilateral	57
Unilateral occlusion with contralateral severe (80%) ICA stenosis	10
Bilateral occlusion	8
Etiology[a]	
Atheroma	53
Spontaneous dissection	12
Traumatic dissection	1
Therapeutic occlusion	5[b]
Siphon[c]	4

[a] The occlusion in the first three groups was located at the origin of the ICA
[b] In three cases this was a dissecting aneurysm of the distal cervical ICA, which could not be technically treated by resection and anastomosis; in two cases it was an intracavernous aneurysm
[c] Three were atheromatous lesions, and one was a moya-moya bilateral occlusion

Table 7. Assessment of the hemodynamic patterns in 75 patients with a chronic ICA occlusion

HR type	First exploration (*n*)		Second exploration (*n*)
I	27	(+ 2)	29
II	4	(+ 2)	6
III	17	(+ 3)	20
IV (HR impairment)	27	(− 7)	20 (27%)
	75		75

Table 8. Assessment of the hemodynamic patterns in 75 patients with a chronic ICA occlusion

Hemodynamic pattern	I	II	III	IV
Patients "eligible" for ECIC bypass	16	0	17	18 (35%)
($n = 51$)				

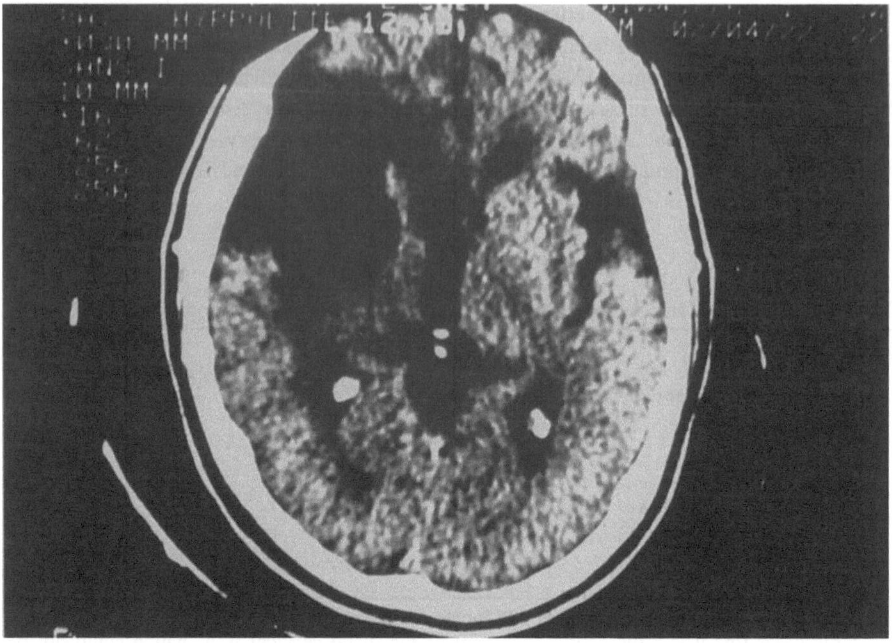

Fig. 2A–D. A case with a large infarction (type II pattern). **A** CT scanner: severe right hemispheric infarction;

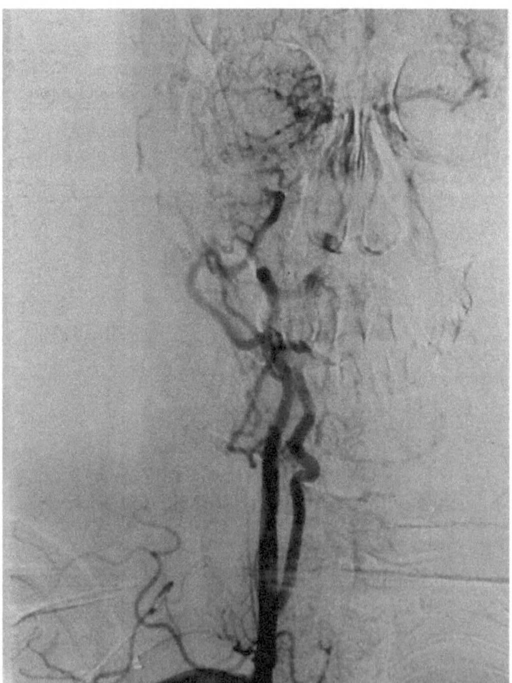

B arteriography: right ICA occlusion;

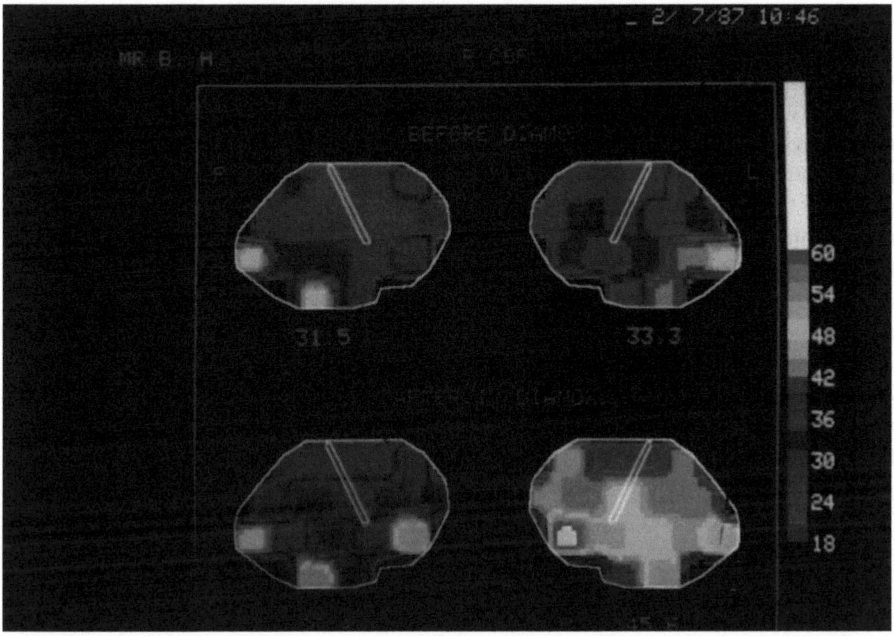

C CBF measurement before and after IV acetazolamide injection: CBF increases only on the left side;

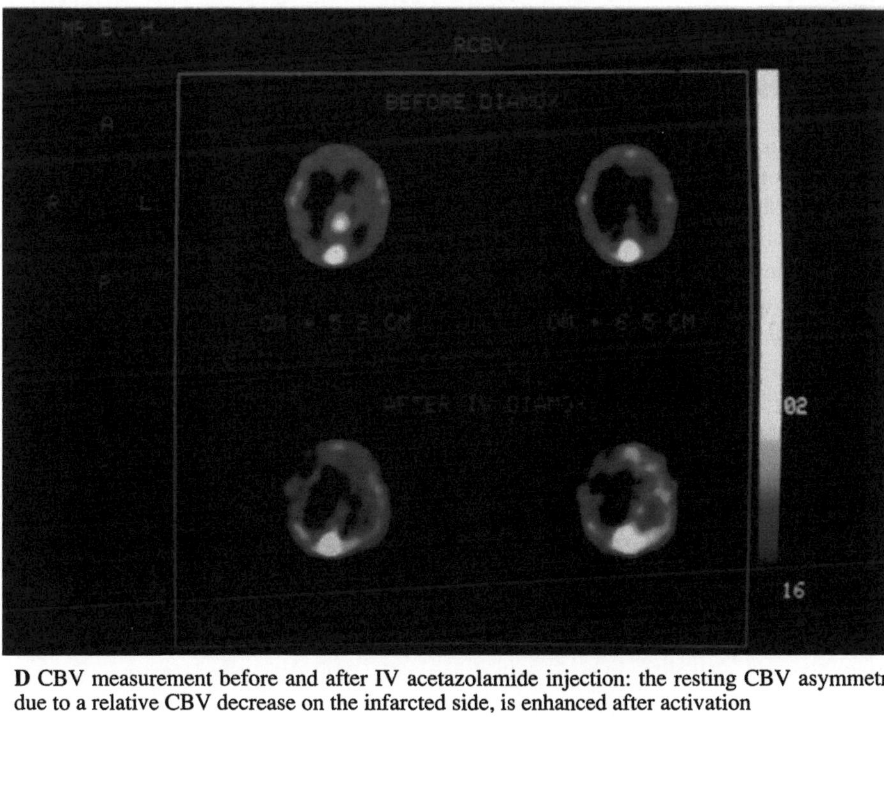

D CBV measurement before and after IV acetazolamide injection: the resting CBV asymmetry, due to a relative CBV decrease on the infarcted side, is enhanced after activation

resting conditions, both CBF and CBV are severely decreased on the lesion side; after acetazolamide injection, the asymmetry is increased for both parameters, since the vasodilation is significant only on the healthy side (Fig. 2). The 51 "eligible" patients were followed-up during a mean period of 24 months. Of the 33 patients with a normal CPP (type I pattern), only 1 developed a delayed ischemic ipsilateral stroke (26 months after the initial hemodynamic assessment), from which he died; another died (after 20 months) from a contralateral stroke, presumably due to an intracranial hematoma; there were no brain ischemic events in the other patients. Of the 18 patients with an impaired CPR (type IV pattern), 4 were not operated on – of whom 2 had a delayed ipsilateral ischemic stroke, 9 and 13 months respectively after the initial assessment; and 14 underwent a uni- or bilateral ECIC bypass. In this latter group, there was a high incidence of perioperative strokes: one had an ipsilateral infarction due to an occlusion of the bypass; another had a patent bypass, but developed a brain stream infarction due to a basilar artery thrombosis 3 days after the operation; the third patient, who had a bypass distal to a cervical ICA occlusion, presented an occlusion of a preoperative severe contralateral siphon stenosis.

From this preliminary study of ICA chronic occlusions, we can suggest that:

– A normal CPR is indicative of a good prognosis as far as the risk of delayed ipsilateral stroke is concerned.

– An impaired CPR is indicative of a higher risk of stroke, not only ipsilateral – with or without surgery, but also in a remote territory in operated patients. It is therefore not clear whether patients with an impaired CPR can benefit from a bypass procedure, and only a prospective and controlled study could address this issue.

Methodological Approach for Comparison of SPECT and PET

Both theoretically and in our clinical experience, it is noteworthy that semiquantitative assessment of the CPR, as performed with the ^{99m}Tc CBV measurements, provided easily understandable results in patients with strictly unilateral ICA lesions and normal brain tissue, but more questionable results in patients with either a bilateral or multiple arterial disease, or with single or multiple brain infarction areas. In the latter populations of patients, symmetrical CBVs could be due to a bilateral autoregulation impairment as well as a normal hemodynamic pattern – and the acetazolamide response is not reproducible enough to be unambiguous in all cases. Even in the former groups, in a few cases there was a discrepancy between both investigations, namely a CBV asymmetry with a normal activated CBF pattern. We therefore decided to carry out absolute quantification of SPECT CBV measurements, and to correlate these with PET CBV measurements in the same patients, in order to validate the former method.

Methods

Using a new-generation, high-resolution PET camera (LETI TTVO3) and the ^{15}O steady-state technique, 14 patients with stenosis or occlusion of the internal carotid artery were studied. Accurate and standardized positioning was obtained so that brain structures could be imaged in seven planes parallel to the glabella-inion (GI) line. One day later, SPECT data were acquired using the Elscint Apex 409 ECT gamma camera. Before the acquisition, the GI line was identified with a point source in order to obtain identical positioning with the two methods. After the intravenous injection of red blood cells (RBCs) labeled in vitro with ^{99m}Tc, SPECT acquisition was performed with the dual-energy window acquisition technique (Jaszczak et al. 1984). Blood samples were taken during SPECT acquisition, and radioactivity of RBCs and plasma were determined in a well counter. The reconstruction of two blood volume images was performed with correction for Compton scatter, as described by Jaszczak et al. (1984) in which 50% of the Compton peak was subtracted from the ^{99m}Tc photoelectric peak. Attenuation correction was performed by the Chang method, in which an attenuation of 0.15 cm was assumed and the head outline taken to be an ellipse. The major axes of two ellipses, determined by PET, were used for the corresponding SPECT images. Calibration of the SPECT system was performed using a skull phantom filled with water and different concentrations of ^{99m}Tc from which aliquots were taken, weighed, and counted. A relationship was then established between the SPECT scans of the phantom and the measured activity in the counter. CBV was calculated according to

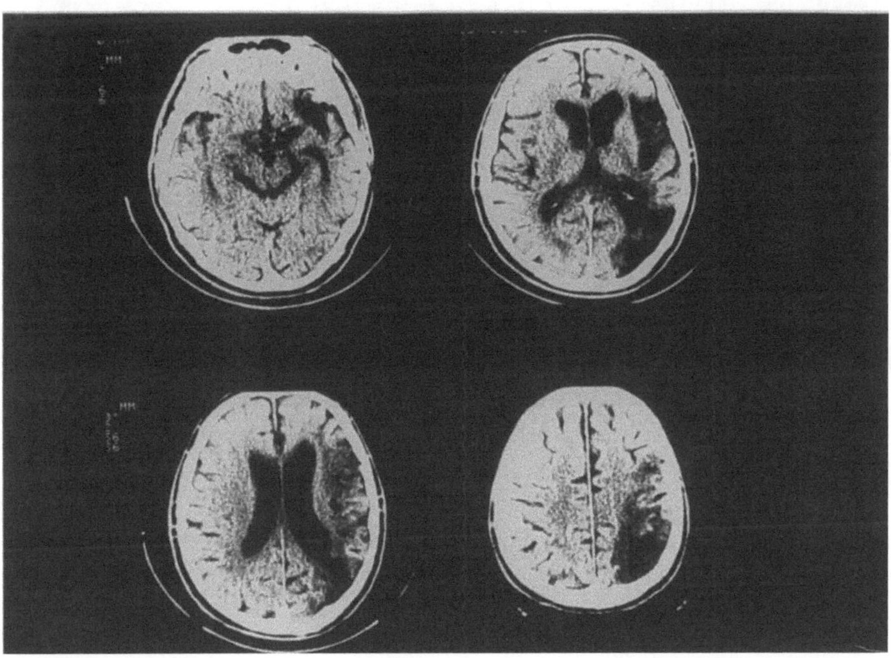

Fig. 3A–C. Comparison of PET and SPECT. **A** CT scanner: left hemispheric infarction;

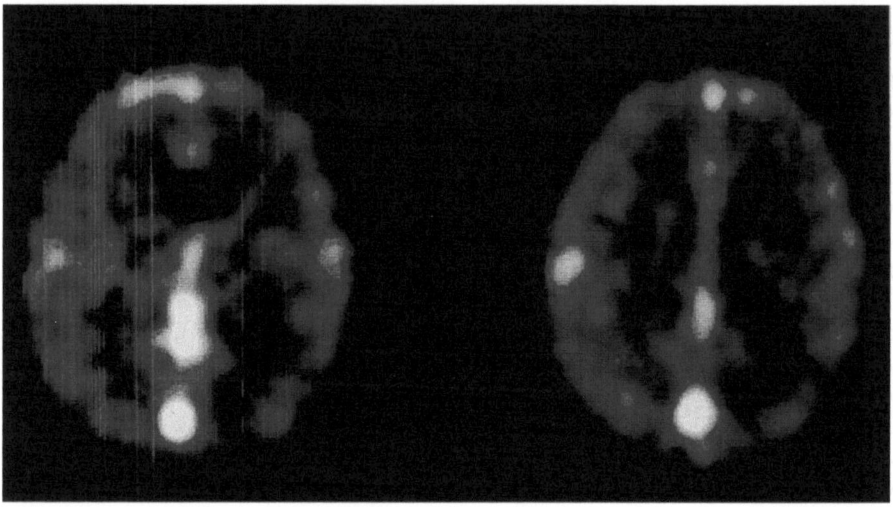

B PET CBV measurement: a left CBV decrease is displayed on slices GI + 44 mm and GI + 56 mm;

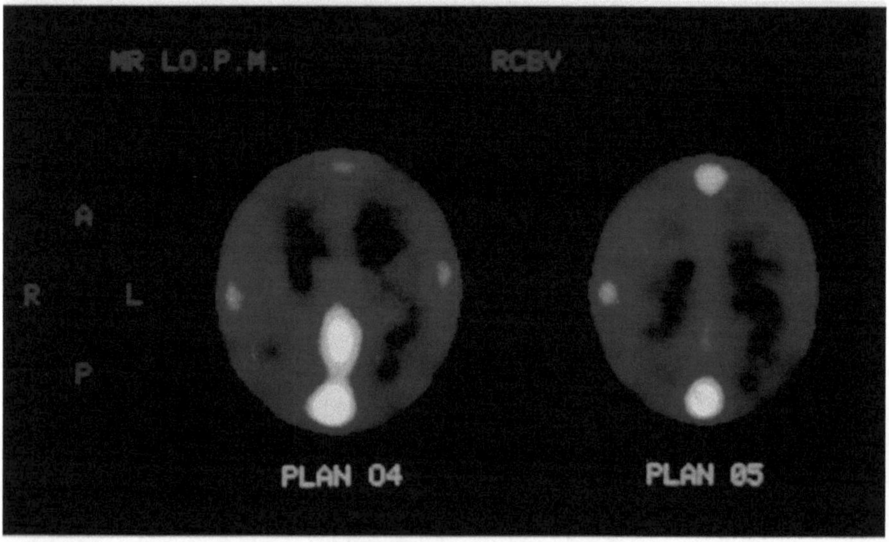

C SPECT CBV measurement: the same CBV pattern is shown at the same slice levels

the equation of Sakai et al. (1983). Four hemispheric ROIs, which excluded vascular structures, were defined at two levels (GI, 44 mm; GI, + 56 mm) of both SPECT and PET images (Fig. 3).

Results

The results for CBV, as measured with ^{99m}Tc RBC, were plotted against those measured with $C^{15}O$. The data were fitted with a linear least-squares analysis (Fig. 4) to yield the equation: $y=0.84x+0.47$. The coefficient correlation was $r=0.88$ ($p<0.001$). The absolute values (mean ± SD) for CBV were as follows: 3.16±0.49 and 2.85±0.45 ml/100 ml (higher and lower hemisphere values respectively, PET method); 3.18±0.46 and 2.86±0.53 ml/100 ml (SPECT). The side-to-side asymmetry was determined as the interhemispheric CBV difference as a percentage of mean CBV. The asymmetry ratios were 0.10±0.07 (PET) and 0.11±0.10 (SPECT).

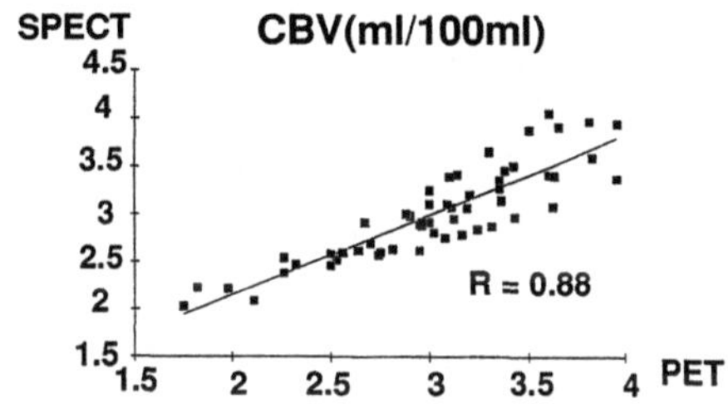

Fig. 4. Correlation between SPECT and PET measurements of CBV

Comments

These data show that SPECT measurement of CBV, when compared with PET determination of the same parameter, is reliable. However, SPECT overestimates low and underestimates high values or CBV. Limited energy resolution, Compton scattering, and attenuation correction were minimized by modification of a published method. The determination of head contours by PET further permitted a reduction in attenuation artifacts. The spatial resolution of the gamma camera was lower than that of the PET system and might influence quantitative SPECT analysis.

Conclusions

From the different results presented in this paper, and from the experience reported by many other groups – working mainly in Germany, Sweden, and Denmark – it is now clear that SPECT assessment of the CPR is a reliable method for determining whether a patient displays a hemodynamic compromise downstream to carotid lesions. Some points, however, must be stressed:

– The measurement of resting CBF by any method is unreliable for such a determination.

– The resting semiquantitative measurement of both CBF and CBV provides consistent results in patients with unilateral disease.

– The dynamic measurements of CBF or CBV before and after IV acetazolamide injection provide similar results, and each could probably be used as a single reliable procedure.

– However, in patients with a bilateral or multiple arterial disease, true quantitative methods are mandatory: the absolute quantitation of brain CBV could provide an alternative or be complementary to activated CBF measurements.

These methods, which can easily be performed in most hospital communities, should be an important adjunct for future prospective studies of the risk of stroke and the benefit of preventive therapeutic procedures in patients with severe ICA obstructive disease.

References

Derlon JM, Bouvard G, Hubert P, Lechevalier B, Dupuy B (1987) Etude hemodynamique des lésions obstructive de l'artère carotide interne; intérêt de la mesure couplée du débit et du volume sanguins régionaux. Rev Neurol (Paris) 143:32–39

Gibbs JM, Leenders KL, Wise JS, Jones T (1984) Evaluation of cerebral perfusion reserve in patients with carotid artery occlusion. Lancet 1:182–186

Jaszczak RJ, Greer KL, Floyd CE, Harris CC, Coleman RE (1984) Improved SPECT quantification using compensation for scattered photons. J Nucl Med 25:893–900

Sakai F, Nakazawa K, Tazaki Y, Kanda N, Kitai N, Hino H, Igarashi H, Shiti K (1983) Evaluation of human cerebral blood volume and hematocrit with single-photon emission computed tomography. J Cereb Blood Flow Metab 3:S160–S161

Schroeder T (1986) Cerebrovascular reactivity to acetazolamide in carotid artery disease. Neurol Res 8:231–236

Schroeder T, Vorstrup S, Lassen NA, Engell HC (1986) Noninvasive Xenon-133 measurements of cerebral blood flow using stationary detector compared with dynamic emission tomography. J Cereb Blood Flow Metab 6:739–746

Cerebral Blood Flow to Cerebral Blood Volume Relationship as a Correlate to Cerebral Perfusion Reserve

U. BUELL, W. REICHE, H. J. KAISER, K. ISENSEE, R. BARES, C. ALTEHOEFER, and E. B. RINGELSTEIN

Introduction

Perfusion reserve is recruited to balance organ perfusion versus systemic changes in blood pressure. Regionally, recruitment is of special interest since it acts (a) to maintain baseline perfusion (or flow) in decreasing perfusion pressure (e.g., beyond a stenosis) or (b) to meet increased metabolic demands of an organ during exercise or any other stimulus (Buell and Schicha 1990). Cerebral perfusion reserve (CPR) is a complex system, comprising cerebral perfusion or blood flow (CBF), cerebral blood volume, blood thixotrophy, adaptions in peripheral hematocrit (Schmid-Schönbein 1988), oxygen carriage, chemical effects, vascular innervation and tone (Aaslid et al. 1989), and hormonal and endothelial factors. The vascular reaction to CO_2, for example, measured with laser Doppler in normal cat brain revealed a 19% increase in pial arteriolar diameter in combination with augmented flow of 70% and flow velocity of 60%. Blood volume increased by 10% (Haberl et al. 1989). In acute or chronic cerebrovascular disease, CPR seems to recruit these determinants in different combinations. For acute disorders, the interactions have been described by Frackowiak and Wise (1983) and, most recently, by Arora et al. (1990). This article considers findings in chronic cerebrovascular disease.

Cerebral Perfusion Reserve in Chronic Cerebrovascular Disease

Since constellations and mechanisms of chronic cerebrovascular disease (CCVD) in man are as yet not reproducible in animal models, such experiments are performed in acute or subacute conditions, e.g., in cats (Kummer et al. 1988): results with normotension (140 torr) showed that a decrease in hematocrit from 35% to 25% caused a sudden increase in rCBF of up to 30%; with hypotension (80 torr) such a decrease did not change the rCBF. Following CO_2 stimulation, capillary recruitment does seem to play a significant role (Kuschinsky, this volume). However, capillaries tend to enlarge in chronic hypoxia. Valid data for CCVD in man, however, have to be obtained from patients.

Cerebral Perfusion Reserve in Patients Determined from Flow Measurements

Numerous groups have measured regional CBF (rCBF) with various protocols (see Table 1) to achieve CPR by comparing baseline flow with the stimulated one, employ-

Table 1. Cerebral perfusion reserve (synonyms: cerebrovascular reserve, vasomotor reserve, vascular reactivity, responsiveness)

In clinical routine determined by

1. Flow labeling (^{133}Xe, ^{99m}Tc-HMPAO, ^{18}F-CH3)
   - Resting state (baseline flow) versus hypercapnia
   - Resting state versus acetazolamide
   - Resting state versus physical movement
2. Blood flow velocity in the middle cerebral artery (transcranial Doppler)
   - Resting state versus hyper- and/or hypocapnia
3. Volume labeling (^{99m}Tc red blood cells or ^{99m}Tc albumin)
   - Resting state versus acetazolamide or hypercapnia
4. Volume labeling (see 3), additional to flow labeling (see 1)
   - Resting state

1, 3, 4, terminal supply area by regional voxels; 2, main stem of the MCA

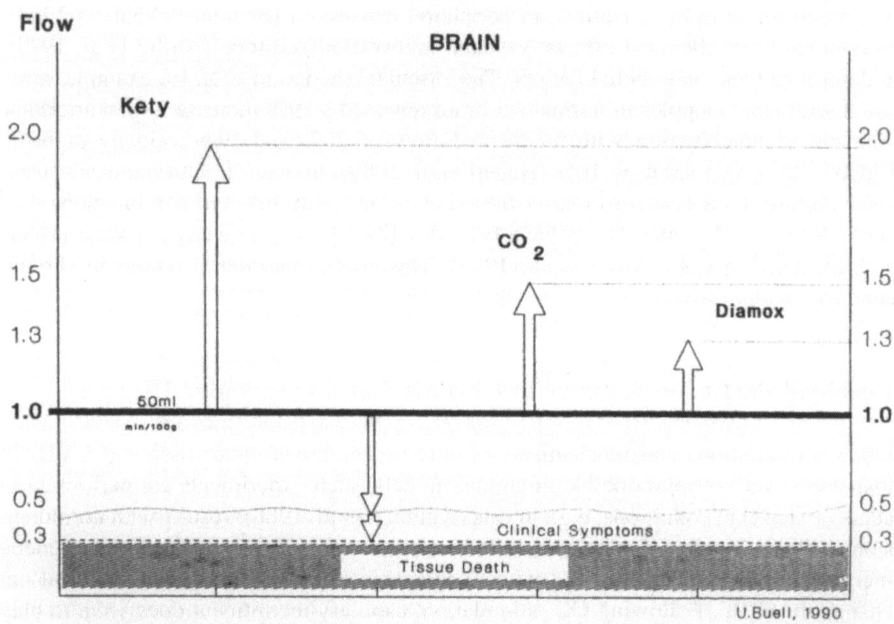

Fig. 1. Flow reserves for brain. If flow reserve is considered as a flow increase over baseline flow, in the multifactoral-determined cerebral vasculature, a maximum of 2.0 is reached. With clinical and/or nuclear protocols (diffusible tracers), in controls 1.5 (CO_2) or less (acetazolamide) is gained for the cerebrum. Physiologically, flow reserve is used to increase flow on demand (cerebrum regionally) but is not employed to keep resting flow normal. Therefore, in the brain, the range to the threshold of low flow beyond which neurological symptoms will be presented is potentially buffered by other factors of the cerebrovascular reserve (e.g., blood volume, hematocrit) or by a metabolic reserve (e.g., oxygen extraction)

Table 2. Results of stimulation of rCBF in controls

Reference	Stimulus	Marker/Method	rCBF increase over baseline[a]
Choksey et al. (1989)	CO_2	^{99m}Tc-HMPAO-SPECT	1.04
Keyeux et al. (1988)	CO_2	^{133}Xe probes	1.25
Reich and Rusinek (1989)	CO_2	^{133}Xe probe array	1.25[b]
			1.15[c]
Levine et al. (1988)	CO_2	^{18}F-CH3 PET	1.61
Schmidt et al. (1988)	CO_2	^{99m}Tc-HMPAO-SPECT	1.28
Ringelstein et al. (1988)	CO_2	Transcranial Doppler	1.52
Bonte et al. (1988)	Acetazolamide	^{133}Xe-SPECT	1.30
Leinsinger et al. (1988)	Acetazolamide	^{133}Xe-SPECT	1.25
Guenther et al. (1986)	Motor	^{133}Xe-SPECT	1.31

[a] Factor
[b] Cortex, young subjects
[c] Cortex, elderly subjects

ing nuclear flow markers (see Table 2) or changes in blood flow velocity in the main stem of the middle cerebral artery (Ringelstein et al. 1988; Aaslid et al. 1989; Kontos 1989). The classical experiment by Kety and Schmidt (1948), performed with a saturation technique and using CO_2 as a dilator stimulus, revealed an rCBF increase of 200% in normals. In contrast, when the usual diffusible nonpolar blood flow tracers are employed, mean flow-increase following carbon dioxide stimulation was only 61%; following acetazolamide (Diamox) administration it was 30% (Table 2, Fig. 1). In addition, Reich and Rusinek (1989) found linear correlations for age versus cerebrovascular reactivity for both cortical gray and subcortical white matter. Thus, as with coronary vascular reserve (Fig. 1), employment of diffusible tracers yields significantly smaller increases than saturation techniques.

Measurable *increase of flow over baseline,* however, does not reflect the mandatory task of flow reserve in CCVD. The desired mechanism is the *maintenance of baseline flow*. On the other hand, increase of flow in the brain is needed and is thus found subsequent to pyhsiological stimulation of neuron activity in regional brain areas. Flow rates match the increased metabolic demand as induced, for example, by motor movement of extremities (Lauritzen et al. 1981; rCBF increase of 31%: Guenther et al. 1986) or by sensory stimulation.

Thus, in the human brain, vascular reserve can only be tested incompletely by way of responses of flow to hypercapnia or to the carboanhydrase inhibitor acetazolamide because mechanisms of basal flow maintenance and further significant determinants remain unchecked. Therefore, other groups have approached this system through monitoring changes of cerebral blood volume (CBV), which plays a significant role (see Powers and Raichle 1985) under conditions of chronic underperfusion.

Cerebral Perfusion Reserve in Patients Determined from Measurements of CBV

Cerebral blood volume, mainly red cell volume, was assessed by nuclear protocols (Table 1; Phelps et al. 1979; Gibbs et al. 1984; Knapp et al. 1986; Sakai et al. 1985;

Sakai and Tazaki 1987; Buell et al. 1988; Toyama et al. 1988, 1990) employing emission computed tomography, either with single photon (SPECT) or with positron emitters (PET). Basic pathopyhsiological mechanisms are listed in Table 3; relevant data for CBF-CBV considerations are given in Table 4. Toyama et al. (1988) found no sig-

Table 3. Basic pathophysiological mechanisms to explain changes in flow-volume relations in cerebral circulation

- Autoregulated perfusion pressure: 70–110 torr
- Assumption: 6% of total brain volume consists of vasculature; of this, 5% represents arterioles (i.e., 0.3% of the brain volume) (for comparison see Friberg, this volume[a])

  If reserve is employed in a chronic state (e.g., with decrease in perfusion pressure, decrease in arterial oxygen transported) within the regulated range:

- Diameter of arterioles may double by active dilation (to 0.6% of brain volume)
- Passive dilation of capillaries and venules (to take away increased blood volume) adds to active dilation
- Peripheral hematocrit (red blood cells) increases by omission of autodilution (network-Fahraeuseffect)

  Thus, CBV by at least three rheological mechanisms augments to values which are potentially measured and imaged by employing radioactive labeled red blood cells and SPECT

[a] Cerebral blood volume is located within arteries, 11%; arterioles, 2%; capillaries, 7%; venules and larger veins, 80%

Table 4. Relevant data for cerebral flow-volume considerations

Normal values	
– Hematocrit	
Central (venous blood), 40%	
Terminal supply area, 20%–30%	
– Oxygen extraction fraction, 44%	
– Regional values:	
Cerebral blood volume,	4.84 ml/100 g
Red blood cell volume,	1.50 ml/100 g
Plasma volume,	3.34 ml/100 g
Mean CBF,	50 ml /100 g/min
Mean flow-to-volume ratio, 10	
Cerebrovascular reserve in action	
– Hematocrit	
Terminal supply area, 30%–40%	
– Oxygen extraction fraction increases to 53%	
– Regional values	
Cerebral blood volume, increase of 12%–50%[a]	
Mean CBF:	normal; decreases after exhaustion of reserve; threshold for reversibility (depending on low-flow time), 23 ml/min/100 g
Mean flow-to-volume ratio; decreases to 6	

Data from Heiss (1983), Gibbs et al. (1984), Sakai et al. (1985); Sakai and Tazati (1987), Gaethgens and Marx (1987), Schmid-Schönbein et al. (1987), Buell et al (1988), and Kanno et al. (1989)

[a] From SPECT protocols, increases up to 93% have been reported (see Fig. 2).

nificant correlation between mean rCBV and age in normal volunteers. Under conditions when CPR is not recruited, CBV is not increased. In various degrees of CCVD (e.g., Fig. 2), all authors, without employing any external stimulus, found the expected increase in regional CBV. In the first stage of CPR employment, indicated by increased CBV, rCBF is maintained at normal (Gibbs et al. 1984; Powers and Raichle 1985; Buell et al. 1988; Toyama et al. 1990). If rCBV is maximally increased, CPR is exhausted.

Since SPECT or PET slices contain CBV data on a pixel basis, simple division by the corresponding CBF image (or vice versa) reveals CPR for each hemisphere up to each hemispheric voxel. Dimensions of these parametric images are 1/s (CBF-to-CBV) or seconds (CBV-to-CBF), thus displaying a correlate to the mean rate of shear or to the transit time, respectively. Therefore, most working groups use these relations and not the original CBV images for diagnostic purposes. In addition, CBV images are governed by the high extracerebral blood volume in sinuses and skull, thus yielding relatively low count rates in the cerebral area. Moreover, CBV was found to be increased locally in sulci enlarged by atrophy, probably reflecting enlarged extracerebral veins (Buell et al. 1990), mimicking exhausted reserve. Thus, a morphological approach has to be added (Kaiser et al. 1990) to rule out such conditions.

Herold et al. (1988), working with CCVD patients, showed a linear relationship of the CBF-to CBV ratio to CO_2 reactivity and a correlation of the results of either method (ratio or CO_2) to the oxygen extraction ratio. These findings were, however,

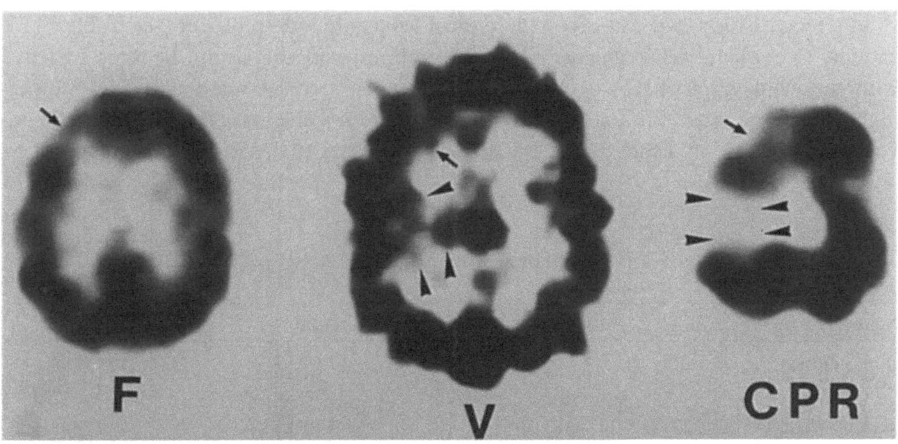

Fig. 2. Fifty-one-year-old male patient with prior (3 weeks) prolonged reversible paresis of the left arm. CT was normal, and Doppler revealed occlusion of the right internal carotid artery. Imaging of flow (^{99m}Tc-HMPAO, *left*), volume (^{99m}Tc red blood cells, *middle*), and reserve (flow/volume, *right*) revealed two findings: (1) small flow deficit *(arrow),* accompanied by increased volume *(arrow),* and exhausted reserve in the frontoparietal part of the right hemisphere *(arrow).* (2) increased volume *(V)* in the parietal parts *(arrowheads);* where flow was still normal, causing a large deficit area in the reserve image. Total hemispheric difference for flow was –4%, for volume +22%, and for CPR –17%. Regional parietal volume increase turned out to be 93%!

obtained from CO_2-stimulated flow over baseline flow versus resting conditions for CBF-to-CBV. Gibbs et al. (1987) and Toyama et al. (1990) showed that increased CBV after extra-intracranial bypass surgery potentially returns to normal.

On the other hand, in normal persons, Celsis (this volume) and Friberg (this volume) reported after administration of acetazolamide a hemispheric increase in CBV (red cells) of 13% up to 30%. Vorstrup (this volume) and Derlon (this volume) found an increase up to 50% by regional evaluation. Considering in normals the flow-to-volume ratio (values of 10–17) as rather constant, an increase in flow has to be combined with an increase in volume within a given range. On the other hand, in pial arterioles, detailed animal experiments with CO_2 as the stimulus revealed a significant difference in flow (+70%) versus volume increase (+10%; Haberl et al. 1989).

It is important to note that CBV measured with technetium-99m-labeled red blood cells represents a different volume than the volume determined by laser Doppler (reflecting total blood cells). If, however, the main portion of the CBV is assumed to be in nonregulated venules and/or larger veins (80% vs. 9% in arterioles and capillaries; Friberg, (this volume)), the question arises of how acetazolamide or CO_2, acting only at the regulated vascular bed, are able to cause such a CBV increase of up to 50%. Cerebral blood volume increase in many protocols reflects the augmented number of red blood cells, i.e., a significant peripheral change in hematocrit (Table 4), contributing to total volume increase. Buell and Schicha (1990), following arguments of Schmidt-Schönbein, postulated a mechanism operating in both capillaries and venules under such conditions: these vessels are assumed to be passively pushed open, a process abandoning increased red cells and volume from the regulated vascular bed (Table 3). Moreover, blood cells or plasma are supposed to attend capillaries in different amounts (H. Schmid-Schönbein, personal communication).

In a recent study, we employed the typical acetazolamide protocol (see Table 5) in patients to evaluate CBV changes in both cerebrum and calvarium. In three patients with various degrees of ICA occlusion, no significant increase was found (Fig. 3). The highest increase was +9% for both CBV ("cerebral" in Table 5) and total cranial blood volume ("cranial" in Table 5, Fig. 3). Similar decreases (to –9% or –11%, respective-

Table 5. Percentage increase[a] in cerebral or cranial blood volume ^{99m}Tc-RBC-SPECT[b]) after administration of acetazolamide[c]

State	Cerebral	Cranial	*n*
ICA stenosis 70%–90%	–9 to +9	–11 to +9	3 vessels, 6 half-slices[e]
ICA occlusion	0 to +6	– 4 to +1	2 vessels, 4 half-slices
ICA normal[d]	–2 to +1	+ 2	1 vessel, 2 half-slices

[a] (density with acetazolamide: density without) –1.0 x 100
[b] 2 pix slices, 64 x 64; density: 1 to 2 x *E* +03
[c] 1 g i.v., SPECT 15 min thereafter
[d] Patient with leuko-araiosis
[e] See Fig. 3

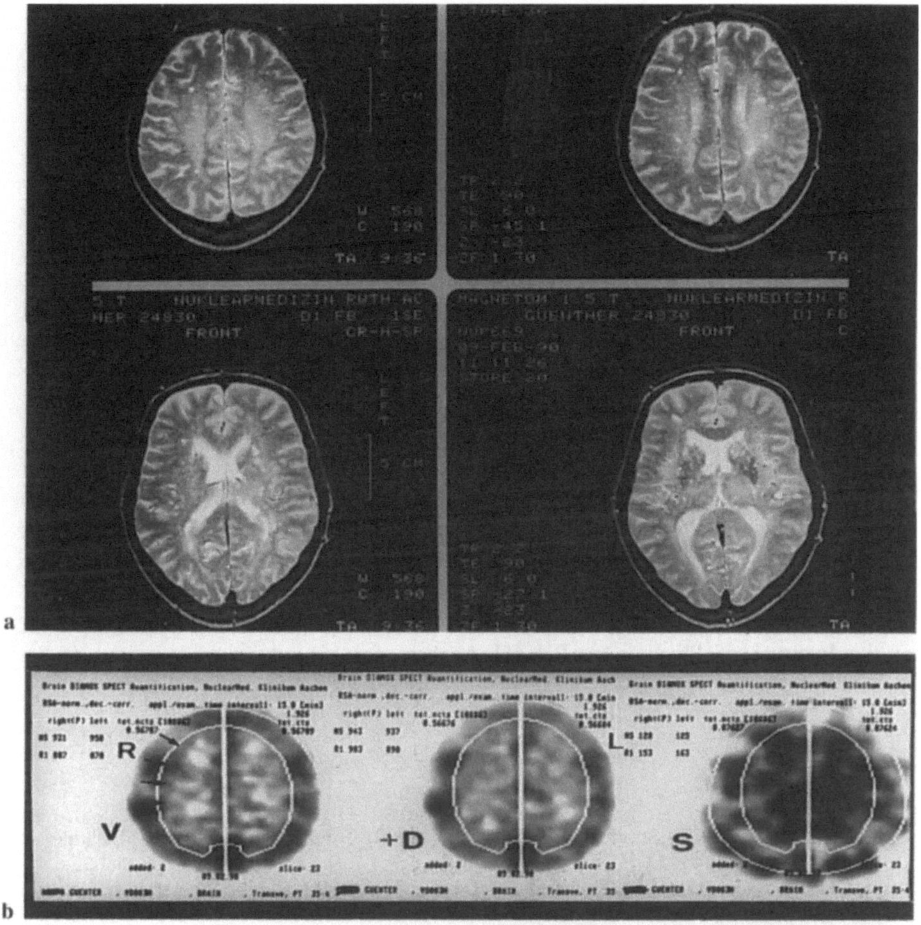

Fig. 3a, b. Sixty-year-old male hypertensive patient with occlusion of the right and a normal left internal carotid artery. No territorial changes in MRI but leuko-araiosis **(a).** Volume images (**b** with ^{99m}Tc-labeled red blood cells) "at rest" *(V, left),* after acetazolamide (+*D*; 1 g i.v., *middle*) and the subtraction image (*S*, acetazolamide minus rest; *right*). Note increased regional blood-volume at rest *(V, arrows)* in the right parietal area. Oval regions separate cerebral from extracerebral (skull) areas. Subtraction revealed few changes with no significant differences for both hemispheres [–4% right side (occluded ICA), +2% left side (open ICA)]

ly) were found. Thus, as expected, there was no systematic response of CBV to acetazolamide in patients with severe CCVD. It is of interest that the patient illustrated in Fig. 3, suffering from leuko-araiosis, failed to react in the hemisphere supported by a normal ICA. Derlin (this volume) found a maximal increase of 15% beyond severe ICA stenoses.

Conclusion

Regional CPR may be assessed by three different examination protocols: (a) CBF or (b) CBV at rest and after stimulation, or (c) the CBF-to-CBV ratio at rest. The latter, imaged by emission computed tomography methods, yields a most powerful tool to assess the regional CPR under baseline conditions, without the problems of standardization for any stimulus protocol. CPR from CBF-to-CBV displays the extent of recruitment of cerebrovascular reserve in its actual rheological state during the effort to maintain the baseline flow by compensating for decreased perfusion pressure or, subsequently, for decreased oxygen transport capacity. CBV (especially red blood cell volume) in normal supply areas reacts to the same stimuli (CO_2, acetazolamide) as CBF and increases regionally up to 50%. Beyond diseased cranial arteries, increases are much lower, e.g., <10%, or are missing. In such patients, an increase in CBV may be a chronic process, potentially representing an increase in peripheral hematocrit, different amounts of cells or plasma attending the capillaries, and/or passive dilation of nonregulated vascular bed or capillary enlargement. Increase in CBV was found to be independent of the individual clinical presentation, which will not occur before CPR is exhausted and a critical threshold of CBF has been reached (Fig. 1).

Acknowledgement. The authors wish to thank Prof. Dr. H. Schmid-Schönbein, Director of the Institute of Physiology, RWTH Aachen, for his advice and review of the manuscript.

References

Aaslid R, Lindegaard KF, Sorteberg W, Nornes H (1989) Cerebral autoregulation dynamics in humans. Stroke 20:45–52

Arora GD, Payne JK, Lowe JL, Kulkarni PV, Devous MD (1990) Regional cerebral hematocrit, mean transit time, blood volume and blood flow in canine acute stroke model (Abstr). J Nucl Med 31:1584

Bonte FJ, Devous MD, Reisch JS (1988) The effect of acetazolamide on regional cerebral blood flow in normal human subjects as measured by SPECT. Invest Radiol 23:564–568

Buell U, Schicha H (1990) Nuclear medicine to image applied pathophysiology: evaluation of reserves by emission computerized tomography (Editorial). Eur J Nucl Med 16:129–135

Buell U, Braun H, Ferbert A, Stirner H, Weiller C, Ringelstein EB (1988) Combined SPECT imaging of regional cerebral blood flow (99m-Tc HMPAO) and blood volume (99m-Tc-RBC) to assess regional cerebral perfusion reserve in patients with cerebrovascular disease. Nuklearmedizin 27:51–56

Buell U, Costa DC, Kirsch G, Moretti JL, van Royen EA, Schober O (1990) The investigation of dementia with SPECT (Review). Nucl Med Commun 11:823–841

Choksey MS, Costa DC, Iannotti F, Ell PJ, Crockard HA (1989) 99Tcm-HMPAO SPECT and cerebral blood flow: a study of CO_2 reactivity. Nucl Med Commun 10:609–618

Frackowiak RSJ, Wise RJS (1983) Positron tomography in ischemic cerebrovascular disease. Neurol Clin 1:183–200

Gaehtgens P, Marx P (1987) Hemorheological aspects of the pathophysiology of cerebral ischemia. J Cereb Blood Flow Metab 7:259–265

Gibbs JM, Wise RJS, Leenders KL, Jones T (1984) Evaluation of cerebral perfusion reserve in patients with carotid-artery occlusion. Lancet 1:310–314

Gibbs JM, Wise RJS, Thomas DJ, Mansfield AO, Ross Ressell RW (1987) Cerebral haemodynamic changes after extracranial-intracranial bypass surgery. J Neurol Neurosurg Psychiatry 50:140–150

Guenther W, Moser E, Mueller-Spahn F, Oefele K, Buell U, Hippius H (1986) Pathological cerebral blood flow during motor function in schizophrenic and endogenous depressed patients. Biol Psychiatry 21:889–899

Haberl RL, Heizer MC, Marmarou A, Ellis EF (1989) Laser Doppler assessment of brain microcirculation: effect of systemic alterations. Am J Physiol 256:H1247–H1254

Heiss WD (1983) Flow thresholds of functional and morphological damage of brain tissue. Stroke 14:329–331

Herold S, Brown MM, Frackowiak RSJ, Mansfield AO, Thomas DJ, Marshall J (1988) Assessment of cerebral haemodynamic reserve: correlation between PET parameters and CO_2 reactivity measured by intravenous 133-xenon injection technique. J Neurol Neurosurg Psychiatry 51:1045–1050

Kaiser HJ, Reiche W, Buell U (1990) A method of adapting and evaluating MRI- and SPECT-tomograms for comparing cerebral morphology and cerebrovascular regulation. Nuklearmedizin 29:13–18

Kanno I, Uemura K, Higano S, Murakami M, Iida H, Miura S, Shishido F, Unugami A, Sayama I (1988) Oxygen extraction fraction at maximally vasodilated tissue in the ischemic brain estimated from the regional CO_2 responsiveness measured by PET. J Cereb Blood Flow Metab 8:227–235

Kety SS, Schmidt CF (1948) The effects of altered arterial tensions of carbon dioxide and oxygen on the cerebral blood flow and carboxide consumption of normal young man. J Clin Invest 27:484–492

Keyeux A, Laterre C, Beckers CH (1988) Resting and hyperkapnic rCBF in patients with unilateral occlusive disease of the internal carotid artery. J Nucl Med 29:311–319

Knapp WH, Kummer R, Kübler W (1986) Imaging of cerebral blood flow-to-volume distribution using SPECT. J Nucl Med 27:465–470

Kontos HA (1989) Validity of cerebral artery blood flow calculations from velocity measurements. Stroke 20:1–3

Kummer R, Scharf J, Back T, Reich H, Machens HG, Wildemann B (1988) Autoregulatory capacity and the effect of isovolemic hemodilution on local cerebral blood flow. Stroke 19:584–597

Lauritzen M, Henriksen L, Lassen NA (1981) Regional cerebral blood flow during rest and skilled hand movements by xenon-133 inhalation and emission computerized tomography. J Cereb Blood Flow Metab 1:385–389

Leinsinger G, Schmiedek P, Kreisig T, Einhäupl K, Bauer W, Moser EA (1988) 133-Xe-DSPECT: Bedeutung der zerebrovaskulären Reservekapazität für Diagnostik und Therapie der chronischen zerebralen Ischämie. Nuklearmedizin 27:127–134

Levine RL, Sunderland JJ, Lagreze HL, Nickels RJ, Rowe BR, Turski PA (1988) Cerebral perfusion reserve indexes determined by fluoromethane PET. Stroke 19:19–27

Phelps ME, Huang SC, Hoffman EJ, Kuhl DE (1979) Validation of tomographic measurement of cerebral blood volume with C-11 labeled carboxy-hemoglobin. J Nucl Med 20:328–334

Powers WJ, Raichle ME (1985) PET and its application to the study of cerebrovascular disease in man. Stroke 16:361–376

Reich T, Rusinek H (1989) Cerebral cortical and white matter reactivity to carbon dioxide. Stroke 20:453–457

Ringelstein EB, Sievers C, Ecker S, Schneider PA, Otis SM (1988) Noninvasive assessment of CO_2-induced cerebral vasomotor response in normal individuals and patients with internal carotid artery occlusion. Stroke 19:963–969

Sakai F, Tazaki Y (1987) Regional cerebral blood flow, volume, and hematocrit measured by SPECT. In: Hartmann A, Kuschinsky W (eds) Cerebral ischemia and hemorheology. Springer, Berlin Heidelberg New York, pp 211–216

Sakai F, Nakazawa K, Tazaki Y, Ishii K, Hino H, Igarashi H, Kanda T (1985) Regional cerebral blood volume and hematocrit measured in normal human volunteers by SPECT. J Cereb Blood Flow Metab 5:207–213

Schmid-Schönbein H (1988) Fluid dynamics and hemorheology in vivo. In: Lowe GDO (ed) Clinical blood rheology. CRC, Boca Raton

Schmid-Schönbein H, Driessen G, Gallasch H (1987) Hemorheology and cerebral infarction: on the role of pathological blood thixotrophy in the pathogenesis of and therapy for states of acute cerebral hypoperfusion. In: Hartmann A, Kuschinsky W (eds) Cerebral ischemia and hemorheology. Springer, Berlin Heidelberg New York, pp 27–50

Schmidt U, Knapp WH, Busse O, Griese H, Vyska K, Minami K, Notohampiprodjo G (1988) Veränderung der cerebralen Aufnahme von Tc-99m-HMPAO in Abhängigkeit vom arteriellen CO_2-Spiegel. Nuklearmedizin 27:27

Toyama H, Takeshita G, Takeuchi A, Anno H, Ejiri K, Katada K, Koga S (1988) Imaging and quantitative analysis of regional cerebral blood volume by ring type SPECT: normal volunteer studies. Kaku Igaku 25:339–344

Toyama H, Takeshita G, Takeuchi A, Anno H, Ejiri K, Maeda H, Katada K, Koga S, Ishiyama N, Kanno T, Yamaoka N (1990) Cerebral hemodynamics in patients with chronic obstructive carotid disease by rCBF, rCBV, and rCBV/rCBF ratio using SPECT. J Nucl Med 31:55–60

Positron Emission Tomography Activation Studies in Neurological Patients

G. Pawlik, G. R. Fink, U. Pietrzyk, M. Grond, and W.-D. Heiss

Introduction

The quantitative imaging of the hemodynamic and metabolic changes occurring in brain regions responding to distinct stimulation or involved in the performance of specific tasks is one of the most intriguing applications of positron emission tomography (PET) (Phelps et al. 1982; Pawlik and Heiss 1989). Depending on the chosen paradigm, PET activation studies can serve many purposes. While elementary and stepwise paradigms are geared primarily at the elucidation of normal functional neuroanatomy, more complex tasks causing widespread activation may be better suited for the assessment of the regional reserve capacity especially in dysfunctional association areas because brain lesions are rarely restricted to primary cortex. Furthermore, even in regions showing no gross structrual abnormality, lesions at the cellular or synaptic level may interfere with the ability to respond to specific stimulation by appropriate neuronal recruitment that cannot be assessed with purely vascular stimuli like forced hypercapnia. This report describes our experience with a few cognitive and behavioral activation paradigms in various common neurological diseases.

In contrast with other functional diagnostic methods yielding information on certain aspects of cerebral hemodynamics only, PET permits the concurrent investigation of cerebral vascular pathophysiology and energy metabolism, thus providing insight into the coupling of neuronal function and substrate supply. Therefore, multivariate PET studies in the resting state may at times even obviate the need for activation studies, as will be illustrated in a selected group of patients with chronic regional ischemia.

Methods

Patients

A total of 120 patients are included in this review. Out of a larger series of patients with *chronic cerebral ischemia* due to high-grade (>80%) atherosclerotic internal carotid artery (ICA) stenosis, a subgroup of 11 were selected because they exhibited significant regional perfusion deficits in the respective supply territory, but showed no gross morphological abnormality on computed tomography (CT) or magnetic resonance imaging (MRI). This group underwent only one multivariate PET study in a resting state.

In 12 patients with symptomatic (6 epileptic seizures, 4 ischemic signs, 2 posthemorrhage deficits) *cerebral angiomas* (8 arteriovenous, 4 venous), both a multivariate resting PET study and another investigation of brain glucose metabolism (CMRgl) during 30-min spontaneous speech were performed on consecutive days.

The other 97 patients had paired PET studies only of CMRgl, at rest and in one or two distinct stimulation conditions. Sixteen patients, who had suffered an *ischemic stroke* in the dominant hemisphere and presented mild to moderate *aphasia* at the postacute stage, were activated using spontaneous speech. Their PET findings were then related to the severity of their aphasic symptoms assessed at least 1 year later. Fourteen *brain tumor* patients (six grade II, four grade III, four grade IV) underwent PET scanning during speech performance for the presurgical localization of their language functions.

For the activation of 21 patients with probable *Alzheimer's disease* according to NINCDS-ADRDA criteria (McKhann et al. 1984), and of 9 age-matched subjects with minor symptoms suggesting an early stage of dementia, an individually difficulty-adjusted continuous visual recognition task was used that required yes/no responses to verbal and nonverbal items presented, in part repeatedly, for 30 min at a rate of one item every 3–6 s.

The same visual recognition paradigm was chosen for the stimulation of 33 patients with EEG-documented temporal lobe *epilepsy,* who also underwent PET scanning during 30-min emotional speech on personal experiences. Another patient with occipital lobe epilepsy had PET studies of cerebral blood flow (CBF) and CMRgl during "spontaneous activation" by persistent, periodic, focal epileptiform discharges. Three seizure-free patients who had undergone total cerebral hemispherectomy in adolescence because of medically intractable, symptomatic epilepsy were studied with PET after 4–36 years during continuous, coordinated limb movements on the paretic side, in order to investigate the brain's capacity for functional recovery following extensive neurosurgery.

Positron Emission Tomography Procedures

For all studies, a Scanditronix PC 384 positron camera (Eriksson et al. 1982) was used that permitted the simultaneous scanning of seven transaxial slices extending from the canthomeatal plane to the supraventricular level, with an in-plane resolution of 7.8 mm at a slice thickness of 11 mm. Each multivariate PET study comprised only these seven tomographic sections, while in studies of CMRgl another set of seven intercalated slices were recorded, thus allowing for subsequent image reconstruction at any desired angle. Prior to the PET study, each patient was familiarized with the procedure, and informed consent was obtained in writing. Images of CMRgl were recorded 30–50 min after i.v. injection of 185 MBq 2[^{18}F]fluorodeoxyglucose (FDG), using a previously described protocol and pixel-by-pixel optimization of rate constants in metabolic quantitation (Heiss et al. 1984; Wienhard et al. 1985). Multivariate PET studies consisted of four separate measurements that were started at intervals of 15–20 min. First, CBF was determined dynamically following the i.v. injection of 1.5 GBq $H_2{}^{15}O$. Next, the kinetics of oxygen in brain tissue were recorded after bolus inhalation of 1.0 GBq $^{15}O_2$ for subsequent computation of the local oxygen extraction fraction (OEF) according to the method of Mintun et al. (1984). This was followed by the static imaging of local cerebral blood volume (CBV) 3–6 min after the rebreathing of 4 GBq $C^{15}O$. CMRgl was measured last. During the entire procedure, the patient remained stable in a comfortable supine position, with eyes closed and head fixed in the scanner gantry. Blood samples were obtained from a radial artery catheter at a rate determined by the respective model for physiological quantitation. In resting and activation studies alike, external stimulation was kept at a minimum; only during performance of the 30-min, continuous visual recognition task did the patients sit in an upright position, with their eyes open.

Image Analysis

Computing operations between the four original measurements of a multivariate PET study, calibrated for the instantaneous substrate and radiotracer concentrations in arterial blood, provided eight quantitative tomographic images for each scanned slice: the cerebral metabolic rate for oxygen ($CMRO_2$), OEF, CBF, CBV, CMRgl, the glucose extraction fraction (GEF), the glucose/oxygen metabolic ratio (CMR%), and the mean vascular transit time (MVTT), equaling the CBV/CBF ratio. These images were displayed slice by slice, and they were evaluated visually in comparison with corresponding CT or MRI scans. Individual CMRgl image data from activation studies were interpolated in three dimensions and then matched to the respective resting data set, thus yielding sets of difference data that could be displayed both as tomographic sections and as cortical projections to the sagittal plane.

In addition to visual image analysis, standard regions of interest (ROIs) were adapted to the individual anatomy, using a semiautomatic computer-assisted procedure (Herholz et al. 1985). These ROIs were then pooled into topographically meaningful areas for further statistical analysis. A categorical similarity-matching algorithm (Pawlik et al. 1986) provided maximum comparability both between a patient's various sets of images and among patient groups.

Descriptive statistics are presented as arithmetic mean ± standard deviation. Regional PET data were analyzed numerically using (repeated measures) analysis of variance. Exact test procedures were used in comparisons of frequencies.

Results

Chronic Cerebral Ischemia

Many high-grade ICA stenoses obviously do not cause cerebral ischemia. If they do, the perfusion deficit need not be limited to the typical arterial supply territory, nor does it necessarily involve the entire carotid irrigation area. At times, even steal effects from the vertebrobasilar system are the only clinical manifestations. This remarkable heterogeneity among patients may be explained in part by anomalies of the individual vascular anatomy, or by intracranial atherosclerosis. CT and MRI scans often reveal no gross morphological abnormality because they are not sensitive enough to demonstrate selective neuronal loss, or because vascular and metabolic mechanisms still can compensate for the decreased perfusion pressure. Therefore, multivariate PET studies may provide the pathophysiological basis for the assessment of the individual risk of hemodynamic stroke. Of course, the risk of cerebral infarction due to other causes, e.g.,

Table 1. Multivariate PET findings in patients with >80% internal carotid artery stenosis and significant regional ischemia in the morphologically intact supply territory

	Hemodynamics			Energy metabolism		
Patient no.	Ischemia	Vasodilation	Prolonged blood transit	Hypo-metabolism	Anaerobic glycolysis	Increased extraction fractions
1	X	X	X	X	X	X
2	X	X	X	X	X	X
3	X	0	X	X	X	X
4	X	0	X	X	X	X
5	X	0	X	X	X	X
6	X	0	X	X	X	X
7	X	0	X	0	0	X
8	X	X	X	X	0	X
9	X	X	X	0	0	X
10	X	X	0	0	0	X
11	X	0	X	X	0	0
% Positive	100	45	91	73	55	91

X/0, present/absent

thromboembolism, cannot be detected by this method, which may be the reason why previous reports were so discouraging (Powers et al. 1989).

The major PET findings in our selected group of patients with chronic regional ischemia are summarized in Table 1. As significant hypoperfusion was a selection criterion, and blood flow velocities are closely related to CBF, the high incidence (10/11) of increased MVTTs was to be expected. The only exception was a patient (# 10) exhibiting both decreases and slight increases in CBF of adjacent subregions, with each flow state being accompanied by proportionate CBV changes. However, in contrast with previous observations on homeostatic hemodynamic mechanisms in cervical occlusive disease (Gibbs et al. 1984), regional cerebral vasodilation was found in less than half the cases (5/11), while GEF and OEF were increased in 10 out of 11 cases. This finding suggests that autoregulation may be severely impaired in many patients with advanced atherosclerosis concurrently involving the large supraaortic and the small cerebral resistance vessels, thus producing a typical misery perfusion syndrome (Baron 1987) demanding therapeutic action. Seven out of ten patients calling on their extraction fractions for metabolic compensation also showed a significant fall in $CMRO_2$ and CMRgl, as illustrated in Fig. 1. In five of those seven cases, regional oxygen consumption was more severely depressed than glucose metabolism, indicating some anaerobic glycolysis. In patient # 11, the absence of an increase in substrate extraction despite dense, hemodynamically uncompensated ischemia suggested substantial neuronal decay in a brain region whose gross morphology appeared intact. The described heterogeneity of multivariate responses was statistically significant (Cochran's Q-test, $P<0.05$).

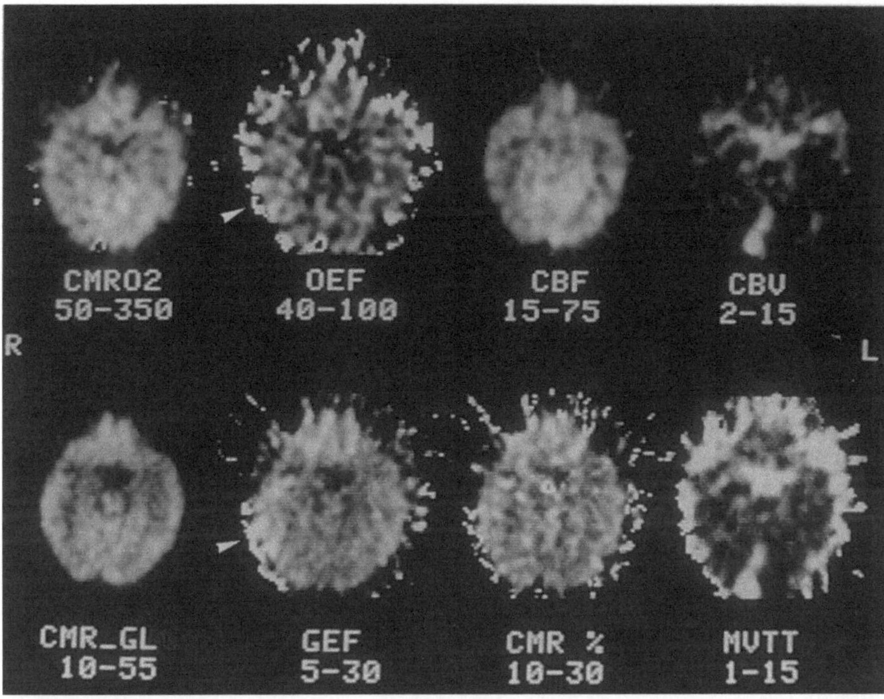

Fig. 1. Multivariate PET images (section across inferior occipital and temporal lobes) of a patient (case # 6 in Table 1) with high-grade stenosis of right ICA, showing hypoperfusion, hypometabolism, and increased extraction fractions *(arrows)* in supply territory of right posterior temporal artery. *R* and *L* indicate right and left side of patient's head, respectively. *Numbers* below the variable names denote the range of values represented by *shades of gray, from black to white.* Units: micromoles/100 g per minute for $CMRO_2$ and CMRgl; percentages for OEF, GEF, CMR%, and CBV; milliliters/100 g per minute for CBF; seconds for MVTT

Ischemic Stroke and Aphasia

Decreases in energy metabolism and blood flow in areas primarily not involved in focal ischemia are generally observed in ischemic stroke as well as in other acute, focal brain lesions (Pawlik et al. 1985; Feeney and Baron 1986). Functional changes occurring in brain regions remote from the primary lesion must be interpreted as deactivation consequent on the interruption of connecting fiber tracts. Dysfunction of tissue adjacent to the infarct, however, may also be due to the loss of particularly vulnerable neurons, caused by short-lasting episodes of ischemia affecting areas much larger than the ultimate infarct (Mies et al. 1983). The clinical implications neither of remote deactivation nor of selective neuronal decay are sufficiently understood, but both may contribute to the patient's persistent neurological deficit, and therefore the degree of resting hypometabolism in conjunction with relative functional unresponsiveness may provide a measure of prognosis.

This hypothesis was tested in moderately aphasic stroke victims, whose CMRgl was investigated with PET in a resting state and during spontaneous speech, respectively.

Eight patients later improved significantly, achieving good or satisfactory language abilities, while the other eight had a poor outcome. In the resting state, all patients' metabolic patterns were characterized by markedly decreased glucose consumption in the ischemic lesion as well as in the entire ipsilateral cerebral hemisphere. This deactivation (Figs. 2, 3) was significantly ($P<0.01$) more prominent in the poor-outcome group (28.2±5.88 μmol/100 g per minute vs. 37.8±4.04 μmol/100 g per minute with good outcome).

During speech, there was a significant ($P<0.0001$) increase in whole-brain metabolism, averaging 18%±11.7%. However, the two groups differed ($P<0.05$) in their activation patterns: Those eventually showing poor functional recovery (Fig. 2) primarily recruited their left cerebellum (7.4±4.96 μmol/100 g per minute vs. 4.7±3.73 μmol/100 g per minute in right cerebellum) and the cerebral hemisphere contralateral to the infarct (6.4±4.52 μmol/100 g per minute vs. 5.0±3.30 μmol/100 g per minute in left cerebrum). In contrast, the patients with good outcome (Fig. 3) activated metabolism in both cerebral (left, 6.3±4.51 μmol/100 g per minute; right, 6.1±4.95 μmol/100 g

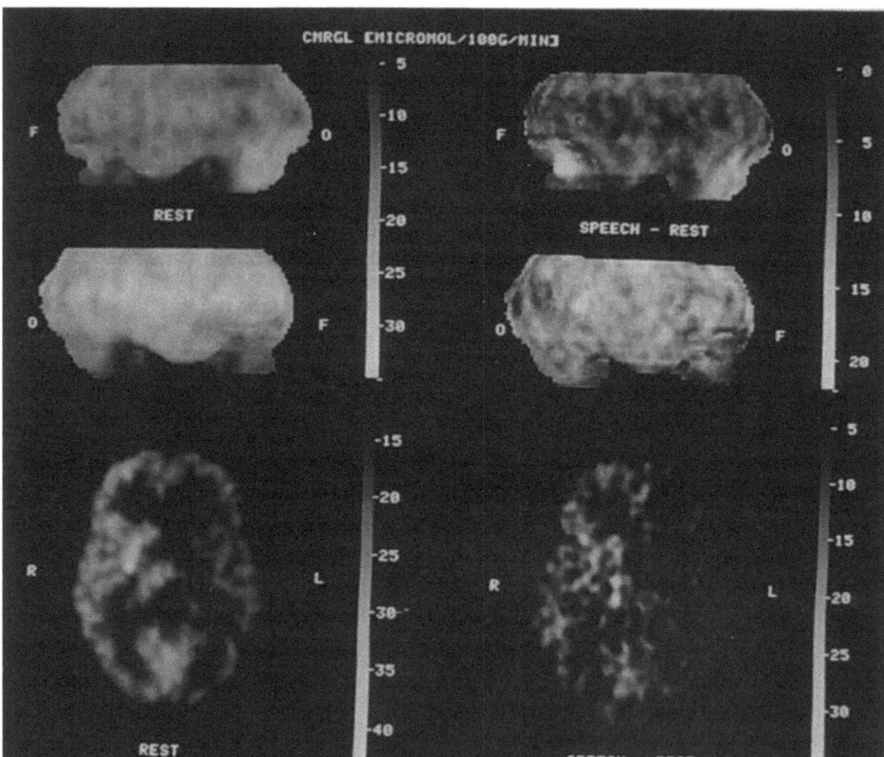

Fig. 2. Left and right lateral views *(upper frames)*, and transaxial PET images *(lower frames)* of CMRgl at rest *(left side)* and of speech-minus-rest metabolic difference *(right side)* of an aphasic stroke patient with poor prognosis. Reference gray scales are calibrated in absolute units. *F* and *O*, frontal and occipital lobe

per minute) and cerebellar hemispheres (left, 10.2±5.09 µmol/100 g per minute; right, 10.7±8.04 µmol/100 g per minute) during task performance, exhibiting some predominance in areas related to language processing in the infarcted dominant hemi-sphere. Those cases with good outcome and bilateral functional recruitment during speech nearly equalized their resting pattern of metabolic cerebellar asymmetry; four patients even reversed it, thus producing a metabolic pattern comparable to the right-greater-than-left cerebellar activation known from studies of healthy speaking volunteers (Pawlik et al. 1987). Furthermore, the two outcome groups differed significantly ($P<0.05$) with respect to the recruitment of their supplementary motor areas, which was observed in seven out of eight good-prognosis candidates, but only in two out of eight patients with poor outcome.

These findings suggest that the capacity for long-term functional recovery from moderate aphasia as a result of cerebral infarction can be estimated in earlier disease stages from the degree of overall metabolic recruitability of spared brain regions in the dominant hemisphere, and from the individual availability of auxiliary neuronal networks. Both parameters in turn seem to depend heavily on a sufficient level of baseline

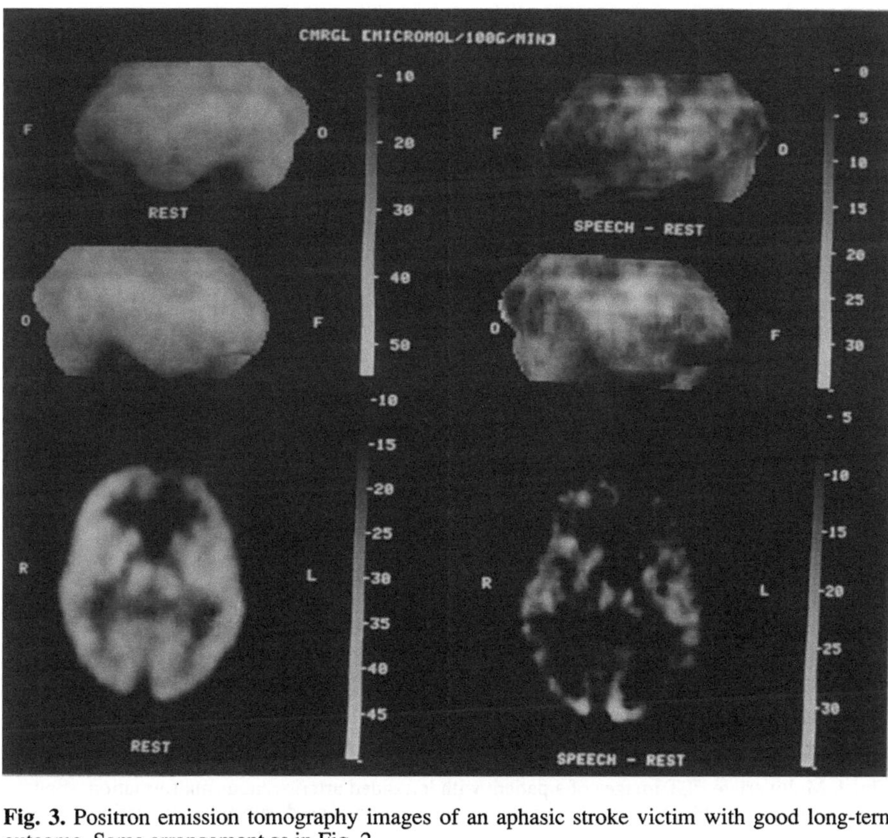

Fig. 3. Positron emission tomography images of an aphasic stroke victim with good long-term outcome. Same arrangement as in Fig. 2

activity, perhaps with very low resting metabolism being indicative of substantial neuronal loss in addition to purely functional deactivation.

Cerebral Angiomas

Patients with larger cerebral angiomas carry an increased risk not only of hemorrhagic stroke but also of epilepsy, and brain tissue adjacent to the vascular malformation may become atrophic either by pressure or by chronic ischemic degeneration due to hemodynamic steal effects. While bleeding angiomas are commonly treated by embolization or surgical resection, the indication for invasive therapy is not as clear with the other angiomas. Particularly in the latter group, however, PET can provide the pathophysiological rationale for surgical intervention – even in cases showing no morphological abnormality outside the angioma on CT or MRI scanning.

In our series of symptomatic patients, multivariate resting PET studies permitted the clear distinction between arteriovenous malformations and venous angiomas in accordance with angiography, because in the former the area of focally increased blood volume consisted of contiguous parts exhibiting either hyperperfusion or prolonged

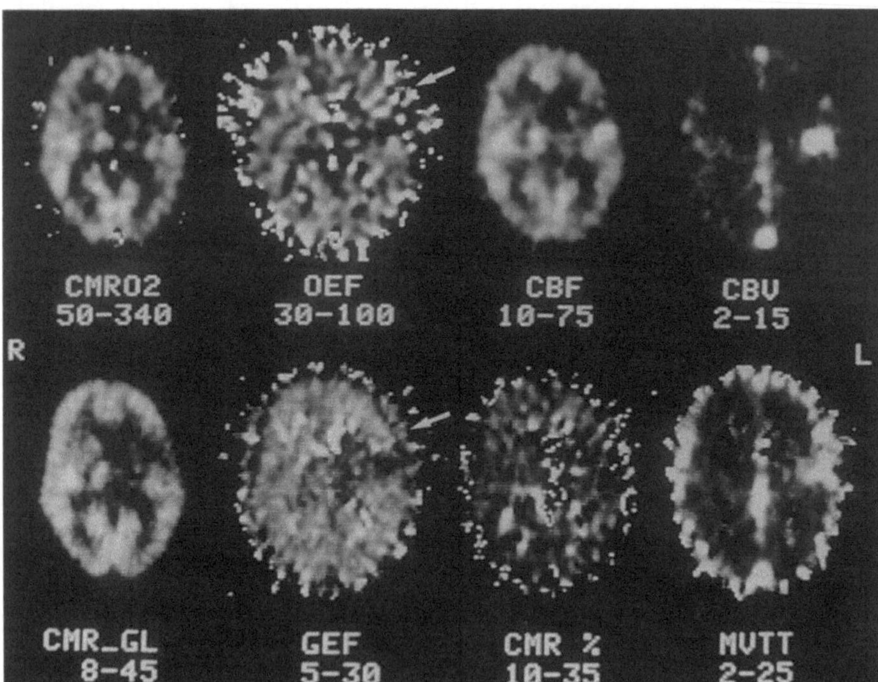

Fig. 4. Multivariate PET images of a patient with left-sided arteriovenous malformation, showing slightly decreased blood flow, hypometabolism, and increased substrate extraction fractions *(arrows)* of adjacent tissue. Same arrangement as in Fig. 1

MVTTs, whereas the latter were characterized by proportionate increases in CBV and MVTT. In contrast with a previous PET study of cerebral arteriovenous malformations (Tyler et al. 1989), revealing only glucose hypometabolism and increased CBF in the ipsilateral hemisphere, we found various functional abnormalities in the brain tissue surrounding the angioma: CBF was decreased in 11 out of 12 cases and 9 of those 11 patients showed concurrent increases in OEF and GEF, respectively, indicating misery perfusion. Energy metabolism was depressed in 11, but signs of anaerobic glycolysis were found only in 4 cases including the 2 with chronic posthemorrhagic state and two epilepsy patients (Fig. 4).

Among the clinical groups, there was no obvious difference in the pattern of physiological abnormalities. During functional activation, 8 out of 12 patients showed a marked lack of metabolic recruitment in the border zone of the angioma, perhaps corresponding with steal-induced, chronic ischemic loss of neurons (Fig. 5).

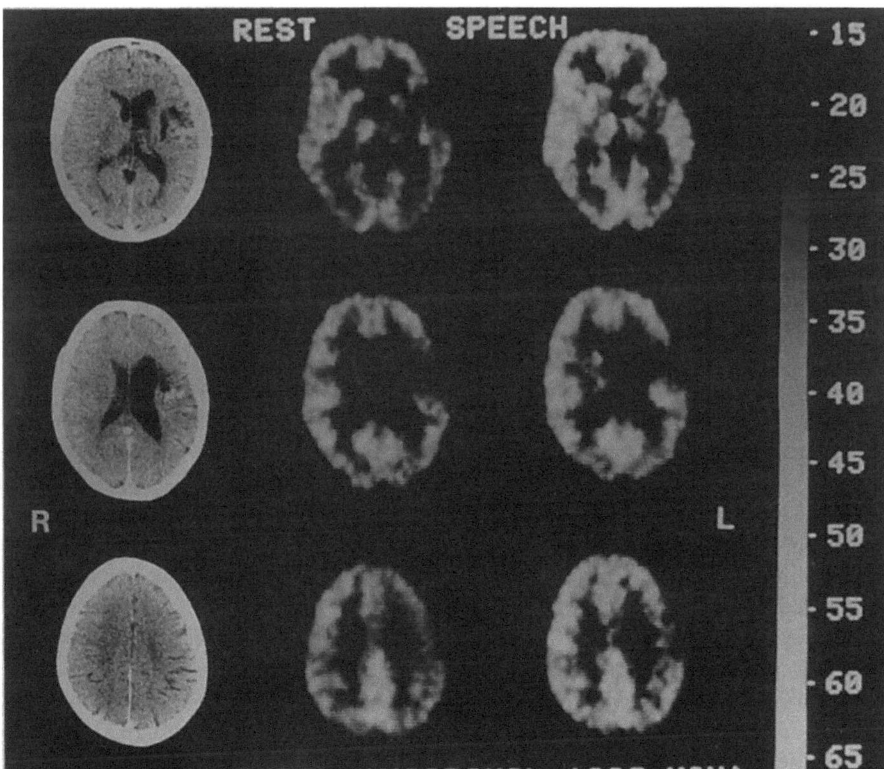

Fig. 5. Computed tomography scans and glucose metabolic PET images obtained in resting state *(middle column)* and during spontaneous speech *(right column)* from the same patient as in Fig. 4. Note the lack of functional recruitment of precentral cortex above the angioma

Brain Tumors

In patients with brain tumors and angiomas alike, one of the factors influencing the decision whether – and how extensively – to perform neurosurgery, is the cerebral localization of language-related functions – particularly in those cases where major postoperative aphasic symptoms are to be expected because of the patient's tumor location in the presumably dominant hemisphere. Another important factor is the degree of malignancy of the tumor that can be estimated fairly reliably with PET (Di Chiro 1986). Therefore, prior to neurosurgery or stereotaxic biopsy, we investigated CMRgl at rest and during spontaneous speech in 14 tumor patients, 8 of whom exhibited some minor language dysfunction.

Glucose consumption was decreased in five out of six grade II tumors, while relative hypermetabolism was found in seven out of eight high-grade tumors, i.e., there was a close correlation (phi=0.71, $P<0.02$) between tumor metabolism and malignancy. During speech, the metabolic activation of Broca's area and premotor cortex was clearly lateralized to the left hemisphere except in one patient with a left frontal glioblastoma, but four patients with tumorous lesions involving their left temporal lobe showed a distinct functional predominance of their right Wernicke-homologous region. Four of the seven patients who did not have their tumor removed were excluded from neurosurgery because their tumors were located in areas relevant to the processing of language. Those patients who did undergo resective neurosurgery because their activation PET scan showed no contraindicative pattern of functional recruitment either remained free from aphasic symptoms ($n=2$) or at least they did not experience a persistent increase in their preexistent language problems ($n=5$).

Focal Epilepsy

Focal areas of epileptogenic dysfunction appear interictally on PET scans as zones of hypometabolism and decreased blood flow, while areas involved in focal seizure onset and spread may show both increased and decreased CMRgl and CBF on ictal PET scans, due in part to measurements of both ictal and postictal effects (Engel 1989). Therefore, concurrent EEG recordings and thorough understanding of the temporal characteristics of the applied PET method are essential for the appropriate interpretation of functional images of epilepsy, which may be regarded as a natural model of abnormal self-stimulation. That effect on the resulting images of different method-dependent temporal resolutions of PET is illustrated in Fig. 6, showing CBF and CMRgl images obtained 25 min apart, during a series of occipital lobe seizures, with focal epileptiform discharges of 4 s duration appearing at intervals of several minutes for the whole scanning period. During the CBF study, a burst of ictal activity was observed only once, 18 s after tracer injection, i.e., at maximum measurement sensitivity. During the subsequent CMRgl study, however, spiking occurred at a time when changes of local metabolism had less effect on the final PET images: 5, 20, 21, 25, and 28 min after tracer injection. Therefore, a focal increase in functional activity was found only on the CBF images.

Ictal PET scans can provide interesting localizing information on epileptic or "epileptized" tissue. However, that area of ictally increased functional activity need not

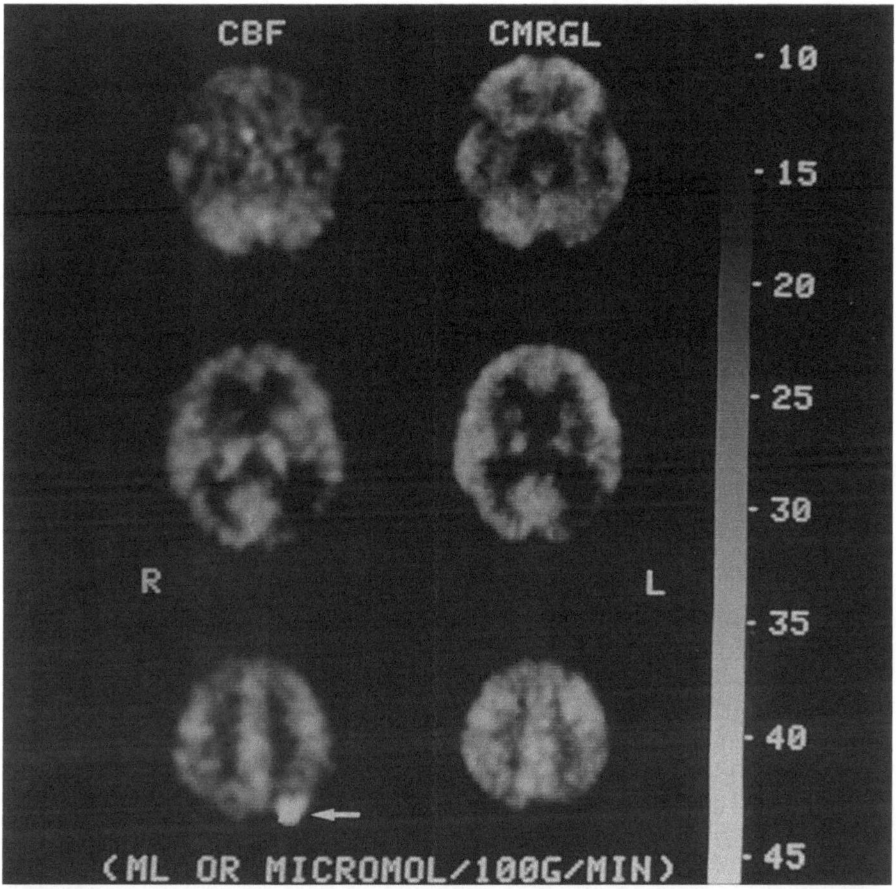

Fig. 6. Blood flow and glucose metabolic PET images obtained during a series of occipital lobe seizures. Because of shorter recording times, only the CBF study shows focally increased activity *(arrow)* at the upper edge of the epileptogenic lesion

necessarily be congruent with the epileptogenic zone, and therefore interictal PET studies are generally considered to be of greater diagnostic value in the presurgical evaluation of focal epilepsy (Engel et al. 1990). Unfortunately, in temporal lobe epilepsy, which is the commonest form of localization-related epilepsy, the epileptogenic area is typically located in a brain region showing low metabolic rates also in healthy resting subjects. Because of inadequate image contrast, the borders of the focus are often too poorly defined as to permit the clear-cut identification of dysfunctional tissue. Hypothesizing that epileptogenic tissue lacks the ability to respond normally to physiological stimulation, we investigated the potential for functional contrast enhancement of two distinct cognitive and behavioral activation paradigms in 33 patients with longstanding epilepsy. According to comprehensive EEG monitoring, their seizures originated consistently from mediobasal foci in the left (n=15) or right (n=18) temporal lobe. PET scanning was performed on three consecutive days, with the order of study conditions being randomized.

In the resting state, the patients' whole-brain CMRgl was only slightly depressed (33±5.1 μmol/100 g per minute) in proportion to their plasma levels of antiepileptic drugs, while the epileptogenic focus showed severe hypometabolism (–33%±11.3%, $P<0.0001$) compared with 60 healthy controls. However, the metabolic contrast with adjacent tissue, e.g., the difference in regional metabolism between midtemporal cortex and focus, was low. Both emotional speech (ES) and continuous visual recognition (CVR) produced comparable, significant($P<0.0001$) metabolic increases in many brain regions (whole brain: ES, 5.9±5.38 μmol/100 g per minute; CVR, 6.1±6.74 μmol/100 g per minute; no significant difference between paradigms), except for the epileptogenic focus where activation was minimal (Fig. 7). Therefore, the CMRgl difference between midtemporal gyrus and focus increased significantly ($P<0.001$), showing clear

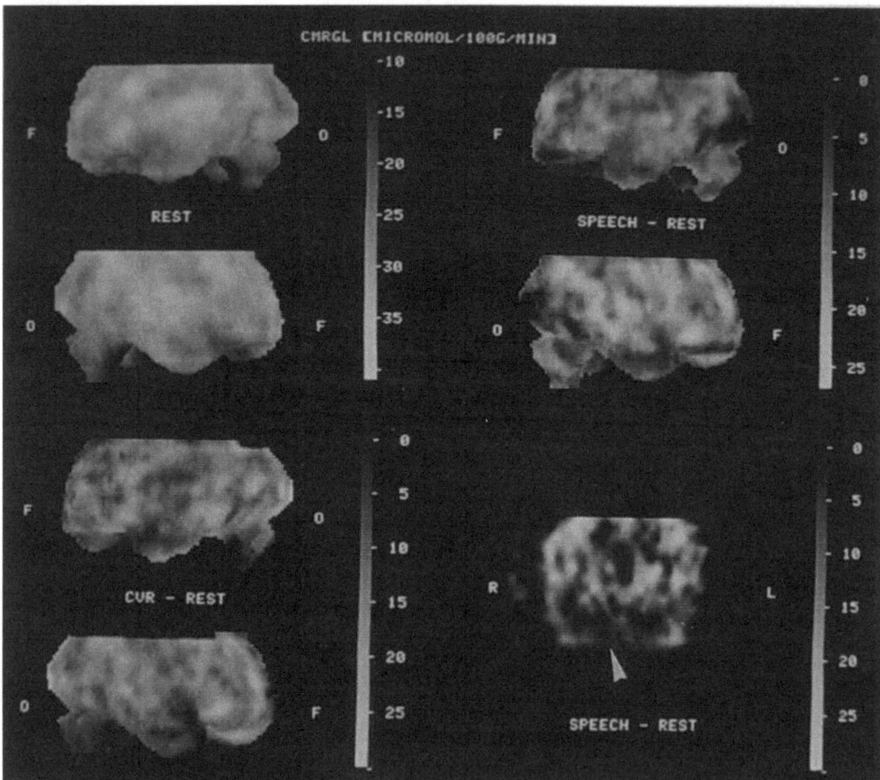

Fig. 7. Left and right lateral views *(upper frames, left lower frame)*, and coronal PET section across anterior temporal lobes, of CMRgl at rest *(left upper frame)*, of CVR-minus-rest metabolic difference *(left lower frame)*, and of speech-minus-rest metabolic difference *(right side of figure)*, of an epilepsy patient, whose seizures consistently originated from his right mediobasal temporal lobe showing a focal lack of functional recruitment during physiological stimulation *(arrow)*. Image orientation and markings as in Fig. 2

superiority of ES over CVR in 23 cases ($P<0.05$), with ES improving the metabolic contrast by 6.2±7.58 µmol/100 g per minute. Concurrently, the visibility of the ipsilateral amygdala on the metabolic images was improved in about half the cases.
Repeated measures ANOVA of these data revealed selective regional effects of the two task conditions, and the lateralized effect of speech, as demonstrated already in the tumor patients described above. Again, with ES, the largest changes occurred in right cerebellum, left thalamus, and left premotor area; with CVR, in primary and secondary visual areas and in both thalami. These findings clearly demonstrate that appropriate psychophysical activation paradigms are not only effective in improving the demarcation of dysfunctional foci, they may also serve to elucidate the distributed networks involved in the higher-order associative processing of complex information.

Even after extensive neurosurgery for epilepsy, the brain retains a remarkable capacity for functional recovery, as we observed with PET in three patients who had undergone total cerebral hemispherectomy (two right, one left) at the ages of 10, 18, and 27 years, respectively, because of medically intractable epilepsy due to unilateral hemisphere damage sustained in infancy or childhood. Their resting CMRgl was in the lower range of normal, showing some regional deactivation of basal temporal and parietal cortical areas. During coordinated, segmental limb movements on the paretic side, major metabolic increases were consistently found in ipsilateral prefrontal, premotor, and parietal association cortex, in basal ganglia, and in both cerebellar hemispheres. On postscanning interviews, all patients reported that they had solved the motor task "by will, internal verbal commands, and imagination." Therefore, a primary motor paradigm had been restructured by the patients to become a mainly associative task.

Alzheimer's Disease

The clinical signs and symptoms of dementias of the Alzheimer type (AD) comprise cognitive and memory deficits that are related to the typical histopathological changes, e.g., neurofibrillary tangles and neuritic plaques, being most prominent in hippocampus and association cortex, where characteristic metabolic decreases are also found. Therefore, PET can be used to support the diagnosis of probable AD (review in Heiss et al. 1989). However, while resting PET studies may reflect primarily structural metabolism, the investigation of stimulation-induced metabolic changes may provide a sensitive and objective measure of the brain's functional reserve capacity. This hypothesis was tested in 30 patients with possible or probable AD, whose MRI scans showed no gross morphological abnormality.

In the resting state, whole-brain CMRgl was similar in the probable AD group and in age-matched controls, but the regional glucose consumption of temporal, parietal, and lateral frontal cortex was typically decreased in AD (Fig. 8). When regional metabolism was related to the severity of dementia, as assessed by means of the global deterioration scale (GDS, Reisberg et al. 1982), analysis of covariance revealed a significant heterogeneity among regional slopes ($P<0.0001$). This difference was largest between the sensorimotor cortex, being virtually unaffected by progressive dementia, and the temporoparietal cortex, showing a strong, linear metabolic decline with advancing clinical stage.

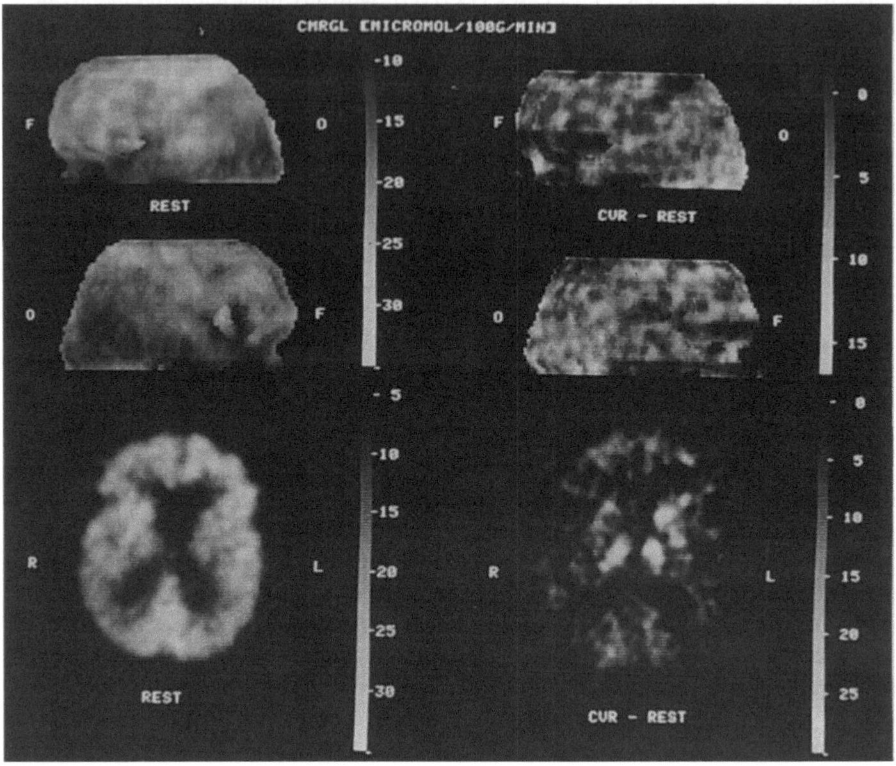

Fig. 8. Resting PET images and CVR-minus-rest metabolic differences of a typical patient with probable Alzheimer's disease. Arrangement as in Fig. 2. Note the lack of functional response, particularly in association cortical areas

Continuous visual recognition produced a large increase in the whole-brain CMRgl of elderly control subjects (6.6±5.66 µmol/100 g per minute), but it had almost no effect ($P<0.05$) in the patients with probable AD (1.5±2.99 µmol/100 g per minute). This was mainly due to the absent response of diseased association areas (Fig. 8). Therefore, in the temporoparietal cortex, a linearly progressive loss ($P<0.02$) of metabolic recruitment at higher GDS scores was found by analysis of covariance (Fig. 9). This finding is in line with the observed relationship between severity of dementia and synaptic density (DeKosky and Scheff 1990), thus supporting the view that activation studies estimate the reserves of functioning neurons.

Conclusions

Pathophysiological mechanisms can be investigated with PET in many ways. While some diseased states, e.g., chronic cerebral ischemia, lend themselves to multivariate studies in a standard resting condition, yielding detailed diagnostic information no

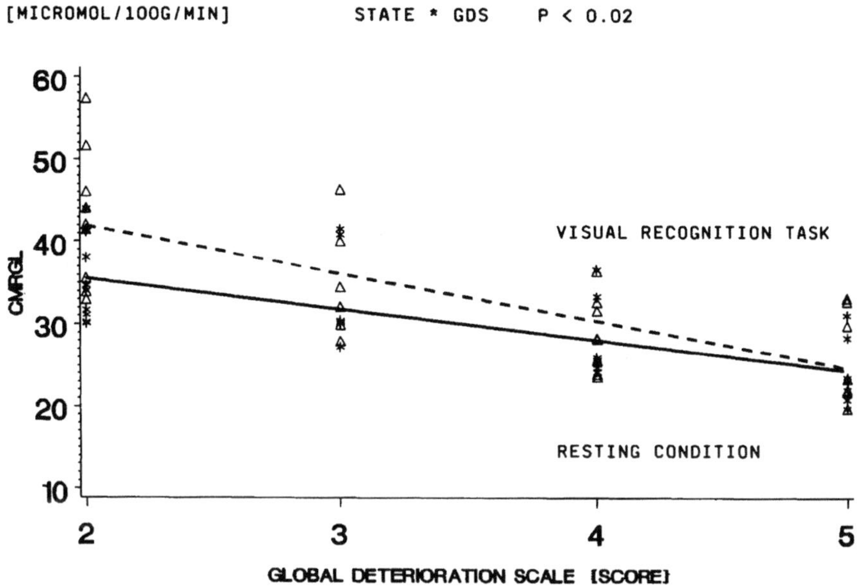

Fig. 9. Relationship between CMRgl of the temporoparietal cortex and GDS score in 30 patients with possible or probable Alzheimer's disease. *Asterisks* indicate individual resting values, *open triangles* the respective measurements during continous visual recognition. Note the significant difference in linear regression slopes

other methodology can provide, others may require only a single measure whose diagnostic value can be improved by distinct stimulation. PET activation paradigms essentially can serve several purposes: They enhance the contrast between dysfunctional areas and normal brain (e.g., in focal epilepsy), they provide an estimate of neuronal recruitment in brain regions where functional impairment is suspected (e.g., in ischemic stroke, angiomas, and Alzheimer's disease), or they elucidate individual networks for the associative processing of neuropsychological tasks (e.g., in aphasia, before, and after resective neurosurgery). The findings of activation studies described in this chapter clearly demonstrate their well-established role in clinical neurology.

References

Baron JC (1987) Ischemic stroke studied by ^{15}O-labeled compounds: misery perfusion and luxury perfusion. In: Heiss WD, Pawlik G, Herholz K, Wienhard K (eds) Clinical efficacy of positron emission tomography. Nijhoff, Dordrecht, pp 15–23

DeKosky ST, Scheff SW (1990) Synapse loss in frontal cortex biopsies in Alzheimer's disease: correlation with cognitive severity. Ann Neurol 27:457–464

DiChiro G (1986) Positron emission tomography using (^{18}F) fluorodeoxyglucose in brain tumors. A powerful diagnostic and prognostic tool. Invest Radiol 22:360–371

Engel J Jr (1989) Seizures and epilepsy. Davis, Philadelphia

Engel J Jr, Henry TR, Risinger MW, Mazziotta JC, Sutherling WW, Levesque MF, Phelps ME (1990) Presurgical evaluation for partial epilepsy: relative contributions of chronic depth-electrode recordings versus FDG-PET and scalp-sphenoidal ictal EEG. Neurology 40:1679–1677

Eriksson L, Bohm C, Kesselberg M, Blomqvist G, Litton J, Widén L, Bergström M, Ericson K, Greitz T (1982) A four ring positron camera system for emission tomography of the brain. IEEE Trans Nucl Sci [New Series] 29:539–543

Feeney DM, Baron JC (1986) Diaschisis. Stroke 17:817–830

Gibbs JM, Wise RJS, Leenders KL, Jones T (1984) Evaluation of cerebral perfusion reserve in patients with carotid-artery occlusion. Lancet 1:310–314

Heiss WD, Pawlik G, Herholz K, Wagner R, Göldner H, Wienhard K (1984) Regional kinetic constants and CMR_{glu} in normal human volunteers determined by dynamic positron emission tomography of (^{18}F)-2-fluoro-2-deoxy-D-glucose. J Cereb Blood Flow Metab 4:212–223

Heiss WD, Herholz K, Pawlik G, Hebold I, Klinkhammer P, Szelies B (1989) PET findings in dementia disorders. Contributions to differential diagnosis and objectivizing of therapeutic effects. Keio J Med 38:111–135

Herholz K, Pawlik G, Wienhard K, Heiss WD (1985) Computer assisted mapping in quantitative analysis of cerebral positron emission tomograms. J Comput Assist Tomogr 9:154–161

McKhann G, Drachman D, Folstein M, Katzman R, Price D, Stadlan EM (1984) Clinical diagnosis of Alzheimer's disease. Neurology (NY) 34:939–944

Mies G, Auer LM, Ebhardt G, Traupe H, Heiss WD (1983) Flow and neuronal density in tissue surrounding chronic infarction. Stroke 14:22–27

Mintun MA, Raichle ME, Martin WRW, Herscovitch P (1984) Brain oxygen utilization measured with 0–15 radiotracers and positron emission tomography. J Nucl Med 25:177–187

Pawlik G, Heiss WD (1989) Positron emission tomography and neuropsychological function. In: Bigler E, Yeo RA, Turkheimer E (eds) Neuropsychological function and brain imaging. Plenum, New York, pp 65–138

Pawlik G, Herholz K, Beil C, Wagner R, Wienhard K, Heiss WD (1985) Remote effects of focal lesions on cerebral blood flow and metabolism. In: Heiss WD (ed) Functional mapping of the brain in vascular disorders. Springer, Berlin Heidelberg New York, pp 59–84

Pawlik G, Herholz K, Wienhard K, Beil C, Heiss WD (1986) Some maximum likelihood methods useful for the regional analysis of dynamic PET data on brain glucose metabolism. In: Bacharach SL (ed) Information processing in medical imaging. Nijhoff, Dordrecht, pp 298–310

Pawlik G, Heiss WD, Beil C, Grünewald G, Herholz K, Wienhard K, Wagner R (1987) Three-dimensional patterns of speech-induced cerebral and cerebellar activation in healthy volunteers and in aphasic stroke patients studied by positron emission tomography of 2(^{18}F)-fluorodeoxyglucose. In: Meyer JS, Lechner H, Reivich M, Ott EO (eds) Cerebral vascular disease 6. Excerpta Medica, Amsterdam, pp 207–210

Phelps ME, Mazziotta JC, Huang SC (1982) Study of cerebral function with positron emission tomography. J Cereb Blood Flow Metab 2:113–162

Powers WJ, Tempel LW, Grubb RL Jr (1989) Influence of cerebral hemodynamics on stroke risk: one-year follow-up of 30 medically treated patients. Ann Neurol 25:325–330

Reisberg B, Ferris SH, DeLeon MJ, Crook T (1982) The global deterioration scale for assessment of primary degenerative dementia. Am J Psychiatry 139:1136–1139

Tyler JL, Leblanc R, Meyer E, Dagher A, Yamamoto YL, Diksic M, Hakim A (1989) Hemodynamic and metabolic effects of cerebral arteriovenous malformations studied by positron emission tomography. Stroke 20:890–898

Wienhard K, Pawlik G, Herholz K, Wagner R, Heiss WD (1985) Estimation of local cerebral utilization by positron emission tomography of (^{18}F)-2-fluoro-2-deoxy-D-glucose: a critical appraisal of optimization procedures. J Cereb Blood Flow Metab 5:115–125

Chapter 3
Stimulation of Cerebral Blood Flow

Chapter 5

Methods for Manipulation of Regional Brain Perfusion, Intracranial Artery Diameter, and Cerebral Blood Volume

L. FRIBERG

Introduction

A number of basically different methods are used to study the human cerebral circulation. No single method can reveal a complete picture of all the intracranial vascular changes and mechanisms which can be induced by physiological or pharmacological stimulation. In that sense each set of findings is linked to the method used.

This chapter will consider some advantages and limitations of the transcranial Doppler technique and methods for measuring regional cerebral blood flow (rCBF) and cerebral blood volume (CBV). Furthermore, some recent results from the application of these methods – alone and in combination – will be reported.

Examination Techniques: What Are We Looking At?

Although all parts of the intracranial vascular system normally work synergistically to facilitate ample blood supply to the brain tissue, there are partly segregated mechanisms regulating different sections of the vascular bed. Each of the clinically accessible examination techniques focuses on one vascular section. The most common methods (Table 1) are of two main categories: (a) those recording signals from the

Table 1. Methods for cerebrovascular studies in man

Methods	Measures	Vessels	Timing
Angiography	Distribution and configuration of vessels	Arteries, veins	(1 sec.)
Transcranial Doppler, TCD	Blood velocity (not flow)	Large arteries	(1 sec.)
CBV (SPECT)	Relative changes	Veins	(10 sec.)
Intraarterial rCBF method	Fast rCBF components, mainly cortical rCBF	Tissue perfusion	(40 sec.)
Stationary detectors	Mixed cortical, white matter and extracranial	Tissue perfusion	(11 min.)
SPECT	Separated cortical and white matter rCBF	Tissue perfusion	(2–4 min.)
PET	rCBF, glucose, and oxygen metabolism	Tissue perfusion Tissue metabolism	(1–3 min.) (45 min.)

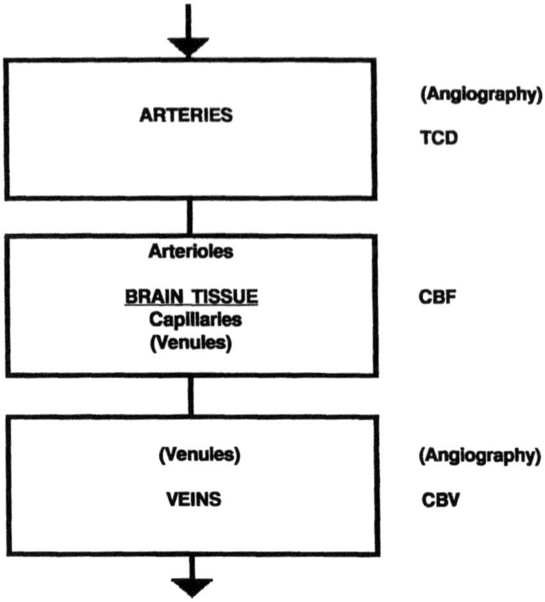

Fig. 1. Vascular sections of the intracranial circulation accessible with different clinical methods

conductance vessels, i.e., the arteries and veins, and (b) those measuring tissue perfusion controlled by the resistance vessels, i.e., the arterioles.

The most common clinically routine examination techniques are cerebral angiography, CBF and CBV measurements most often performed with single photon emission computerized tomography (SPECT), and transcranial Doppler (TCD) sonography. From measured changes in one vascular section one can attempt to make qualified estimates of changes in connected sections (Fig. 1).

Angiography

Although cerebral angiography is still the routine examination that reveals the site and extension of pathological changes of the larger vessels, it only gives sparse information about the resulting hemodynamic changes – if any. Normally a reduction of the diameter of the larger arteries has to exceed 75% before brain tissue flow is affected.

Transcranial Doppler Sonography

With the TCD technique it is possible to monitor the blood velocity (distance/time)in the large intracranial arteries (Aaslid 1986). The methods offers a high temporal resolution, but used as the sole technique it can *not* provide information about absolute flow rate (volume/time) in the intracranial arteries as information about the arterial diameter is not accessible. However, if TCD recordings are combined with simultaneous quantified rCBF measurements of flow in the suppy territories of the studied artery (e.g., the middle cerebral artery, MCA), it is possible to estimate relative changes in the diameter of the large supplying artery (Friberg 1989).

Regional Cerebral Blood Flow

Blood flow tracers for rCBF techniques all diffuse from vessels into brain tissue and therefore actually indicate tissue perfusion. Depending on the type of flow tracer, CBF is measured during tracer uptake, as the amount of retained tracer, or during clearance of tracer.

Using xenon-133 and a stationary detector system for determination of regional CBF can cause some problems when interpreting the results (Obrist and Wilkinson 1990). The detectors "look through" several extra- and intracranial compartments, and blood flow changes in one compartment (e.g., temporal muscle) can affect the calculation of blood flow in another compartment (e.g., cerebral cortex) even though the blood flow in the latter compartment is unchanged (Friberg et al., 1986). If rCBF is reduced in a part of one hemisphere, the "look through phenomenon" causes considerable detection of isotope clearance from the contralateral hemisphere (Bolmsjö 1984). However, the stationary detector method is very suitable for detection of global CBF changes (taking mean values from all detectors), e.g., when studying effects of pharmaceutical compounds on the brain tissue perfusion.

Due to its tomographic characteristics, the SPECT technique can provide a fairly good separation between the different kinetic compartments. This enables differentiation between tracer clearance from gray and white matter and extracranial structures to be excluded. SPECT visualizes the rCBF patterns in several transversal slice levels with a spatial resolution of about 10–13 mm in the plane. rCBF can be quantified when using a fast rotating multihead SPECT system and xenon-133 inhalation or i.v. injection. The 4-min measurements can be repeated many times in the same subject at 20- to 30-min intervals. This provides good possibilities for studying *induced* changes in rCBF.

Recently another type of blood flow tracer has been introduced for clinical application with SPECT; the technetium-99m-labeled retained blood flow tracer. After intravenous injection the lipophilic form of the tracer ^{99m}Tc-hexamethyl-propyleramine oxim (HMPAO) is distributed like the blood flow, is taken up by the brain tissue, and is converted intracellularly to a nondiffusible hydrophilic substance, all within 2 min of the injection (Neirinckx et al 1988). This tracer type makes it possible to obtain a "frozen" rCBF picture. The actual SPECT scanning can take place several hours after the injection. The SPECT recording will still represent the rCBF distribution at the time of injection. However, there are certain drawbacks associated with retained tracer rCBF recordings. It is not possible to quantify absolutely rCBF (blood volume/tissue weight/time), but it is possible to perform semiquantitative rCBF calculations (Andersen et al. 1988; Lassen et al. 1988). Furthermore, as the tracer is fixed within the brain and the amount of radiation only declines with the physical decay of the isotope (^{99m}Tc, $T_{1/2}$=6 h, it is difficult to perform multiple repeated measurements during the course of a treatment.

Recently, however, a method with *two* separate ^{99m}Tc-HMPAO injections and SPECT scannings was used successfully with less than an hour's interval between the injections (Rubin et al. 1991). In clinical investigations this means that it is possible to carry out one more rCBF examination to evaluate the development of this disease or the effect of the treatment. In patients initially studied with ^{99m}Tc-HMPAO it is also possible to perform close follow-up examinations with subsequent ^{133}Xe (81 keV) and ^{99m}Tc (140 keV). It is even possible to perform simultaneous detection of both radionuclides (Holm et al. 1990).

Cerebral Blood Volume

After labeling erythrocytes with ^{99m}Tc (Kelbaek 1986), it is possible with SPECT to carry out continuous relative measurements of the intravascular blood content of the brain vessels. About 80% of the blood is in the veins and only about 7% is in the capillaries; the CBV recordings reflect mainly venous changes.

Induced Intracranial Hemodynamic Changes

In principle it is possible to alter rCBF in two ways in the normal brain:

1. Neuronal activity can be provoked by sensory stimulation or by letting the subject internally activate brain regions related to the "brain work" task. This is the genuine kind of physiological or functional activation test which normally results in activation of several regions; a pattern of focal CBF changes. In the normal brain there is a close coupling between regional oxygen metabolism and rCBF (Raichle et al. 1976; Lebrun-Grandié et al. 1983; Roland et al. 1987). Therefore, changes in rCBF reflect changes in regional neuronal activity and the rCBF methods can be used in functional mapping of the human brain (Friberg and Roland 1988; Lassen et al. 1991).
2. The second method of altering rCBF in the normal brain is to manipulate rCBF pharmacologically, either by administering drugs possessing direct vascular effects or by giving drugs which primarily affect the neuronal activity, resulting secondarily in rCBF changes. This type of test should not be referred to as "activation," but should preferably be termed *pharmacological manipulation,* as it does not directly involve brain-work.

Physiological Activation

The rCBF methods have provided opportunities to perform physiological activation studies of the working human brain. To some extent it has been possible to explore the organization of smaller cortical regions participating in brain work. The most interesting, but also the most difficult, studies to perform are the activation studies of higher cortical functions unique to the human race: language functions and thinking.

The cortical activation patterns seen during language processing and speech show that higher cortical functions unique to man have many participating cortical fields localized within the uncommitted cortex, i.e., cortex not predetermined to handle primary sensory and motor functions. Although language is generally considered to be a lateralized function, the general picture is that of bilateral activation of many symmetrically located regions, but with a left-sided preponderance of the rCBF responses (Friberg and Roland 1988). Activation studies by way of sensory stimulation have shown that the subject's profound attention toward the incoming stimulus is very influential on the degree of cerebral activation, which has been termed "tuning" of cortex (Roland 1981).

Pure intrinsic brain work can increase rCBF by 15%–30% in large regions in the frontal and parietal lobes, resulting in up to 11%–14% increases in global CBF (Roland and Friberg 1985). At the other end of the normal physiological scale, deep sleep (stages III, IV) causes a global CBF decrease of 15%–30% (Madsen et al. 1990a). During rapid eye movement sleep (REM) there is no significant global CBF change compared with the awake resting condition although there is a distinct frontal to posterior redistribution of rCBF (Madsen et al. 1991a, b).

Even with the TCD technique it is possible to see marked fluctuations of velocity in one posterior cerebral artery synchronous with presentation of visual stimuli (Conrad and Klingelhöfer 1989). Assuming that the large artery caliber was unchanged during this stimulation procedure, the velocity alterations reflected changes in brain tissue perfusion.

These fairly large rCBF responses that physiological activation (e.g., intrinsic brain work or verbalization) can cause should be kept in mind whenever rCBF pictures are evaluated for clinical reasons.

Pharmacological Manipulation

Only during extreme conditions is CBF subject to changes in the systemic circulation, also those induced systemically by pharmaceutical compounds. This is due to the extraordinarily powerful autoregulatory capability of the brain on the level of the arterioles. However, some drugs given in appropriate doses exert a local effect on the cerebral arteriolar tone and can induce pronounced changes in global CBF.

Indirect Pharmacological Manipulation

Indirect pharmacological manipulation of CBF in man is almost exclusively performed by administering drugs with the ability to inhibit neuronal activity or transmission. This reduces the metabolism of the nervous tissue, secondarily causing a CBF reduction. Of course it also provokes development of neurological symptoms. Drugs like barbiturates, benzodiazepines, and other anesthesiological compounds have the ability to cause indirect CBF reduction. During complete inhibition the normal resting rCBF pattern of hyperfrontality disappears and there is a uniform global CBF reduction down to values around 25–30 ml/ 100 g per minute (Roland and Friberg 1988). This might therefore be considered the "true" resting CBF level for supplying healthy but inactive gray matter tissue. Indirectly induced CBF reduction is seen during the performance of a Wada-test. Unilateral intracarotid injection of 200 mg amybarbital promptly causes flattening of EEG, contralateral hemiparesis, and a CBF decrease of >50% with a delay of 25–30 s, a time interval which represents the actual "metabolic delay" of the vascular response.

Direct Pharmacological Manipulation

Acetazolamide increases CBF by 60% by dilating the resistance vessels (Vorstrup et al. 1984). The acetazolamide (Diamox) test is now a clinical routine procedure for determination of local feeding capacity in many patients with cerebrovascular diseases. The direct manipulation of CBF does not affect cerebral function in normal man and is therefore not normally associated with development of neurological symptoms.

Cerebral Blood Flow During Prolonged Pharmacological Treatment

Prolonged oral treatment with a 1-g daily acetazolamide dose caused an acute CBF increase of 40%, but CBFs were quickly adapted and after two days the CBF had

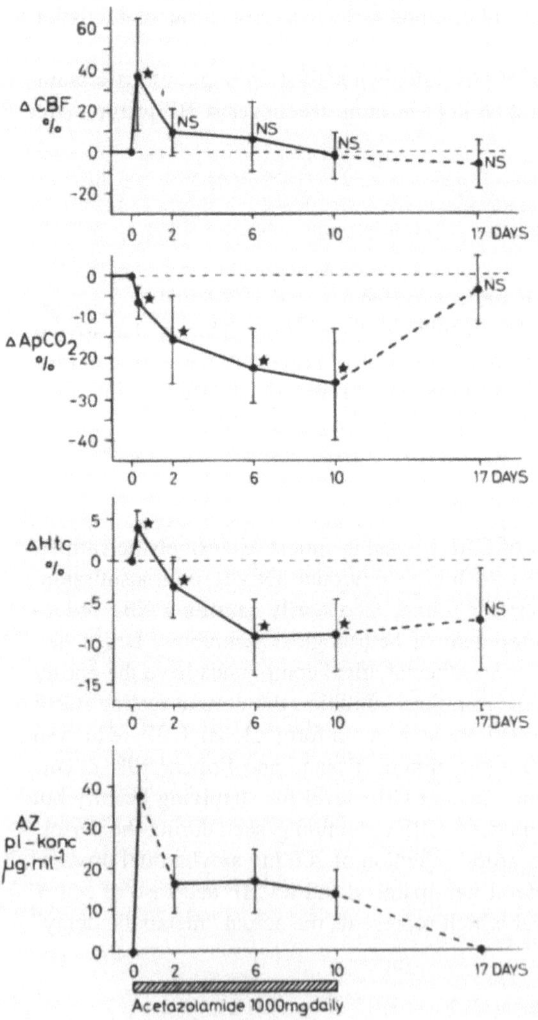

Fig. 2. Mean changes in CBF alveolar carbon droxile (A pCO_2), hematocrit *(Hct)* in percentage of the control values from eight subjects. Bottom, Mean plasma concentrations of acetazolamide *(AZ)*. *Bars* indicate SD. Statistically significant, $p<0.05$; *NS*, not significant, , $p>0.05$. (From Friberg et al. 1990, with permission)

Table 2. Suggested effects of acute and prolonged acetazolamide treatment on H^+ concentration and physiological effects shown in a schematic form. (From Friberg et al. 1990, with permission)

	Changes in brain [H^+]			Physiological effects		
	Arterial	Extra cellular	Intra-cellular	Arterial PCO_2	CBF	Venti-lation
Short-term	→	↑↑	→	→	↑↑	→
Day 2	→	→	↑	↓	→	↑
Day 10	→	→	↑↑	↓↓	→	↑↑

→ = unchanged
↑ and ↑↑ = slight and pronounced increase
↓ and ↓↓ = slight and pronounced decrease

returned to control values where it remained for the next 8 days of treatment (Friberg et al. 1990). Over the same period acetazolamide gradually induced mild hyperventilation, and after 10 days $PaCO_2$ was reduced down to 70% of the control value (Fig. 2). As illustrated in Table 2 it has been suggested that short-term administration of acetazolamide causes slight extracelluar acidosis in the brain, inducing arteriolar dilatation. The normalization of CBF but gradually decreasing $PaCO_2$ during continued treatment suggests normalization of extracelluar pH, but a decrease in intracellular pH, causing an increased ventilatory drive (Friberg et al. 1990).

Intravenous injection of theophylline causes an immediate 10%–30% decrease in CBF, but during subsequent prolonged oral treatment with sustained release theophylline (10 mg/kg daily) CBF gradually returned to control values (Jensen et al. 1987). Also theophylline gradually induced slight hypoventilation and after 17 days $PaCO_2$ was reduced to about 90% of the control value. The CBF seems to adapt fairly quickly to the changes induced by short-term administration of acetazolamide and theophylline. However, preliminary results from a recent study of the prolonged effect of indomethacin seem to indicate that the marked (down to 50%) CBF decrease can be sustained by i.v. infusion or repeated i.v. injections (Jensen et al., unpublished results). This principle of treatment might be applicable in acute neurosurgical patients with head trauma, where CBF (and CBV, see below) might be reduced in the awake patient, which are presently treated with sedation and artificial hyperventilation in order to obtain the same CBF/CBV effect on the brain.

Combination of TCD, CBF, and CBV Measurements

With modern SPECT equipment, it is possible to perform dual isotope scanning (Holm et al. 1990). In this way rCBV (^{99m}Tc) and rCBF (^{133}Xe) can be measured simultaneously. At the same time one or two small TCD probes can be fixated to the head without causing interference with the SPECT equipment. By using this setup one can obtain simultaneous information from all parts of the intracranial vascular system as illustrated in Fig. 1. With this method we have found that a short-term acetazolamide-induced rCBF increase of 40% is associated with a CBV increase of 30% in the MCA supply territories. Indomethacin reduced MCA rCBF by 40% and MCA rCBV by 15%. The velocity in the MCA changed in proportion to the rCBF changes.

During experimental nitroglycerin-induced headache, Iversen et al. (1989) simultaneously recorded rCBF velocity in the MCA and CBV. Nitroglycerin did not affect rCBF in the MCA supply territory when the induced headache occured, CBV increased and but there was a significant 20% decrease in blood velocity in the corresponding MCA which is in the order of magnitude also found by Dahl et al. (1989). The lack of rCBF change but decrease in velocity indicates that the headache under these circumstances was related to large artery dilatation and that this might explain some of the migraine mechanisms (Friberg 1991). In a very recent report on combined rCBF and TCD measurements in migraine patients, it has actually been confirmed that unilateral migraine pain is associated with large artery dilatation on the headache side (Friberg et al. 1991).

References

Aaslid R (1986) Transcranial Doppler sonography. Springer, Berlin Heidelberg New York

Andersen AR, Friberg HH, Schmidt JF, Hasselbalch SG (1988) Quantitative measurements of cerebral blood flow using SPECT and 99m-T*c-d, l*-Hm-PAO compared to xenon-133. J Cereb Blood Flow Metab 8:S69–S81

Bolmsjö MS (1984) Hemisphere cross talk and signal overlapping in bilateral regional cerebral blood flow measurements using Xe-133. Eur J Nucl Med 9:1–5

Conrad B, Klingelhöfer J (1989) Dynamics of regional cerebral blood flow for various visual stimuli. Exp Brain Res 77:437–441

Dahl A, Rassel D, Nyberg-Hansen R, Rootwelt K (1989) Effect of nitroglycerine on cerebral circulation measured by transcranial Doppler and SPECT blood flow studies. Stroke 20:1733–1736

Friberg L (1989) Effects of a new 5-HT1-like receptor agonist, GR43175, on the regional brain tissue perfusion and intra-cerebral artery tone regulation in healthy volunteers. Cephalalgia [Suppl 10] 9:359–360

Friberg L (1991) Cerebral blood flow changes in migraine: methods, observations and hypothesis. J Neurol 238:S12–S17

Friberg L, Roland PE (1988) Functional activation and inhibition of regional cerebral blood flow and metabolism. In: Olesen J, Edvinsson L (eds) Basic mechanisms of headache. Elsevier, Amsterdam, pp 89–98

Friberg L, Kastrup J, Hansen M, Bülow J (1986) Cerebral effects of scalp cooling and extracerebral contribution to calculated blood flow values using the intravenous 133-Xe technique. Scand J Clin Lab Invest 46:375–379

Friberg L, Kastrup J, Rizzi D, Jensen JB, Lassen NA (1990 Cerebral blood flow and end tidal pCO2 during prolonged acetazolamide treatment in man. Am J Physiol H954–H959

Friberg L, Olesen J, Iversen H, Sperling B (1991) Migraine pain associated with middle cerebral artery dilatation: reversal by sumatriptan. Lancet 338:13–17

Holm S, Friberg L, Iversen HK, Lassen NA (1990) Dual energy brain SPECT – methods and applications. In: Schmidt HAE, Chambron J (eds) Nuclear medicine: quantiative analysis in imaging and function. Schattauer, Stuttgart, pp 11–13

Iversen HK, Holm S, Friberg L (1989) Intracranial hemodynamics during intravenous nitroglycerine infusion. Cephalalgia [Suppl 10] 9:84–85

Jensen JB, Friberg L, Chiara SD, Lassen NA (1987) Changes in CBF during acute and prolonged administration of theophylline. J Cereb Blood Flow Metab [Suppl 1] 7:S276

Kelbaek H (1986) Technetium-99m labeling of red blood cells: in vitro evaluation of a new approach. J Nucl Med 27:1770–1773

Lassen NA, Andersen AR, Friberg L, Paulson OB (1988) The retention of [99mTc]-d, l-HMPAO in the human brain after intracarotid bolus injection: a kinetic analysis. J Cereb Blood Flow Metab 8.S13–S22

Lassen NA, Ingvar DH, Raichle ME, Friberg L (eds) (1991) Brain work and mental activity: Quantitative studies with radioactive tracers. Munksgaard, Copenhagen, pp 1–443.

Lebrun-Grandil'e P, Baron J-C, Soussaline F, Loch'h C, Sastre J, Bousser M-G (1983) Coupling between regional cerebral blood flow and oxygen utilization in the normal human brain. Arch Neurol 40:230–236

Madsen PL, Schmidts JF, Wildschiødtz G, Friberg L, Holm S, Vorstrup S, Lassen NA (1991a) Cerebral O2 metabolism and cerebral blood flow in humans during deep and rapid eye movement sleep. J Appl Physiol 70:2597–2601

Madsen PL, Holm S, Vorstrup S, Friberg L, Lassen NA, Wildschiødtz G (1991b) Human regional cerebral blood flow during rapid eye movement sleep 7 Cereb Blood Flow Metab II:502–507

Neirinckx RD, Burke JF, Harrison RC, Forster AM, Andersen AR, Lassen NA (1988) The retention mechanism of technetium-99m-HM-PAO: intracellular reaction with glutathione. J Cereb Blood Flow Metab 8:S4–S12

Obrist WD, Wilkinson WE (1990) Regional cerebral blood flow measurement in humans by Xenon-133 clearance. Cerebrovasc brain Metab Rev 2:283–327

Raichle ME, Grubb RL, Gado MH, Eichling JO, Ter-Pogossian MM (1976) Correlation between regional cerebral blood flow and oxidative metabolism. Arch Neurol 33:523–526

Roland PE (1981) Somatotopic tuning of the postcentral gyrus during focal attention in man. A regional cerebral blood flow study. J Neurophysiol 46:744–754

Roland PE, Friberg L (1985) Localization of cortical areas activated by thinking. J Neurophysiol 53:1219–1243

Roland PE, Friberg L (1988) The effect of the GABA-A agonist THIP on regional cortical blood flow in humans. A new test of hemispheric dominance. J Cereb Blood Flow Metab 8:314–323

Roland PE, Eriksson L, Stone-Elander S, Widen L (1987) Does mental activity change oxidative metabolism of the brain? J Neurosci 7:2373

Rubin P, Holm S, Friberg L, Videbaek P, Andersen HS, Bjerg-Bentsen B, Strømsø N, Larsen JK, Lassen NA, Hemmingsen R (1991) Altered modulation of prefrontal and subcortical brain activity in newly diagnosed schizophrenia and schizophreniform disorder: a regional cerebral blood flow study. Arch Gen Psychiatr 48: 987–995.

Vorstrup S, Henriksen L, Paulson OB (1984) Effect of acetazolamide on cerebral blood flow and cerebral metabolic rate for oxygen. J Clin Invest 74:1634–1639

Carbon Dioxide and Oxygen Reactivity in Cerebral Circulation

R. VON KUMMER and T. BACK

Introduction

Brain function and tissue integrity are highly dependent on a continuous oxygen (O_2) supply and clearance of carbon dioxide (CO_2). The brain can be affected not only by low flow due to low perfusion pressure, but also by a decrease in arterial oxygen content (aO_2C) or high arterial CO_2 tension. To hold cerebral blood flow (CBF), cerebral O_2 transport rate (the product of CBF and aO_2C), and CO_2 clearance (the ratio $PaCO_2$/CBF) constant, autoregulatory mechanisms of cerebral circulation alter the resistance of cerebral vessels. This occurs within certain limits, described as autoregulatory capacity, vasodilatory capacity, or perfusion reserve.

Since measurement of CBF is possible, it is well known that changes in the arterial tension of O_2 (PaO_2) and carbon dioxide ($PaCO_2$) affect CBF (Gibbs et al. 1935; Kety and Schmidt 1948). However, the quantitative relationship between $PaCO_2$ and CBF has not yet been well described. Moreover, the concept of O_2 reactivity is not widely known. Therefore, it is worthwhile reviewing experimental data on the influence of aO_2C and $PaCO_2$ on CBF.

CO_2 Reactivity

It has often been confirmed that $PaCO_2$ is a prominent factor of circulatory control in the CNS. An increase in $PaCO_2$ produces marked vasodilation of the cerebral vasculature, and a reduction in $PaCO_2$ a profound vasoconstriction. Recently, changes in $PaCO_2$ and transcranial Doppler ultrasound have been used to determine cerebral perfusion reserve (Ringelstein et al. 1988; Widder 1985). To explain the response of CBF to alteration in $PaCO_2$, the mechanism of vasoreaction should be known. First it is necessary to find out what CO_2 reactivity means in quantitative terms. When CO_2 reactivity is defined quantitatively, we can study whether it is uniform or not in the CNS. If the vascular response to changes in $PaCO_2$ is heterogeneous, we will need to know the local conditions which alter CO_2 reactivity.

Quantitation of CO_2 Reactivity

The method of CBF measurement found its first application in a study of the cerebral circulatory effects of altered arterial tensions of CO_2 and O_2. In seven normal young men, Kety and Schmidt (1948) measured an increase in mean CBF from 53 to 93 ml

100 g^{-1} min^{-1}, when mean $PaCO_2$ was elevated from 43 to 52 mmHg. The positive correlation between CBF and $PaCO_2$ values showed an exponential slope: The higher the $PaCO_2$ the steeper the increase in CBF.

Absolute CO_2 Reactivity

Since then various methods have been used to describe the CBF-$PaCO_2$ relationship. Absolute CO_2 reactivity is defined as the absolute change in CBF per change in $PaCO_2$ expressed as ml 100 g^{-1} min^{-1} $mmHg^{-1}$. To determine absolute CO_2 reactivity, CBF has to be measured at least twice at the same site in the same individual under steady state conditions except for variance of $PaCO_2$ (Ackerman et al. 1973; von Kummer 1984). If the global CBF of different individuals is correlated with the corresponding $PaCO_2$, the slope of the regression line will hardly define CO_2 reactivity quantitatively, because CBF may be influenced by other conditions than $PaCO_2$. This may explain the somewhat contradictory findings in studies where the slope of the regression line was found to be exponential (Kety and Schmidt 1948; Olesen et al. 1971; Tominagon et al. 1974; Waltz 1970) as well as linear (Alexander et al. 1964, Grubb et al. 1974; Reivich 1964) when $PaCO_2$ was altered within 20–80 mmHg. Absolute CO_2 reactivity varied in the series of Kety and Schmidt (1948) between 2.1 and 8.7 ml 100 g^{-1} min^{-1} $mmHg^{-1}$ with a mean of 4.58±1.96 ml 100 g^{-1} min^{-1} $mmHg^{-1}$. Alexander et al. (1984) defined the CBF to $PaCO_2$ relationship in man by the expression CBF=1.37 $PaCO_2$ – 5.08. Olesen et al. (1971) measured the response of CBF to change in $PaCO_2$ in patients. Recalculation of their data gives an absolute CO_2 reactivity between 0.75 and 4.59 ml 100 g^{-1} min^{-1} $mmHg^{-1}$ (mean: 2.02±1.03 ml 100 g^{-1} min^{-1} $mmHg^{-1}$).

Relative CO_2 Reactivity

According to Harper and Glass (1965), relative CO_2 reactivity is defined as the percentage change in CBF_{40} divided by the $PaCO_2$ difference from 40 mmHg when CBF_{40} is the CBF occurring at a definite $PaCO_2$ of 40 mmHg. Using this definition, Harper and Glass (1965) found a 100% increase in CBF when raising the $PaCO_2$ from 40 to 80 mmHg in dogs under normotensive conditions. This means a relative CO_2 reactivity of 2.5%/mmHg which is in good agreement with the findings of others (Flohr et al. 1969; von Kummer 1984). Without defining the 100% value, the correlation between percentage CBF change and $PaCO_2$ change will give unreliable and noncomparable data (Ackerman et al. 1973). The percentage change of "resting" or "basal" CBF has been reported to be 6% (Tominaga et al. 1974), 4% (Olesen et al. 1971), between 1% and 4% (Ackerman et al. 1973), between 3.4% and 4.5% (Shapiro et al 1965), between 2.6% and 3.9% (Mayer et al. 1980), and between 2% and 3.4% (Symon et al. 1973) per millimeter of mercury change in $PaCO_2$.

Is CO_2 Reactivity Uniform Within the CNS?

To determine local CO_2 reactivity at various sites within the CNS, CBF has to be measured locally and the definition of CO_2 reactivity must be clear. CO_2 reactivity cannot be independently assessed when CBF is calculated from the two-compartmental model of isotope clearance because of a shift into the fast-clearing compartments at low flow rates (Iliff et al. 1974). Symon et al. (1973) determined CO_2 reactivity by local CBF measurement with hydrogen clearance. They did, however, calculate percentage CBF increase in relation to undefined "basal flow." Using the same method of CBF measurement, Fieschi et al. (1969) found CO_2 reactivity to vary between 1.85 and 7.47 ml 100 g^{-1} min^{-1} $mmHg^{-1}$ in the caudate nucleaus of cats. Flohr et al. (1969) studied CO_2 reactivity in various parts of the cat's CNS by means of the [^{131}I]albumin method. They observed considerable differences in absolute CO_2 reactivity, with the lowest value of 0.54 ml 100 g^{-1} min^{-1} $mmHg^{-1}$ in the thoracic cord and the highest of 3.05 ml 100 g^{-1} min^{-1} $mmHg^{-1}$ in the prosencephalon. Our own study of local CO_2 reactivity in the cat's brain revealed differences in absolute CO_2 reactivity between 0.4 and 2.8 ml 100 g^{-1} min^{-1} $mmHg^{-1}$ (von Kummer 1984). Relative CO_2 reactivity, however, was rather uniform at 2.37%±1.70%/mmHg in the cortex, 2.17%±1.30%/mmHg in the caudate nucleus, and 2.64%±1.08%/mmHg in the subcortical white matter (von Kummer 1984). Calculation of the data of Flohr et al. (1969) showed relative CO_2 reactivity between 2.47% and 3.72%/mmHg. Griffiths (1973) measured spinal cord CO_2 reactivity in dogs, finding absolute values between 0.20 and 0.96 ml 100 g^{-1} min^{-1} $mmHg^{-1}$ (mean: 0.39±0.21) and 100% increase in CBF in relation to CBF_{40} when the $PaCO_2$ was raised from 40 to 85 mmHg. That is a relative CO_2 reactivity of 2.22%/mmHg.

Which Local Condition Determines CO_2 Reactivity?

Obviously relative CO_2 reactivity is rather uniform within the CNS. Then, absolute local CO_2 reactivity must be a function of local CBF. Correlating absolute local CO_2 reactivity with local CBF, we found a linear relationship, the equation of the regression line being $y=0.02x+0.22$, and the correlation coefficient being $r=0.71$ ($p<0.01$) (von Kummer 1984).

We conclude from these observations that local CO_2 reactivity is mainly determined by local flow, meaning local CO_2 reactivity is a function of capillary density. Changes in $PaCO_2$ homogeneously affect the vessels of the CNS. The change in local CBF then depends on the perfusion reserve of the local vascular network. This concept fits well with the finding of missing capillary recruitment during hypercapnia (Goebel et al. 1989).

Cerebral O_2 Reactivity

There is experimental evidence to add to the current concepts of CBF regulation the concept of "oxygen reactivity." While CO_2 reactivity represents the second mechanism of the breathing brain, the clearance of metabolic products such as H^+ ions and CO_2, the term "O_2 reactivity" describes a regulatory mechanism maintaining constant oxygen delivery into the brain. It represents the regulation of "cerebral inspiration."

Experimental Evidence

It is a well-known phenomenon that circulation in general is sensitive to changes in the number of oxygenated red cells perfusing a certain tissue volume per time. The O_2 transport rate can be expressed as the product of blood flow and arterial O_2 content. As O_2 availability changes, local blood flow regulation is induced.

In current physiology, two theories are used to explain local adaption of flow: the vasodilator theory and the oxygen demand theory for blood flow control. The first postulates the leak of local vasodilators, preferably adenosine, in conditions of compromised O_2 transport to restore sufficient flow. This theory is mainly based on investigations of coronal heart arteries and was transferred to cerebral circulation (Guyton 1986). A second theory assumes that precapillary sphincter tone is dependent directly on local O_2 availability. With decreasing O_2 concentration, the rate of open precapillary sphincters rises because smooth muscle activity is thought to be a primarily O_2-consuming process (Duling 1977). A change in vascular tone is involved in both theories.

Vasodilation increases CBF. Therefore, CBF measurements can be used to elicit cerebrovascular responses to alterations of arterial blood gases. Shinozuka et al. (1989) demonstrated in rats that local CBF was a function of arterial PaO_2 when $PaCO_2$ was held constant. CBF also increases when oxygen-binding capacity is reduced by exposure to carbon monoxide (Paulson et al. 1973). Viscosity changes withouth an alteration of arterial O_2 content do not markedly influence CBF (Borgström et al. 1975).

Both hypoxia and hypercapnia enhance CBF by vasodilating resistance vessels and/or recruitment of capillary channels. Metzger et al. (1971) tried to differentiate the effects of hypoxia and hypercapnia on local tissue PO_2 (PtO_2) in rats. Short-lasting changes in PaO_2 (reduction) and $PaCO_2$ (increase) via alterations of the respirated gas mixture evoked a fast reaction of PtO_2. In hypoxia the prompt depression of PtO_2 was followed by an overshoot to values above the basic one, when inspiratory O_2 concentration was as low as 3%–5%. With simultaneous application of both hypoxia and hypercapnia for 1 min, the sudden drop in PtO_2 was compensated after 1 min by a vasodilatory response resulting again in an overshoot of the local O_2 concentration (Metzger et al. 1971). Thus, the reactivity of cerebral vessels to hypoxia depends on the depth of hypoxia. Obviously, the time course of the cerebrovascular response is different under hypoxic conditions.

In another series, a short period of hyperoxia was applied. PtO_2 rose mainly in brain areas with initially high PtO_2 values, i.e., at the arterial end of the capillary network. In contrast, initially low PtO_2 values representing the venous capillary site remained unchanged (Metzger et al. 1971). Here, the increase in O_2 content via hyperoxia was already compensated by a vasoconstrictory depression of flow.

In conclusion, cerebral O_2 reactivity is a regulatory mechanism of cerebral vessels being directly triggered by changes in arterial O_2 content. With an arterial O_2 tension below 50 mmHg, progressive vasodilation occurs to maintain constant O_2 transport.

Quantitation of Cerebral O_2 Reactivity

To study the effect of varying arterial O_2 content on cerebral O_2 reactivity, we performed hemodilution in cats (von Kummer et al. 1990). Hemodilution induced a compensatory vasodilation to regulate reduced O_2 content by increasing CBF. With impaired perfusion reserve, lowering arterial O_2 content did not enhance CBF. Then, hemodilution decreased O_2 transport rate to critical levels (von Kummer et al. 1990). This example can be used to determine cerebral O_2 reactivity quantitatively. Absolute O_2 reactivity is defined as the ratio between the inverse absolute changes in CBF and arterial O_2 content. It is expressed as the equation:

Absolute $O_2R = \triangle CBF / \triangle$ art. O_2 content (ml g^{-1} min^{-1})

Relative O_2 reactivity, in consequence, is defined as the ratio between the percentage changes in CBF and arterial O_2 content. This value relates to a basic CBF value measured with normal arterial O_2 content (in cats 16–18 ml/100 ml). In our study, replacement of 20% total blood volume with dextran 40 increased CBF from 46 to 59 ml 100 g^{-1} min^{-1}, and reduced arterial O_2 content from 16.9 to 10.8 ml/100 ml. Absolute O_2 reactivity was calculated to be 2.1 ml/g^{-1} min^{-1}, relative O_2 reactivity being 4.6%. This means that a reduction in arterial O_2 content by 1 ml/100 ml blood results in a CBF increase by 2.1 ml 100 g^{-1} min^{-1}. We demonstrated that with an impaired perfusion reserve O_2 reactivity was abolished (von Kummer et al. 1990).

Pressure Autoregulation, O_2 Autoregulation, and Metabolism

The regulation of constant CBF with varying cerebral perfusion pressure has been well studied. In various clinical situations, such as anemia or pulmonary insufficiency, regulation of constant O_2 transport is vital to compensate alterations of actual cerebral O_2 delivery. Bicher (1974) and Taguchi et al. (1984) termed this phenomenon brain oxygen autoregulation. It could be shown that the range of constant PtO_2 was significantly wider than the limits of pressure autoregulation, indicating that oxygen autoregulation still can be intact when perfusion reserve is exhausted (Taguchi et al. 1984).

The primary underlying mechanism is what we defined as O_2 reactivity. As mediator for the regulation of vascular tone, the local adenosine concentration could be responsible, or local PtO_2 itself as suggested by the O_2 demand theory. The meaning of localized PaO_2-sensitive responses is underlined by the inhomogeneity of the PO_2 field in brain tissue. Cortical PtO_2 in rabbits ranged from 5 to 20 mmHg, revealing sharp differences within small distances (Smith et al. 1977). If it is true that local O_2 utilization promotes local O_2 delivery by mainly passive diffusion mechanisms, the inhomogeneity of the PaO_2 represents actual metabolic activity. Yet, it is unclear whether this inhomogeneity of PtO_2 is paralleled by that of cerebral O_2 reactivity.

Clinical Relevance of O_2 Reactivity

Oxygen reactivity is, in a physiological sense, a protective reflex to hypoxia and hyperoxia originating from various causes. The condition of hyperoxia is of clinical significance in pediatrics: retrolental fibroplasia is a typical complication of hyperoxic treatment (Silverman 1977). Tissue hypoxia following cerebral ischemia certainly is the more frequent condition that O_2 reactivity is involved in. Pressure autoregulation and CO_2 reactivity are severely disturbed in ischemic tissue. In the surrounding tissue, called penumbra, electrical function is impaired, but morphological integrity is preserved (Astrup et al. 1981).

In penumbral zones, flow is reduced, autoregulation abolished, but CO_2 reactivity can be partially preserved (Nakagawa et al. 1981; Symon et al. 1975). Ross Russell et al. (1970) demonstrated that in focal ischemic tissue the area with ebolished pressure autoregulation is larger than that with impaired CO_2 reactivity. It will be of great importance to know whether O_2 reactivity is at least partially intact in the penumbra where CBF can be enhanced by hypercapnia. Following MCA occlusion, the extracerebral proximal vessel resistance is elevated, but pial arterial pressure falls (Date et al 1984). In this situation, the vasoreactivity of the collaterals is of great relevance for the outcome and perfusion of ischemic tissue. The impairment of O_2 utilization correlates better with the final extent of tissue necrosis than the decrease in CBF (Baron et al. 1984), which could indicate that O_2 reactivity is at least partially preserved in low-flow regions, compensating decreased O_2 delivery.

When perfusion reserve (autoregulatory capacity) is exhausted, oxygen reserve is still present as long as O_2 extraction is not complete. Local acidosis (e.g., lactate) increases O_2 extraction (Bohr effect), and increases cerebral vasodilation to a higher extent than pressure autoregulation can increase vessel diameter (Date et al. 1984).

Conclusions

Oxygen reactivity is a measure of the regulatory ability of "cerebral inspiration." We can differentiate O_2 reactivity from CO_2 reactivity and pressure autoregulation: Pressure autoregulation of CBF is a mainly myogenic, generalized response of extra- and intracerebral vessels to alterations in intraluminal pressure (Hossmann 1989). CO_2 reactivity takes place at the distal precapillary vascular segment (resistance vessels), reflecting the clearance function of brain metabolism. Cerebral O_2 reactivity serves as a regulatory mechanism, also being located in the parenchymal vascular segment.

The function of cerebral O_2 reactivity can be demonstraded best in pathophysiological situations when CBF does not reflect actual O_2 transport into the brain: (a) In anemic disease or iatrogenic anemia (e.g., infusion therapy, hemodilution) CBF is high, but O_2 content is diminished. (b) In polycythemia or exsiccosis CBF is low, but Hc and O_2 content elevated. (c) In early phases of ischemic stroke CBF is uncoupled from metabolism. Here, we need further experimental studies to define the functional role of cerebral O_2 reactivity in stroke.

It is well known that hematocrit as well as O_2 transport rate is a function of vessel diameter. The capillary to systemic hematocrit ratio seems to be a dynamic parameter which can change under pathophysiological conditions (Todd et al. 1991). Therefore, it is difficult to predict what will happen to local cerebral O_2 delivery and reactivity in cerebrovascular disease. Further investigations are needed to establish the full meaning of this mechanism which regulates constant O_2 supply and sufficient CO_2 release in brain.

References

Ackermann RH, Zilkha E, Bull JWD, Du Boulay GH, Marshall J, Ross Russel RW, Symon L (1973) The relationship of the CO_2-reactivity of cerebral vessels to blood pressure and mean resting blood flow. Neurology (Minneap) 23:21–26

Alexander SC, Wollman H, Cohen PJ, Chase PE, Behar M (1964) Cerebrovascular response to $PaCO_2$ during halothane anesthesia in man. J Appl Physiol 19:561–565

Astrup JB, Siesjö B, Symon L (1981) Thresholds in cerebral ischemia – the ischemic penumbra. Stroke 12:723–725

Baron JC, Rougemont MG, Soussaline F, Bustany P, Crouzel C, Bousser MG, Comar D (1984) Local interrelationships of cerebral oxygen consumption and glucose utilization in normal subjects and in ischemic stroke patients: a positron tomography study. J Cereb Blood Flow Metab 4:140–149

Bicher HI (1974) Brain oxygen autoregulation: a protective reflex to hypoxia? Microvasc Res 8:291–313

Borgström L, Johannsson H, Siesjö BK (1975) The influence of acute normovolemic anemia on cerebral blood flow and oxygen consumption of anesthetized rats. Acta Physiol Scand 93:505–514

Date H, Hossmann KA, Shima T (1984) Effect of middle cerebral artery compression on pial artery pressure, blood flow, and electrophysiological function of cerebral cortex of cats. J Cereb Blood Flow Metab 4:593–598

Duling B (1977) Oxygen, metabolism, and microcirculatory regulation. In: Kaley G, Altura BM (eds) Microcirculation; vol. 2. University Park Press, Baltimore, p 176

Fieschi C, Bozzao L, Agnoli A, Nardini M, Bartolini A (1969) The hydrogen method of measuring local blood flow in subcortical structures of the brain: including a comparative study with the 14-antipyrin method. Exp Brain Res 7:111–119

Flohr HW, Brock M, Christ R, Heipertz R, Pöll W (1969) Arterial PCO_2 and blood flow in different parts of the central nervous system of the anesthetized rat. In. Brock M, Fieschi C, Ingvar DH (eds) Cerebral blood flow. Springer, Berlin Heidelberg New York, pp 86–88

Gibbs FA, Gibbs EL, Lennox WG (1935) Changes in human cerebral blood flow consequent on alterations in blood gases. Am J Physiol 111:557–563

Göbel U, Klein B, Schröck H, Kuschinsky W (1989) Lack of capillary recruitment in the brains of awake rats during hypercapnia. J Cereb Blood Flow Metab 9:491–499

Griffiths JR (1973) Spinal cord flow in dogs: the effect of blood gases. J Neurol Neurosurg Psychiatry 36:42–49

Grubb RL, Raichle ME, Eichling JO, Ter-Pergossian MM (1974) The effects in changes in $PaCO_2$ on cerebral blood volume, blood flow, and vascular mean transit time. Stroke 5:630–639

Guyton AC (1986) Textbook of medical physiology. Saunders, Philadelphia, pp 232–234

Harper AM, Glass HJ (1965) Effects of alteration in the arterial carbon dioxide tension on the blood flow through the cerebral cortex at normal and low arterial blood pressure. J Neurol Neurosurg Psychiatry 28:449–452

Hossmann KA (1989) Pathophysiology of cerebral infarction. In: Vinken PJ, Bruyn GW, Klawans HC (eds) Handbook of clinical neurology, vol 6. Elsevier/North-Holland, Amsterdam, p 114

Iliff LD, Zilkha E, DuBoulay GH, Marshall J, Ross Russell RW, Symon L (1974) Cerebrovascular CO_2 reactivity of the fast and slow clearing compartments. Stroke 5:607–611

Kety SS, Schmidt CF (1948) The effects of altered arterial tensions of carbon dioxide and oxygen on cerebral blood flow and cerebral oxygen consumption of normal young men. J Clin Invest 27:484–492

Metzger H, Erdmann W, Thews G (1971) Effect of short periods hypoxia, hyperoxia, and hypercapnia on brain O_2-supply. J Appl Physiol 31(5):751–759

Meyer JS, Hayman LA, Yamamoto M, Sakai F, Nakajima S (1980) Local CBF measured by CT after stable xenon inhalation. AJNR 1:213–225

Nakagawa Y, Yamamoto YL, Meyer E, Hodge CP, Feindel W (1981) Effects of hypercapnia on enhancement of decreased perfusion flow in non-infarcted brain tissues. Stroke 12(1):85–92

Olesen J, Paulson OB, Lassen NA (1971) Regional cerebral blood flow in man determined by the initial slope of the clearance of intraarterially injected 133-Xe. Stroke 2:519–540
Paulson OB, Parving HH, Olesen J, Skinhoj E (1973) Influence of carbon monoxide and of hemodilution on cerebral blood flow and blood gases in man. J Appl Physiol 35:111–116
Reivich m (1964) Arterial PCO_2 and cerebral hemodynamics. Am J Physiol 206:25–35
Ringelstein EB, Sievers C, Ecker S, Schneider PA, Otis SM (1988) Noninvasive assessment of CO_2-induced cerebral vasomotor response in normal individuals and patients with internal carotid artery occlusions. Stroke 19:963–969
Ross Russell RW, Simcock JP, Wilkinson MS, Frears CC (1970) The effect of blood pressure changes on the leptomeningeal circulation of the rabbit. Brain 93:491–504
Shapiro W, Wasserman AJ, Patterson JL (1965) Human cerebrovascular response time to elevation of arterial carbon dioxide tension. Arch neurol 13:130–138
Shinozuka T, Nemoto EM, Winter PM (1989) Mechanisms of cerebrovascular O_2-sensitivity from hyperoxia to moderate hypoxia in the rat. J Cereb Blood Flow Metab 9:187–195
Silverman WA (1977) The lesson of retrolental fibroplasia. Sci Am 236(6):100
Smith RH, Guilbeau, Reneau DD (1977) The oxygen tension field within a discrete volume of cerebral cortex. Microvasc Res 13:233–240
Symon L, Pasztor E, Dorsch NWC, Branston NM (1973) Physiologic responses of local areas of the cerebral circulation in experimental primates determined by the method of hydrogen clearance. Stroke 4:632–642
Symon L, Crockard HA, Dorsch NWC, Branston NM, Juhasz J (1975) Local cerebral blood flow and vascular reactivity in a chronic stable stroke in baboons. Stroke 6:482–492
Taguchi Y, Kaminogo M, Austin GM (1984) Autoregulation of cortical blood flow and oxygen tension in the rabbit. Neurol Res 6:159–162
Todd MM, Weeks JB, Warner DS (1991) The effects of hemodilution on the relationships between cerebral blood flow, blood volume, and cerebral tissue hematocrit. J Cereb Blood Flow Metab 11 [Suppl. 2]:S85
Tominaga S, Strandgaard S, Uemura K, Ito K, Kutsuzawa T, Lassen NA, Nakamura T (1974) Cerebrovascular CO_2 reactivity in normotensive and hypertensive man. Stroke 7:507–510
Von Kummer R (1984) Local vascular response to change in carbon dioxide tension. Long term observation in the cat's brain by means of the hydrogen clearance technique. Stroke 15:108–114
Von Kummer R, Back T, Scharf J (1990) Impairment of autoregulatory capacity and the effect of hemodilution on cerebral blood flow and oxygen transport. Stroke [Suppl. 1] 21(8):I126
Waltz AG (1970) Effect of $PaCO_2$ on blood flow and microvasculature of ischemic and nonischemic cerebral cortex. Stroke 1:27–37
Widder B (1985) The CO_2 test for the diagnosis of hemodynamically critical carotid artery stenosis with Doppler sonography. Dtsch Med Wochenschr 110(40):1553

Noninvasive Testing of Vasomotor Reserve*

E. B. Ringelstein

Introduction

Critically reduced *perfusion pressure* in the brain arteries may lead to ischemic damage in certain vulnerable areas (Bogousslavsky and Regli 1986; Leblanc et al. 1987; Ringelstein et al. 1983; Yamaguchi et al. 1979; Zülch 1961). The perfusion pressure of the brain cannot, however, be measured directly in man. *Indirect parameters* are the regional cerebral blood flow (rCBF) versus regional cerebral blood volume (rCBV) ratio (Gibbs et al. 1984), or the oxygen extraction ratio (Gibbs et al. 1984; Kanno et al. 1988; Levine et al. 1988) documented either by SPECT or by PET imaging. Another approach is to measure the reactivity of the cerebral vasculature to vasodilating stimuli (CO_2, acetazolamide). This may be done by measuring an increase in blood flow or blood flow velocity by either rCBF techniques or transcranial Doppler sonography (TCD) (Kanno et al. 1988; Norrving et al. 1982; Ringelstein et al. 1988; Wodarz 1980; see also Dahl et al. and Haberl et al. in this volume).

The TCD technique delivers flow velocity data with a poor spatial, but a unique temporal, resolution (Aaslid 1987; Ringelstein et al. 1988). If measured intraindividually, changes in flow velocity reflect true changes in blood flow volume (Kirkham et al. 1986). This is why TCD measurements can be used as a nonradioactive and simple technique to evaluate *cerebral vasomotor reactivity (VMR)*. Further prerequisites for TCD application and its theoretical background have been detailed elsewhere (Arnolds and von Reutern 1986; Ringelstein et al. 1988, 1990; Ringelstein 1988). This chapter deals with the clinical application and validation of the CO_2 reactivity measurement in various models and subtypes of patients (Ringelstein 1991).

Examination Technique

During application or reduction of CO_2, modulation of blood flow velocity was measured by TCD within the proximal middle cerebral artery (MCA) at insonation depths of 50–55 mm with each subject at rest and supine. Simultaneously, the end-tidal CO_2 volume percentage (CO_2 vol%) was recorded by an infrared CO_2 analyzer (Capnolog,

* This project was in part supported by Verein zur Bekämpfung der Gefäßkrankheiten e.V., Engelskirchen.

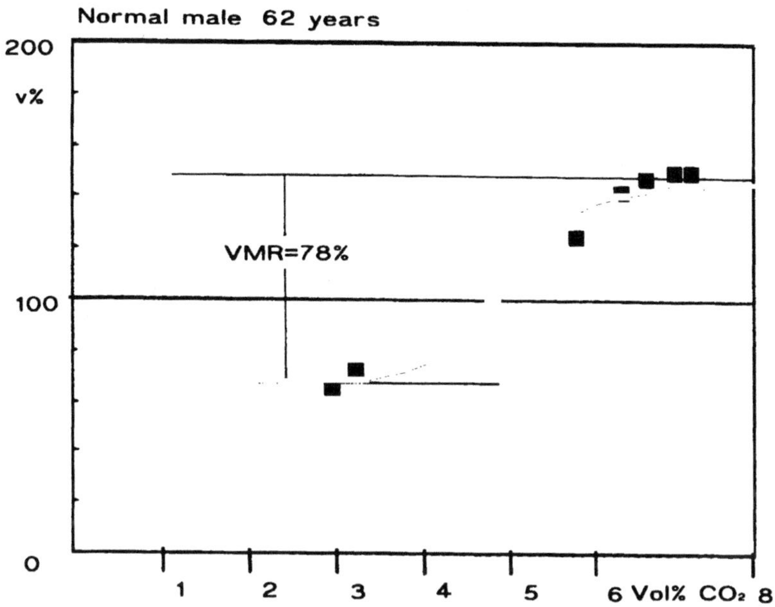

Fig. 1. Normal S-shaped curve of flow velocity changes reflecting vasomotor reactivity (VMR) of the middle cerebral artery (MCA) territory. Flow velocity (V) at rest within the MCA is set at 100%. During hyper- and hypocapnia, flow velocity increases or decreases to an upper and lower plateau. Abscissa, end-tidal CO_2 volume percentage. The distance between the plateaus represents the VMR value within this particular MCA territory (delta V, 78%) (curve fitting according to a tangent hyperbolic function). (From Ringelstein et al. 1991a)

Datex Instrumentarium OY, Helsinki, Finland), and blood pressure and heart rate were also monitored noninvasive (Dinamap Ergometer, Criticon, IMC, Tampa, Florida, United States). After reaching steady states in mean MCA blood flow velocity *and* end-tidal CO_2 vol% values under normocapnia, oxygen with CO_2 concentrations of 6%, 5%, 4%, 3%, and 2% was given for 2–3 min each. Subsequently, three or four increasing intensities of hyperventilation were used to produce hypocapnia. During each steady state period, a sequence of approximately 20 cardiac cycles was recorded on tape, and was analyzed off-line for a precise determination of mean blood flow velocities. Flow velocity during inhalation of room air was set 100% and was compared with percentage changes in mean blood flow during hyper- and hypocapina. Relative blood flow velocity changes were plotted against the corresponding end-tidal CO_2 vol%. Data were subjected to curve fitting. A tangent hypobolic function gave the best fit. The distance between the resulting asymptotes of the curve was considered to reflect the individual vasomotor reactivity of the MCA territory under study, and was called CO_2-induced cerebral vasomotor reactivity (Fig. 1).

Findings in Normal Volunteers

Forty healthy adults clinically and sonographically free of cerebrovascular disease were studied (mean age, 51 years; range, 20–75 years). The VMR of each individual was taken to calculate the overall mean VMR of the cohort, which was 86%±16%. The intraindividual reproducibility of vasomotor reactivity measurements within the MCA territory was less than 10% for ten measurements on ten different days (Ringelstein et al. 1988). On average, blood flow velocity within the normal MCA increased by 52.5% during hypercapnia and decreased by 35.3% during hypocapnia.

These findings agree precisely with previous data from animal experiments, as well as ultrasound and rCBF measurements in man (Breslau et al. 1982; Harper and Glass 1966; Kety and Schmidt 1948; Kindt et al. 1969; Yonas et al. 1987; Young and Appen 1981).

Clinical Models

Findings in Unilateral and Bilateral ICA Occlusions

In 40 symptomatic (N=28) and asymptomatic (N=12) patients with *unilateral* ICA occlusions, VMR on the occluded side was significantly lower (mean 45%, median 50%) than on the nonoccluded side (mean ±SD 68%±13%; p<0.0001). On the nonoccluded side, VMR was also significantly lower than would be expected from normal individuals (68%±13% vs. 86%±16%, p<0.01). The curve of an illustrative case with severely reduced VMR is given in Fig. 2.

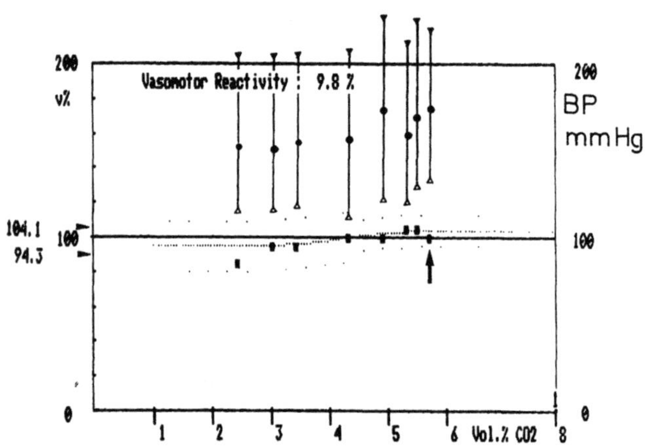

Fig. 2. Vasomotor reactivity and blood pressure during CO_2 testing in a 44-year-old patient with unilateral internal carotid artery occlusion. Despite a slight increase in arterial blood pressure (BP), blood flow velocity within middle cerebral artery (MCA) decreased during 5% CO_2 inhalation (arrow), indicating some degree of intracerebral steal. Vasomotor reactivity was nearly lost. Residual vasomotor reactivity of 9.8% was mainly due to vasoconstrictor response during hypocapnia, which was less severely affected. These findings indicate severe low-flow conditions within the MCA territory under study. (*Circle*, mean BP; *closed triangle*, systolic BP; *open triangle*, diastolic BP). The patient had suffered repeated hypostatic transient ischemic attacks, and computed tomography demonstrated a typical low-flow infarction within the centrum semiovale. (V%, relative blood flow velocity; *vol% CO_2*, end-tidal carbon dioxide volume percentage. (From Ringelstein et al. 1988)

Cerebral vasomotor reactivity was significantly lower in symptomatic than in asymptomatic patients (mean 68%; median 42% vs. mean ±SD 63%±16%; $p<0.006$). The most striking finding was that all patients with either low-flow-induced infarctions on CT (*N*=5) or chronic ischemic ophthalmopathy of the ipsilateral eye (Copetto et al. 1985, Zülch 1961) (*N*=2) and/or repeated hypostatic transient ischemic attacks (TIAs) (Caplan and Sergay 1976) (*N*=2) had VMR values of less than 38%. This was less than 3 standard deviations below the normal control. A VMR of 38% seems to be a threshold below which the risk of ischemic complications of the brain or eye increases abruptly.

Similar findings were seen in 15 patients with *bilateral* ICA occlusions (for details see Ringelstein et al. 1988). The most remarkable finding, however, was a normal or nearly normal vasomotor reactivity in two of these patients despite bilateral ICA occlusions. VMR values on the right or left side were 77% or 78% and 68% or 76%, respectively.

Very few patients showed paradoxical reactions to CO_2 stimulation with a decrease in blood flow velocity during hypercapnia. This was interpreted as an intracerebral transfer of blood from the affected to the nonaffected hemisphere (Fig. 2).

The above-described findings underline the validity of the CO_2 stimulation test from a clinical point of view. All findings were in the expected direction, and differences were always statistically highly significant for comparison of subgroups. Findings also demonstrate that in the individual case a prediction of the hemodynamic impact of even very severe or bilateral extracranial occlusive disease on intracranial hemodynamics is not possible from the angiological findings alone. Due to compensatory capabilities of the circle of Willis or extracranial collateral pathways, a (nearly) normal cerebral perfusion pressure can be maintained even in patients with bilateral internal carotid artery occlusions. The TCD-based measurement of CO_2-induced cerebral vasomotor reactivity enables the individual risk of hemodynamic compromise due to extracranial occlusive disease to be predicted reliably. This is confirmed by the close relationship between clinical findings and VMR values.

Findings in ICA Stenoses

A series of 135 patients with ICA stenoses of varying severities were subdivided into groups with 60%, 70%, 80%, 90%, and subtotal lumen narrowing. Findings were compared with data from 32 patients with complete ICA occlusions and with normal controls. There was a clear-cut dependency of vasomotor reactivity on the degree of the ICA lesion (Fig. 3). As soon as the degree of ICA stenoses reached 80% of the cross-sectional area reduction, the decrease in mean VMR became statistically significantly different from that of normal controls ($p=0.053$).

These findings again demonstrate the clinical validity of the above-described transcranial Doppler technique for the measurement of VMR. The broad overlap of VMR values in subgroups of patients again underlines that the degree of extracranial lesion alone does not allow its impact on intracranial blood flow to be predicted in the individual case. The presence of a hemodynamically significant extracranial lesion is only one of several prerequisites for the production of a critical drop in cerebral perfusion pressure. As will be shown below, the circle of Willis plays the key role in the patho-

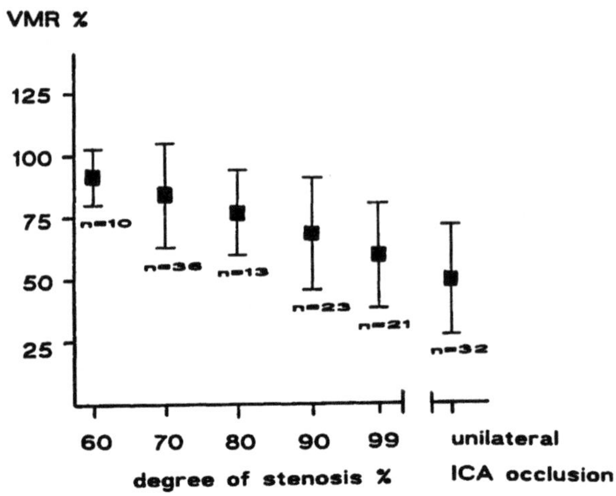

Fig. 3. Dependency of cerebral vasomotor reactivity (VMR) within the MCA distribution on the degree of ipsilateral internal carotid artery lesion. As compared with normal controls (*N*=40; mean ±SD=86%±16%, not shown here), reduction in vasomotor reactivity was statistically significant as soon as the degree of ICA stenosis reached 80% lumen narrowing (*p*=0.053). Note the broad scatter of values within each subgroup

physiology of low-flow induced brain ischemia (Keunen et al. 1989; Ringelstein et al. 1991b).

Cerebral Vasomotor Reactivity Before and After Carotid Endarterectomy

A series of 31 patients were investigated 3 days before, and 10–20 days after, carotid endarterectomy. Patients had ICA stenoses of at least 80% lumen narrowing. The overall increase in VMR after carotid endarterectomy was highly significant with preoperative VMR values of 67%±23% and postoperative values of 85.7%±16% ($p<0.0001$)

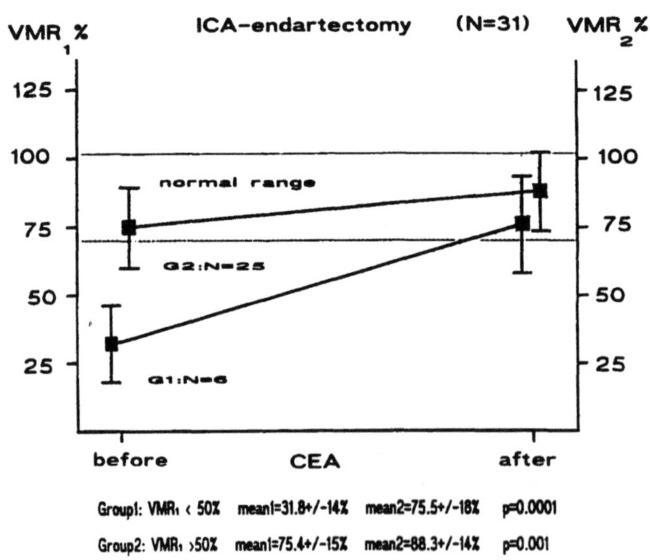

Fig. 4. Improvement of VMR after internal carotid artery endarterectomy. Patients were subdivided into two groups, one with a preoperative VMR of <50% (G1) and another with a VMR >50% (G2). The improvement in VMR was statistically highly significant in both subgroups, but more pronounced in the former

(Fig. 4). In a considerable number of patients, however, the postoperative increase in vasomotor reactivity was not very spectacular. Their VMR values had already been close to or even within the lower normal range before endarterectomy. By contrast, in patients with preoperatively low (<50%) VMR values, carotid endarterectomy dramatically improved vasomotor reactivity.

Patients subjected to carotid endarterectomy provide an ideal opportunity to investigate the effects of removal of extracranial occlusive disease on cerebral perfusion pressure. From a statistical point of view, even minor improvements in VMR after carotid endarterectomy may be „significant" in a formal sense. A clinically relevant improvement, however, can only be achieved in those few cases with a preoperatively critically reduced VMR beyond the aforementioned threshold of 38%. Our findings confirm that in the majority of cases carotid endarterectomy is a procedure for removing a source of embolism, and not so much for improving CBF.

Long-term Observations on VMR in Extracranial Occlusive Disease

The author is not aware of any report in the literature about changes of vasomotor reactivity over time. A series of 32 patients with ICA occlusions were followed-up over a period of 1.5 years, with VMR measurements every 6 months. There was an overall gradual improvement of VMR over time, predominantly during the first 6 months (mean initial VMR 49.8%±22%, mean follow-up VMR, 61%±22%; p<0.001). This tendency was particularly pronounced in patients whose VMR values had been low initially. Only exceptionally did individuals show persistence of an exhausted cerebrovascular reserve or even worsening during the observation period (Fig. 5).

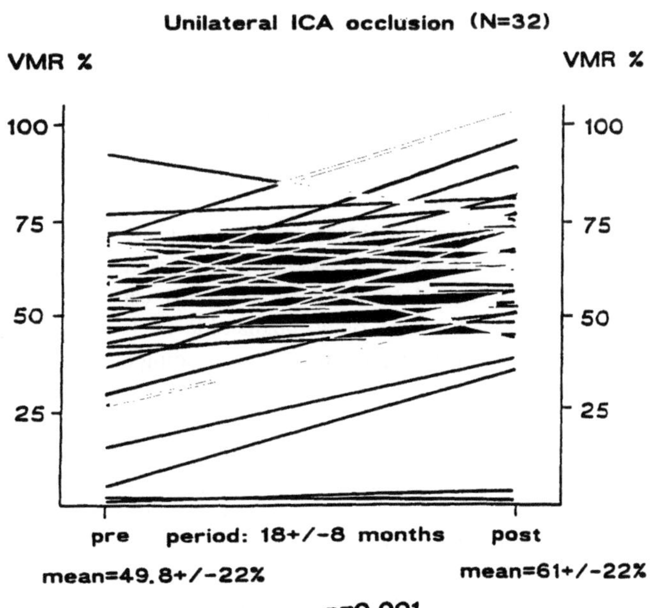

Fig. 5. Spontaneous course of VMR over time in patients with chronic ICA occlusions (*N*=32). Over a period of 18±8 months, the mean VMR increased highly significantly from 49.8%±22% to 61%±22%, p <0.001. In a few individuals, however, no improvement occured at all (lower two lines) or the VMR even deteriorated (also two cases)

These observations are of clinical interest. Obviously, in the majority of cases, a severely curtailed cerebrovascular reserve improves spontaneously without any specific treatment. Extracranial-intracranial bypass surgery would not be justified despite severe hemodynamic compromise. I am not aware of any clinical or laboratory test which would allow the selection of those few cases without spontaneous improvement of their exhausted VMR. While improvement of VMR over time may be explained by gradual augmentation of the initially activated natural collateral pathways (comparable to the increasing transport capacity of an EC/IC bypass within the first few weeks or months), the reasons for a persistently low VMR, or even worsening in perfusion reserve, remain unclear.

Measurements of VMR by Means of CO_2 Versus Acetazolamide Stimulation

To measure the CO_2 responsiveness by hyper- and hypocapnia requires the patient's cooperation. In cases with chronic obstructive lung disease, congestive heart failure, and severe malaise, patients would not tolerate the stress of CO_2 breathing or the labor of hyperventilation. Acetazolamide is a compound which dilates the brain resistance arteries by carboanhydrase inhibition and subsequent tissue acidosis. Acetazolamide can be administered with no cooperation by the patient, which makes it an interesting compound to test cerebrovascular reserve in the acute state of brain diseases.

We applied both methods, the above-described CO_2 technique and supramaximal vasodilation by injection of 1 g acetazolamide, to a series of 93 MCA territories (N=47 patients). They had been shown to suffer from various degrees of extracranial occlusive disease (Ringelstein et al. 1991a).

The correlation coefficient of the linear regression between both parameters was 0.7 and was highly significantly different from zero. Both parameters were able to differentiate significantly between subgroups with bilateral high-grade lesions, unilateral high-grade lesions, or low-grade stenoses (Fig. 6). In different angiological subgroups (see legend of Fig. 6), acetazolamide was even slightly superior to the CO_2 technique. Discriminant regression analysis was used to determine which parameter would best reclassify patients to the aforementioned angiological subgroups by means of VMR. Both stimulation techniques did equally well, and 54 of 93 hemispheres were correctly reclassified by each.

Findings indicate that acetazolamide is a useful compound for the testing of cerebral vasomotor reactivity in patients with extracranial occlusive disease. It cannot be used, however, to evaluate the *vasoconstrictive* capabilities of the cerebral vasculature. A potential disadvantage of acetazolamide is its elevation of intracranial pressure, which limits its usage in patients with impending brain swelling.

Cerebral Vasomotor Reactivity , the Configuration of the Circle of Willis, and the Extent and Type of Brain Infarctions

To test the hypothesis that cerebral VMR is significantly more reduced in patients with hemispheric low-flow infarctions than in brain infarctions due to arterio-arterial embolism, a series of 64 consecutive patients with internal carotid artery occlusions were studied. The configuration of the circle of Willis was also determined by TCD using

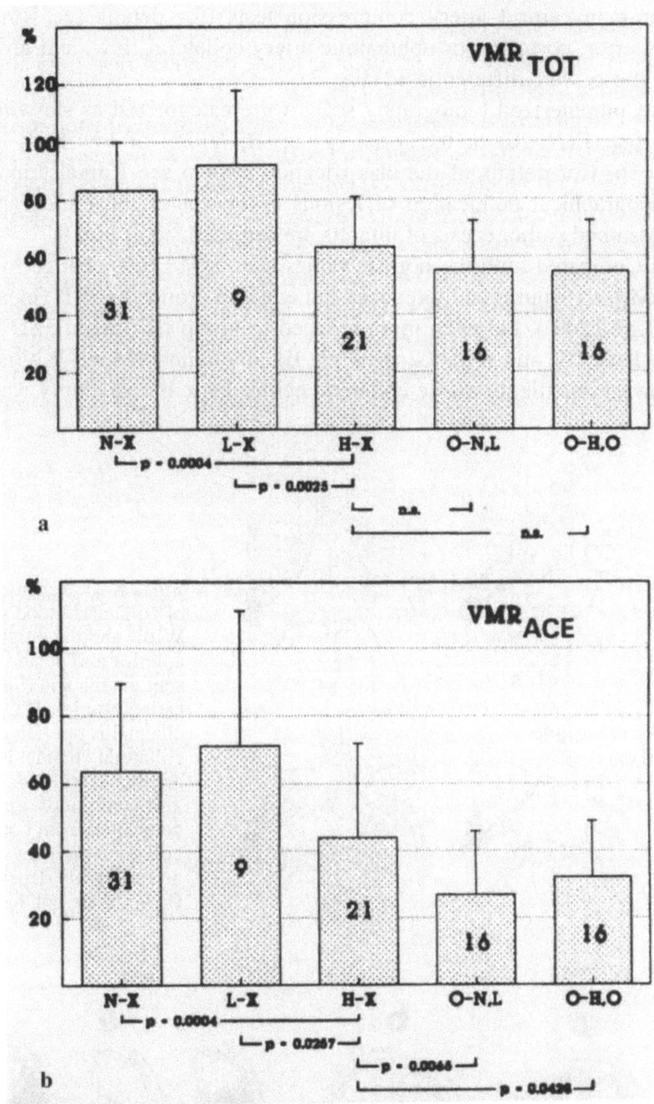

Fig. 6a, b. Ability of acetazolamide-induced VMR (VMR^{ACE}) and CO_2-induced VMR (VMR^{TOT}) to differentiate between angiolo gical subgroups. **a** Stimulation with hyper- and hypocapnia (= the total VMR) was able to differentiate between normal carotid arteries or low-grade carotid lesions and high-grade carotid lesions. VRM^{TOT} failed, however, to show significant differences between patients with high-grade carotid lesions and those with internal carotid artery occlusions. **b** Stimulation with acetazolamide (= VMR^{ACE}). Significant and highly significant differences in VMR^{ACE} were observed between patients with normal ICAs or low-grade ICA stenoses and those with high-grade lesions, and also between high-grade lesions and internal carotid artery occlusions. Explanation of labels of subgroups: N–X, ipsilateral normal, contralateral any ICA findings from normal to any degree of occlusion; L–X, ipsilateral <80% stenosis, contralateral any findings from normal to any degree of occlusion; H–X, ipsilateral >or=80% stenosis contralateral any findings from normal to any degree of occlusion; O–NL, ipsilateral occlusion, contralateral <80% stenosis or normal; O–HO, ipsilateral occlusion, contralateral occlusion or >/=80% stenosis. (From Ringelstein et al. 1991a)

common carotid artery compression tests (for details see Ringelstein et al. 1988). Anterior, posterior, or ophthalmic artery collateral flow, and absence or combinations of these, were differentiated (Fig. 7).

Computerized tomography scans were categorized as showing either no infarction (group I; N=20) or territorial (group II; N=28) or low-flow infarctions (group III; N=16) (for details of the classification system see Ringelstein et al. 1983). Site and topographical delineation of lesions on computerized tomography, terminology, and presumed pathogenesis of infarcts are summarized in Fig. 8.

Compared with the normal values (i.e., 86%±16% change in MCA flow velocity), VMR was significantly reduced but equal in groups I and II (means ±SD, 48.3%±14%; 49.5%±20%), but even more reduced in group III (mean, ±SD 27.6%±22%; $p<0.006$ in I vs. III, and $p<0.002$ in II vs. III, one-tailed Mann-Whitney-U-test). VMR was lowest in patients whose collateral hemispheric blood supply was from the ophthalmic

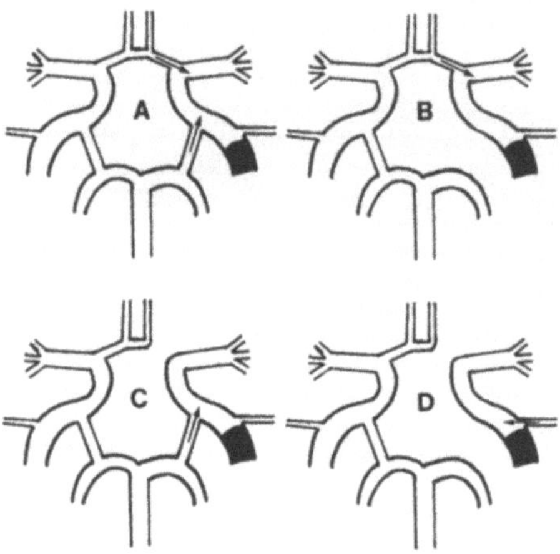

Fig. 7A–D. Schematic drawings of the types of collateral blood supply via the circle of Willis and the ophthalmic artery. **A** Both anterior and posterior cross-filling are present via the anterior and posterior communicating arteries. **B** Only the anterior collateral channel is operative. **C** Only the posterior collateral channel is operative, while the anterior circulation is disconnected. **D** The "isolated middle cerebral artery" is disconnected from both anterior and posterior collateral pathways of the circle of Willis and is mainly dependent on retrograde blood flow via the ophthalmic artery

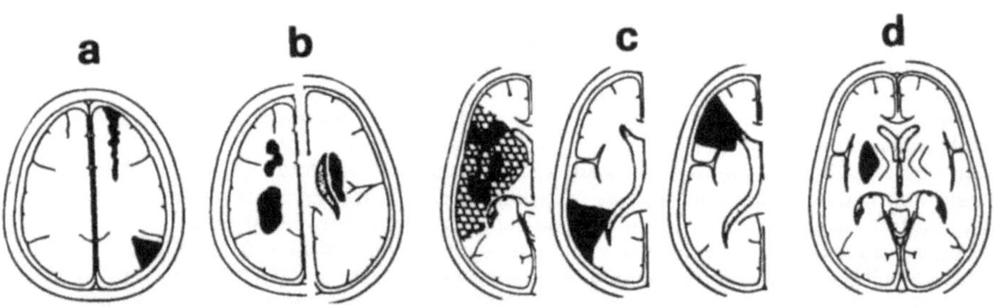

Fig. 8a–d: Brain infarctions due to internal carotid artery occlusion. **a, b** Hemodynamically induced infarctions with predominantly cortical, extraterritorial or b strikingly subcortical location (a=watershed infarction, borderline infarction; b=terminal supply area infarction, terminal zone infarction, deep low-flow infarction). **c** Thromboembolic, pial artery territory infarctions of various size with cortical-subcortical extension (hatched zone indicates partial infarction). **d** Large striatocapsular infarct restricted to the basal ganglia reflecting the subcortical type of thromboembolic infarction. (Modified from Ringelstein et al. 1983)

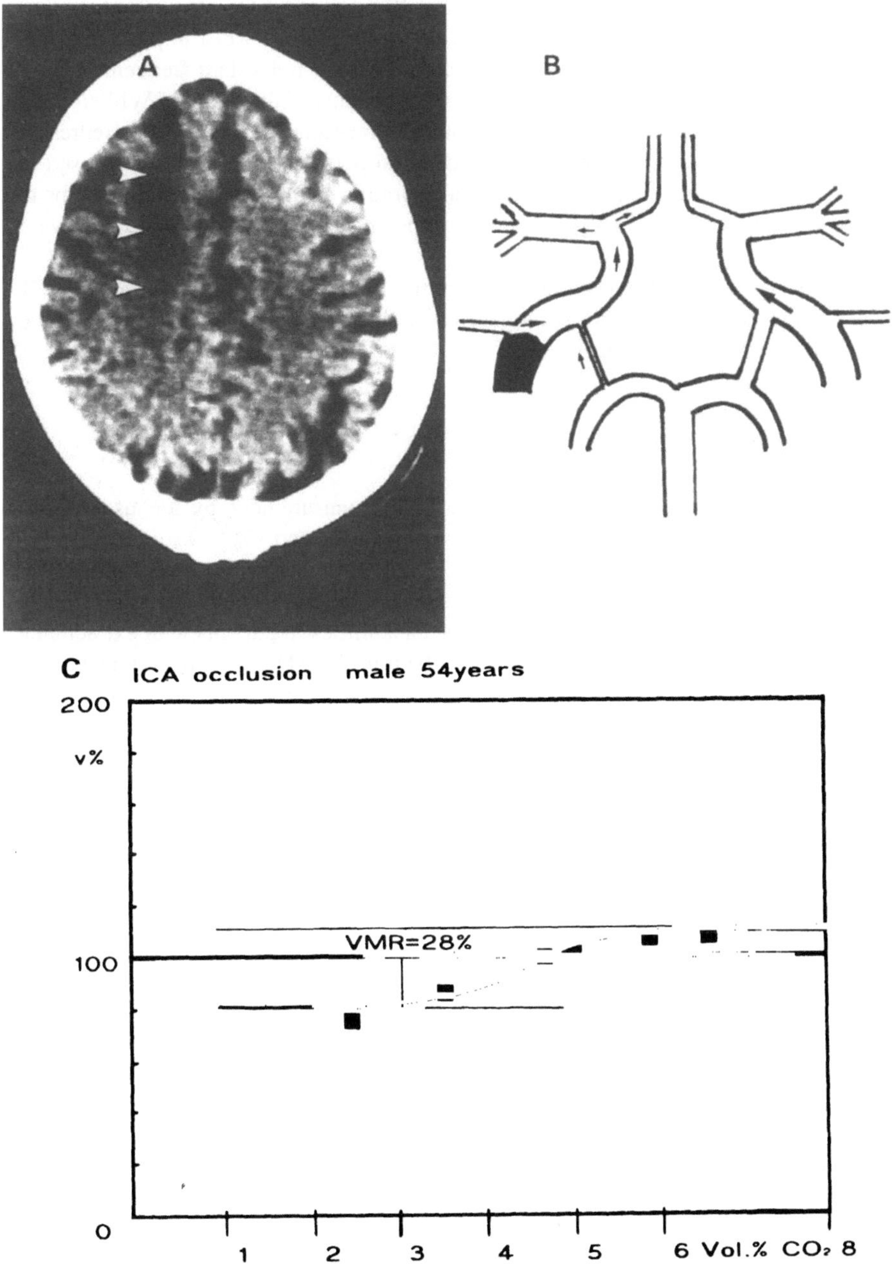

Fig. 9A–C Illustrative case of subgroup III (male, 54 years, right-sided ICA occlusion, left-sided hemiparesis, ischemic ophthalmopathy *on the right*). **A** Frontoparasagittal watershed infarction (arrowheads). **B** Transcranial Doppler sonography revealed a high-velocity retrograde flow within the ophthalmic artery, absence of anterior cross-filling, and only minimal collateral blood flow via the posterior communicating artery *on the right*. **C** Cerebral VMR was severely reduced to 28%

artery alone (mean VMR ±SD=27%±21%) (Fig. 9) as opposed to patients with a complete or nearly complete circle of Willis (mean VMR ±SD=52%±15%; p=0.002; one-tailed Mann-Whitney-U-test). Low-flow infarctions were much less frequent in patients with collateral blood flow via the regular components of the circle of Willis.

Findings indicate that low-flow infarctions in extracranial ICA occlusions represent brain damage due to a critical reduction in cerebral perfusion pressure, as opposed to thromboembolically induced lesions. The configuration of the circle of Willis seems to play the key role, while a history of systemic hypotension turned out to be less relevant in our series.

Findings also support the view that the pattern of hemispheric infarction seen on CT delivers important clues to the pathogenesis of the stroke (Ringelstein et al. 1983, 1989; Valk 1980; Widder et al. 1986).

Summarizing Conclusions

The above-described technique of cerebral VMR measurement by means of TCD sonography allows for the assessment of the vasodilative and vasoconstrictive capabilities of the cerebral vasculature. While CO_2 is the most frequently used stimulus for both vasodilation and vasoconstriction, acetazolamide can exclusively, but equally reliably, be used to evaluate the vasodilatative capabilities in patients with extracranial occlusive disease. Whether these findings can be transferred to other pathological conditions remains to be demonstrated. A major disadvantage of the TCD technique is its poor spatial resolution. VMR values can only be given for the whole vascular territory under study (mostly the entire MCA territory).

Data from a normal control group have been produced, which demonstrates a fairly low standard deviation. Furthermore, findings in pathological conditions drastically differed from normal control and were always in the expected direction in various clinical models. The consistency of these findings demonstrates the validity of TCD-based VMR measurements in cerebrovascular occlusive disease. Most interestingly, empirical findings were also completely in line with our theoretical expectations in different configurations of the circle of Willis and in different types of brain infarction (hemodynamically induced low-flow infarctions versus thromboembolically induced territorial infarctions). This strongly supports the view that cerebrovascular reactivity, in fact, reflects cerebral perfusion pressure. There is also strong support for the presumption that CO_2 or acetazolamide-induced VMR reflects the true pressure-dependent cerebral autoregulation.

The above-described techniques are of practical value in that they enable patients to be identified and selected with a high risk of low-flow induced brain ischemia. As soon as the VMR is lower than three standard deviations below normal mean values, the risk of cerebral or ophthalmic ischemic compromise increases abruptly. This knowledge has already influenced therapeutic decisions in our department. In subtotal yet asymptomatic internal carotid artery stenosis with a VMR value of <38%, we prefer carotid endarterectomy. We also use this technique to select very few patients for EC/IC bypass surgery. Whether this is truly beneficial for the patients, however, remains to be demonstrated by prospective studies.

Acetazolamide turned out to be reliable for measuring cerebrovascular reactivity if the doses were high enough. This compound may considerably facilitate VMR evaluation in uncooperative patients. It may, however, have adverse effects in those with elevated intracranial pressure. Despite its technical and methodological simplicity, TCD-based evaluation of cerebrovascular reactivity is a valuable new tool for the solution of actual scientific and clinical problems in stroke pathophysiology.

Acknowledgement The author wishes to thank Dres. Sabine van Eyck, Andreas Holling, Irene Mertens, Matthias Weckesser, and Susanne Weckesser for long-term scientific cooperation and support, and Christiane Göbel-Dizinger, Vera Schappeler, Gabriele Tietz and Waltraud Schumacher, vascular technicians, for their assistance.

References

Aaslid R (1987) Visually evoked dynamic blood flow response of the human cerebral circulation. Stroke 18:771–775

Arnolds BJ, von Reutern GM (1986) Transcranial Doppler sonography. Examination technique and normal reference values. Ultrasound Med Biol 12:115–123

Bogousslavsky J, Regli F (1986) Unilateral watershed cerebral infarcts. Neurology 36:373–377

Breslau PJ, Knox R, Fell G, Greene FM, Thiele BL, Strandness BE Jr (1982) Effect of carbon dioxide on flow patterns in normal extracranial arteries. J Surg Res 32:97–103

Caplan LR, Sergay S (1976) Positional cerebral ischemia. J Neurol Neurosurg Psychiatry 39:385–391

Copetto JR, Wand M, Bear L, Sciarra R (1985) Neovascular glaucoma and carotid artery obstructive disease. Am J Ophthalmol 99:567–570

Gibbs JM, Wise RJS, Leenders KL, Jones T (1984) Evaluation of cerebral perfusion reserve in patients with carotid-artery occlusion. Lancet 1:310–314

Harper AM, Glass HI (1966) Effect of alteration in the arterial carbon dioxide tension on the blood flow to the cerebral cortex at normal and low arterial blood pressure. J Neurol Neurosurg Psychiatry 28:449–452

Kanno I, Uemura K, Higano S, Murakami M, Ieda H, Miura S, Shishido F, Inugami A, Sayama I (1988) Oxygen extraction fraction at maximally vasodilated tissue in the ischemic brain estimated from the regional CO_2-responsiveness measured by positron emission tomography. J Cereb Blood Flow Metab 8:227–235

Kety SS, Schmidt CF (1948) The effects of altered arterial tensions of carbon dioxide and oxygen on cerebral blood flow and cerebral oxygen consumption of normal young men. J Clin Invest 27:448–492

Keunen RWM, Ackerstaff RGA, Stegeman DF, Schulte, BPM (1989) The impact of internal carotid artery occlusion and of the integrity of the circle of Willis on cerebral vasomotor reactivity – a transcranial Doppler study. In: Meyer JS, et al. (eds) Cerebral vascular disease. Elsevier, Amsterdam, pp 85–88

Kindt GW, Humans JR, Convey LW (1969) The use of ultrasound to determine cerebral arterial reserve. J Neurosurg 31:544–549

Kirkham FJ, Padayachee TS, Parsons S, Seargeant LS, House RF, Gosling RG (1986) Transcranial measurement of blood flow velocities in the basal cerebral arteries using pulsed Doppler ultrasound: velocity as an index of flow. Ultrasound Med Biol 12:15–21

Leblanc R, Yamamoto YL, Tyler JL, Dikscic M, Hakim A (1987) Borderzone ischemia. Ann Neurol 22:707–713

Levine RL, Sunderland JJ, Lagreze HL, Nickles RJ, Rowe BR, Turski PA (1988) Cerebral perfusion reserve indexes determined by fluoromethane positron emission scanning. Stroke 19:19–27

Norrving B, Nilsson B, Risberg J (1982) rCBF in patients with carotid occlusion – resting and hypercapnic flow related to collateral pattern. Stroke 13:155–162
Ringelstein EB, Zeumer H, Angelou D (1983) The pathogenesis of strokes from internal carotid artery occlusion. Diagnostic and therapeutic implications. Stroke 14:867–875
Ringelstein EB, Sievers C, Ecker S, Schneider PA, Otis SM (1988) Non-invasive assessment of CO_2-induced cerebral vasomotor response in normal individuals and patients with internal carotid artery occlusions. Stroke 19:936–969
Ringelstein EB (1989) A practical guide to transcranial Doppler sonography. In: Weinberger J (ed) Non-invasive assessment of the cerebral circulation in cerebrovascular disease. Frontiers of clinical neuroscience theories. Liss, New York, pp 75–121
Ringelstein EB, Koschorke S, Holling A, Thron A, Lambertz H, Minale C (1989) Computerized tomography patterns of proven embolic brain infarctions. Ann Neurol 26:759–765
Ringelstein EB, Kahlscheuer B, Niggemeyer E, Otis SM (1990) Transcranial Doppler sonography: anatomical landmarks and normal velocity values. Ultrasound Med Biol 16:745–761
Ringelstein EB, van Eyck S, Mertens I (1991a) Evaluation of cerebral vasomotor reactivity by various vasodilating stimuli: comparison of CO2 with acetazolamide. J Cereb Blood Flow Metab (in press)
Ringelstein EB, Weiller C, Weckesser M, Weckesser S (1991b) Cerebral vasomotor reactivity is significantly reduced in low-flow as compared to thromboembolic infarctions: the key role of the circle of Willis. J Neurol Sci (in press)
Ringelstein EB (1991) Physiologic testing of vasomotor reserve. In: Newell DW, Aaslid R (eds) Transcranial Doppler sonograpy. Clinical aspects. Raven, New York (in press)
Valk J (1980) Computed tomography and cerebral infarctions. Raven, New York
Weiller C, Ringelstein EB, Reiche W, Büll U (1991) Clinical and hemodynamical aspects of low-flow infarcts. Stroke 22:1117–1123
Widder B, Paulat K, Hackspacher J, Mayr E (1986) Transcranial Doppler CO_2-test for the detection of hemodynamically critical carotid artery stenosis and occlusions. Eur Arch Psychiatry Neurol Sci 236:162–168
Wodarz R (1980) Watershed infarctions and computed tomography: topographic study in cases with stenosis or occlusion of the carotid artery. Neuroradiology 19:245–248
Yamaguchi F, Meyer JS, Sakai F, Yamamoto M (1979) Normal human aging and cerebral vasoconstrictive responses to hypocapnia. J Neurol Sci 44:87–94
Yonas H, Gurr D, Latchav RE, Wolfson SD Jr (1987) Xenon computed tomographic blood flow mapping. In: Wood JH (ed) Cerebral blood flow. Physiologic and clinical aspects. McGraw-Hill, New York, pp 220–245
Young LH, Appen RE (1981) Ischemic oculopathy: a manifestation of carotid artery disease. Arch Neurol 38:358–361
Zülch KJ (1961) Die Pathogenese von Massenblutungen und Erweichungen unter besonderer Berücksichtigung klinischer Gesichtspunkte. Acta Neurochir [Suppl] (Wien) 7:51–117

Identification of Hemodynamic Patients for EC–IC Bypass Surgery

S. Vorstrup, J. Schmidt, G. Waldemar, J. Haase, and O. B. Paulson

Introduction

Recurrent ischemic symptoms from a hemisphere where the internal carotid artery (ICA) is occluded are either embolic or hemodynamic. Distinguishing between these two etiologies is not possible on clinical grounds alone, although multiple, brief attacks including limb shaking are suggestive of hemodynamic origin (Levine et al. 1989). In particular, when the symptoms occur in relation to orthostatic changes, a clinical suspicion of an inadequate regional flow arises. Nevertheless, in most of these patients the setting of clinical symptoms alone and even when supplemented by angiography and CT will not identify the hemodynamic cases, and additional studies are needed. Measurement of CBF during CO_2 inhalation (Levine et al. 1989; Norrving et al. 1982) or after intravenous administration of acetazolamide (Vorstrup et al. 1986) has been used to evaluate the cerebral vasodilatory capacity. The development of positron emission tomography has permitted concomitant measurement of CBF, oxygen extraction fraction, and cerebral metabolism for oxygen ($CMRO_2$), which identifies critically perfused areas during baseline conditions. In addition, measurement of CBF and cerebral blood volume (CB) can be applied for this purpose (Gibbs et al. 1984).

The results of the large multicenter extracranial-intracranial (EC-IC) bypass trial (EC-IC Bypass Study Group 1985) showed no long-term preventive clinical effect of surgery compared with medical therapy in patients having transient ischemic attacks (TIAs) or minor stroke ipsilateral to an occluded ICA. Since then, prophylactic EC–IC bypass surgery has become much less common. However, whether EC–IC bypass surgery could be beneficial in the small, hemodynamically threatened subgroup is still an open question.

The aim of the present study was to identify this subset of patients by CBF measurements during an autoregulatory stress test in order to mimick everyday life.

Material and Methods

Four patients (3 men, 1 woman) have so far been included in this study on the basis of clinical symptoms, angiography, and CBF studies, including measurements of the regional vasodilatory capacity using acetazolamide (Diamox). Acetazolamide has a strong vasodilatory effect upon the cerebral vessels, quite comparable to CO_2 inhalation (Vorstrup 1988). In normally perfused regions, acetazolamide will induce a CBF

Table 1. Clinical data and results of angiography, CT, and Doppler examination of the extracranial vessels

Patient	Age/sex (years)	Clinical data (No., duration)	Neurological findings between attacks	Angiography	CT scan	Doppler
1	49/M	Nonfluent aphasia (10, min) Right hemiparesis (20, min)	NL	L ICA occluded, R ICA small plaque	NL	L ICA occluded, Retrograde ophthalmic flow
2	69/F	Orthostatic R hemiparesis and nonfluent aphasia (multiple, min)	NL	L ICA occluded	Small deepseated L lacunar infarct	Not done
3	36/M	Paresthesia of L hand and face (20,5–45 min)	NL	Severe stenosis of R MCA after lenticulostriate arteries	NL	NL
4	67/M	L hemiparesis	Moderate L hemiparesis leg > arm	Bilateral ICA occlusion	Two infarcts in R hemisphere	Not done

R, right; L, Left; NL, normal; ICA, internal carotid artery

increase of about 30%. However, in regions with a reduced perfusion pressure, as is the case in the hemisphere ipsilateral to an ICA occlusion with poor collateral supply, only a slight or no CBF increase will be seen, as the vessels already at rest are maximally dilated in order to preserve flow (Vorstrup et al. 1986). Thus, in hemodynamic cases, a marked asymmetrical flow-response is induced during the stress test. Studies on regional CBF autoregulation were performed in these selected cases.

Table 1 gives the clinical findings and results of angiography and CT in the four patients. CBF was measured by xenon-133 inhalation and single photon emission tomography (Tomomatic 64). After a baseline study, 1 g acetazolamide was administered intravenously, and CBF measured again 20 min later. On a separate day, the baseline study was repeated, after which the mean arterial blood pressure (MAP) was increased approximately 30% by continuous intravenous norepinephrine infusion, and CBF was measured during steady state. To reduce MAP, a combination of lower body suction and trimethaphane camphosulfonas (Arfonad) infusion was used. MAP was reduced gradually to about 20%–30% of the baseline level. The CBF studies were evaluated by calculating both the absolute flow values and the regional flow distribution as estimated by *D*, the interhemispheric side-to-side asymmetry index for a given region of interest. *D* is defined as the absolute side difference taken as a percentage of the higher value.

Results

Regional CBF Autoregulation Test. During increased MAP, inconsistent findings in both absolute flow values and *D* were found. During MAP reduction, all four patients showed a further CBF decrease in the low-flow area, which caused marked enhancement of the side-to-side asymmetry in three cases. In the last case having bilateral ICA occlusions, the low-flow areas were in both frontal areas. Neurological deficits were not elicited during the studies.

Extracranial-intracranial bypass surgery was performed without complications in three patients, while one suffered a perioperative ischemic infarct.

Discussion

The clinical course after occlusion of one ICA depends on the collateral circulation, which is predominantly supplied by the contralateral ICA and the posterior circulation through the circle of Willis. If adequate compensatory flow is provided, and if distal embolization at the time of ICA occlusion does not occur, the ICA occlusion is generally well tolerated without acute ischemic manifestations. The subsequent narrowing of the collaterals by atherosclerotic processes will gradually lead to a reduction of the regional perfusion pressure and eventually rCBF. In some cases, this will cause intermittent focal neurological deficits on a hemodynamic basis. Evidently, the number of patients with such a clinical course is quite rare, probably amounting to 10%–15% of patients with occlusive cerebrovascular disease (Powers et al. 1989).

The present study was undertaken to document our earlier findings with the acetazolamide test (Vorstrup et al. 1986; Vorstrup 1988). Patients were included only if the test was suggestive of a low regional perfusion pressure, i.e., only a slight or no CBF increase was observed in the symptomatic region (in some cases, CBF decreased even further due to an intracerebral steal effect). We thereafter proceeded with CBF studies on regional CBF autoregulation by increasing and decreasing MAP.

Four patients have been studied. Consistent findings were obtained during reduction of MAP as a significant reduction in focal CBF was seen in all four cases. This confirmed that CBF in this region was belong the lower limit of CBF autoregulation. This was observed despite marked hyperventilation in two patients.

During increasing MAP the findings were less consistent. Two patients showed a moderate but favorable redistribution of flow toward the hypoperfused areas, while the other two showed a reduction in CBF. Although it was expected that CBF in the hypoperfused areas was pressure passive and would respond to a systemic MAP increase, transmission of an increased pressure through the restricted collaterals may not be possible.

Three of the patients have undergone uncomplicated EC–IC bypass surgery. In one patient EC–IC bypass surgery was complicated by an ischemic stroke, causing aphasia and a moderate hemiparesis. Only some language deficits remained at the 6-month follow-up. In this patient the regional perfusion pressure in the middle cerebral artery territory was measured perioperatively, and was reduced to 29% of the systemic MAP (normally, the pressure in this region is equal to the systemic pressure, i.e., 100%).

However, the patient's TIAs did not reoccur and, despite a permanent flow defect due to infarction of the brain tissue, rCBF increased, as did the flow response at the postoperative acetazolamide test. This case underscores how fragile these hemodynamic patients are. Although a surgical approach appears to be the correct treatment, these patients undoubtedly run a much higher perioperative risk of ischemic deficit. Particular care of the systemic blood pressure should be taken pre-, peri- and postoperatively, as prolonged hypotension will cause permanent ischemic damage.

Based on these limited observations, the results of the autoregulatory stress test during hypotension seem to agree well with the findings during acetazolamide test. Although a reduction of the arterial blood pressure would appear to be more physiological, the test procedure is more tedious and time-consuming. The advantage of the acetazolamide test is its easy use and application, with no major side effects. It is not possible from this small series to draw any conclusions which test should be preferred.

The major question which remains to be answered is how to treat these hemodynamically threatened patients. As the perioperative complication rate is high, EC–IC bypass surgery will only be indicated if the procedure improves the prognosis considerably. The question can only be answered by a new randomized clinical trial with carefully selected cases.

References

EC-IC Bypass Study Group (1985) Failure of extracranial-intracranial arterial bypass to reduce the risk of ischemic stroke. Results of an international randomized trial. N Engl J Med 313:1191–1200

Gibbs JM, Leenders KL, Wise RJS, Jones T (1984) Evaluation of cerebral perfusion reserve in patients with carotid artery occlusion. Lancet 1:310–314

Levine RL, Lagreze HL, Dobkin JA, Hanson JM, Satter MR, Rowe BR, Nickles RJ (1989) Cerebral vasocapacitance and TIAs. Neurology 39:25–29

Norrving B, Nilsson B, Risberg J (1982) rCBF in patients with carotid occlusion: resting and hypercapnic flow related to collateral flow pattern. Stroke 13:155–162

Powers WJ, Tempel LW, Grubb RL (1989) Influence of cerebral hemodynamics on stroke risk: one-year follow-up of 30 medically treated patients. Ann Neurol 25:325–330

Vorstrup, S, Brun B, Lassen NA (1986) Evaluation of the cerebral vasodilatory capacity by the acetazolamide test before EC–IC bypass surgery in patients with occlusion of the internal carotid artery. Stroke 17:1291–1298

Vorstrup S (1988) Tomographic cerebral blood flow measurements in patients with ischemic cerebrovascular disease and evaluation of the vasodilatory capacity by the acetazolamide test. Acta Neurol Scand [Suppl 114] 77:1–48

Effect of Blood Pressure on Cerebral Blood Flow and Infarct Size: Haemodynamic Considerations

A. D. MENDELOW, R. D. STRACHAN, P. J. KANE, I. CHAMBERS, W. FITCH, D. I. GRAHAM, and U. TUOR

Introduction

The phenomenon of autoregulation is well known in the presence of a normal cerebral circulation (Harper 1966). However, in pathological states this autoregulation is often lost. With occlusive stroke Denny-Brown (1951) was the first to suggest that increasing the blood pressure may limit ischaemic brain damage. Subsequent studies (Wise et al. 1972) confirmed his original observations. Similarly, in subarachnoid haemorrhage (SAH) hypertensive treatment has been shown to reverse postoperative ischaemic deficits (Kassell et al. 1982). In head injury, where ischaemic brain damage (IBD) is found in the majority of patients who die (Graham et al. 1989), it has also been shown that the policy of maintaining a higher than normal cerebral perfusion pressure (CPP) is associated with a better outcome (McGraw 1989). The phenomenon of autoregulation cannot therefore be relied upon to maintain cerebral blood flow (CBF) once the cerebral circulation has become disordered.

The aim of the experimental studies presented here was to quantify the effect of hypotension on CBF and infarct size following large vessel occlusion.

Material and Methods

Three different experimental models were used in these studies:

1. Middle cerebral artery (MCA) occlusion in the rat
2. Internal carotid artery (ICA) occlusion in the rat
3. Internal carotid artery occlusion and stenosis in the baboon

General Preparation

All studies were performed in animals anaesthetized with halothane (0.5%–1.5%) in a mixture of nitrous oxide and oxygen, 70:30.

Blood Pressure

Blood pressure was monitored continuously via a femoral arterial line. Haemorrhagic hypotension was achieved by withdrawal and, where necessary, infusion of arterial blood through a contralateral femoral arterial line. In the rat MCA occlusion model a software-controlled infusion/withdrawal pump was connected to a computerized pressure monitoring system to maintain a constant pressure (Chambers et al. 1991).

Ventilation

All animals were ventilated and blood gases were maintained within normal physiological limits. Continuous end expiratory carbon dioxide monitoring with a capnograph was used to ensure a constant level of $PaCO_2$.

Vascular Occlusion

In the rat MCA occlusion model the MCA was exposed via a craniectomy and the proximal MCA was occluded with diathermy (Tamura et al. 1981). In the rat and baboon ICA occlusion models, the ICA was occluded in the nack after ligating the external carotid artery and its branches. In the baboon a 90% ICA stenosis was produced in a separate group of animals by partial ligature of the ICA.

Measurement of CBF

In the rat MCA occlusion model CBF was measured from four platinum electrodes using the hydrogen clearance method (Young 1980). In the rat and baboon ICA occlusion and stenosis models, CBF was measured using carbon-14 iodo-antipyrine autoradiography (Sakurada et al. 1988; Tuor et al. 1986). In the baboon ICA model CBF was also measured at different levels of mean arterial blood pressure using the intra-arterial xenon-133 clearance method (Fitch et al. 1978).

Measurement of Ischaemic Brain Damage

In the rat MCA occlusion model infarct size was measured by the triphenyl tetrazolium chloride (TTC) perfusion technique (Park et al. 1989). In the rat and baboon ICA occlusion model the amount of IBD was measured by light microscopy after FAM fixation (40% formaldehyde/glacial acetic acid/absolute methanol = 1:1:8).

Protocols

Rat MCA Occlusion Model

After MCA occlusion, MABP was reduced to 70 mmHg for 30 min using the computerized infusion/withdrawal pump. The blood pressure was then returned to normal levels for 4 h. In control animals with MCA occlusion BP was maintained within normal limits for the whole 4-h occlusion period.

Rat ICA Occlusion model

Haemorrhagic hypotension (40–50 mmHg) was induced for 15 min, and CBF was then measured. In the neuropathology studies BP was restored to normal after 30 min and maintained at that level for 2 h, after which perfusion fixation with FAM was used to prepare the brains for light microscopy. In control animals the BP was maintained within normal limits throughout. In a further series of controls haemorrhagic hypotension was induced without internal carotid occlusion.

Baboon ICA Occlusion and Stenosis Model

Haemorrhagic hypotension was induced by 10-mmHg decrements and CBF was measured with xenon-133 at each level. Carbon-14 iodo-antipyrine (IAP) autoradiographic CBF was measured at the lowest level of BP (30 mmHg). Transcardiac perfusion fixation with FAM was used for the light microscopy studies after a similar series of decrements at 30 mmHg. In control and 90% internal carotid stenosis animals, haemorrhagic hypotension was induced in the same way.

Results

Middle Cerebral Artery Occlusion in the Rat

The Blood pressure was maintained constant at 70 (± 1) mmHg while all other physiological parameters were maintained within normal limits. Compared with the normotensive controls (MABP = 101 ± 4 mmHg) there was a significant reduction in CBF in

Table 1. Cerebral blood flow (ml 100 g^{-1} min^{-1}) in four regions after right MCA occlusion in normotensive and hypotensive rats

Group	Electrode position				Mean BP (mmHg ± SE)
	Right frontal	Right parietal	Left frontal	Left parietal	
Normotensive (*n* = 7)	41.5 ± 2.8	38.2 ± 3.5	60.1 ± 6.0	59.1 ± 4.4	101.4 ± 3.6
Hypotensive (*n* = 6)	28.0* ± 4.4	26.5* ± 2.5	44.9 ± 3.6	43.8* ± 2.3	69.8* ± 1.3

* = $p < 0.05$ (between normotensive and hypotensive animals)

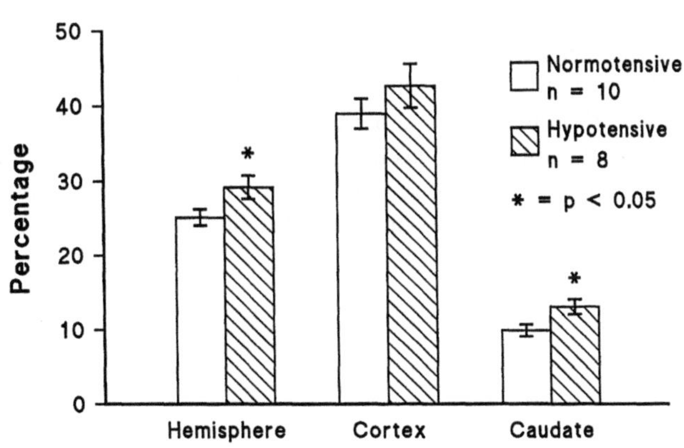

Fig. 1. Infarct size (percentage) measured by TTC perfusion in normotensive and hypotensive (70 mmHg) rats following right MCA occlusion

Table 2. Brain specific gravity following right MCA occlusion in normotensive and hypotensive rats

Group	Side	Cortex	White matter	Caudate	Cerebellum
Normotensive	Right	1.0493*	1.0466	1.0445	1.0532
BP = 101.4		± 0.0011	± 0.0009	± 0.0010	± 0.0008
± 3.6 mmHg*	Left	1.0526	1.0499	1.0528	1.0523
($n = 7$)		± 0.0007	± 0.0011	± 0.0012	± 0.0011
Hypotensive	Right	1.0455	1.0477	1.0448	1.0526
BP = 69.8		± 0.0013	± 0.0006	± 0.0017	± 0.0018
± 1.3 mmHg*	Left	1.0508	1.0465	1.0507	1.0530
($n = 6$)		± 0.0008	± 0.0008	± 0.0010	± 0.0009

* $p < 0.05$ (between normotensive and hypotensive animals)

the right frontal and parietal regions (Table 1) during the 30 min of occlusion. The infarct size (as measured at 9 mm anterior to the interaural line) was significantly larger in the ipsilateral hemisphere of hypotensive animals, mainly because of a significant increase in size of the lesion in the caudate nucleaus (Fig. 1). The degree of brain oedema in the cortex following MCA occlusion with hypotension was significantly greater than in the normotensive group (Table 2).

Carotid Occlusion and Hypotension in the Rat

Cerebral blood flow with carbon-14 IAP autoradiography at 45 mmHg was significantly lower in the deeper layers of the cerebral cortex following carotid occlusion compared with hypotensive animals with patent internal carotid arteries (Figs. 2, 3). This pattern was evident in both the frontal and visual cortex of the ipsilateral hemisphere (Fig. 4). Neuropathological examination demonstrated IBD in the deeper layers of the cortex where CBF was lowest.

Carotid Occlusion and Stenosis with Haemorrhagic Hypotension in Baboons

Cerebral blood flow measurement with xenon-133 at each decrement of MABP in normal animals did not differ significantly from those with a 90% ispilateral internal carotid stenosis (Fig. 5). By contrast there was an ipsilateral loss of autoregulation in animals with IC occlusion (Fig. 6). CBF measured with carbon-14 IAP autoradiography at 30 mmHg showed a reduction in CBF in the arterial boundary zones following ICA occlusion which was not present with hypotension alone (Fig. 7). Neuropathological studies demonstrated IBD in the arterial boundery zone between the anterior and middle cerebral arteries on both sides, but especially on the side of the ICA occlusion.

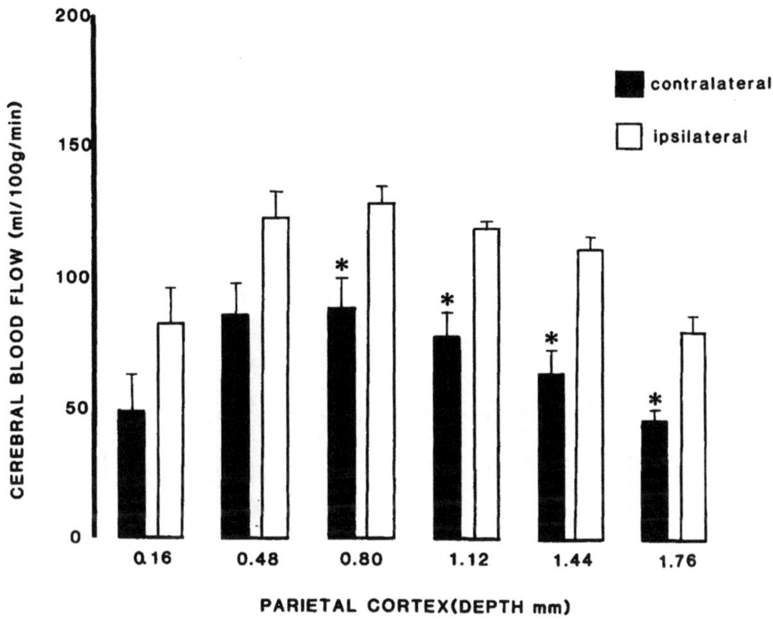

Fig. 2. Cerebral blood flow determined by carbon-14 autoradiography with hypotension and internal carotid occlusion in the rat. * indicates a significant difference (P<0.05) between ipsilateral and contralateral hemispheres

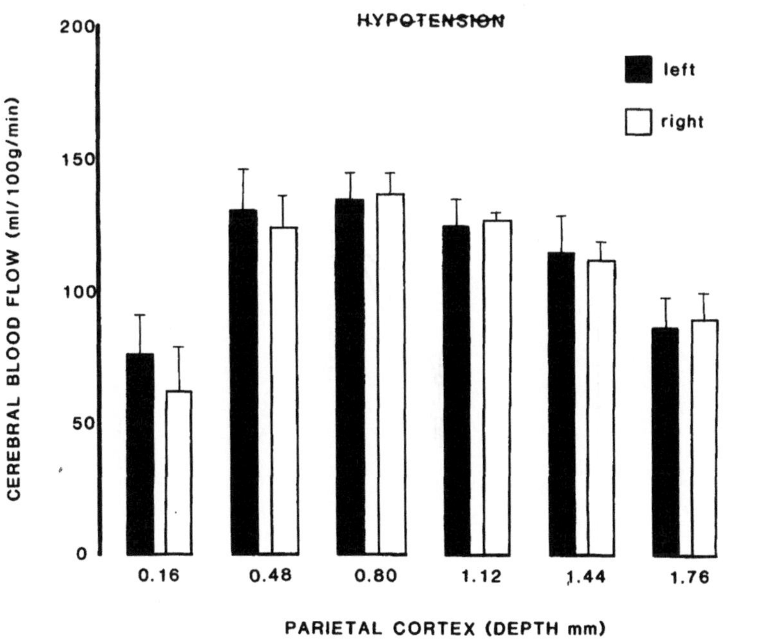

Fig. 3. Cerebral blood flow determined by carbon-14 autoradiography with hypotension and patent internal carotid arteries

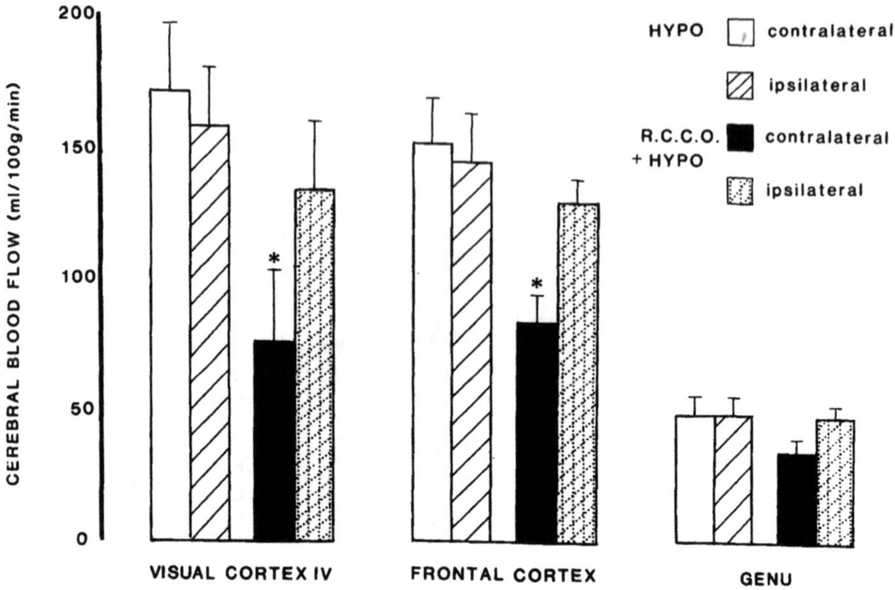

Fig. 4. Cerebral blood flow with carbon-14 autoradiography in rats with hypotension and internal carotid occlusion compared with normal animals with hypotension: different cortical areas. * indicates a significant difference (P<0.05) between ipsilateral and contralateral hemispheres

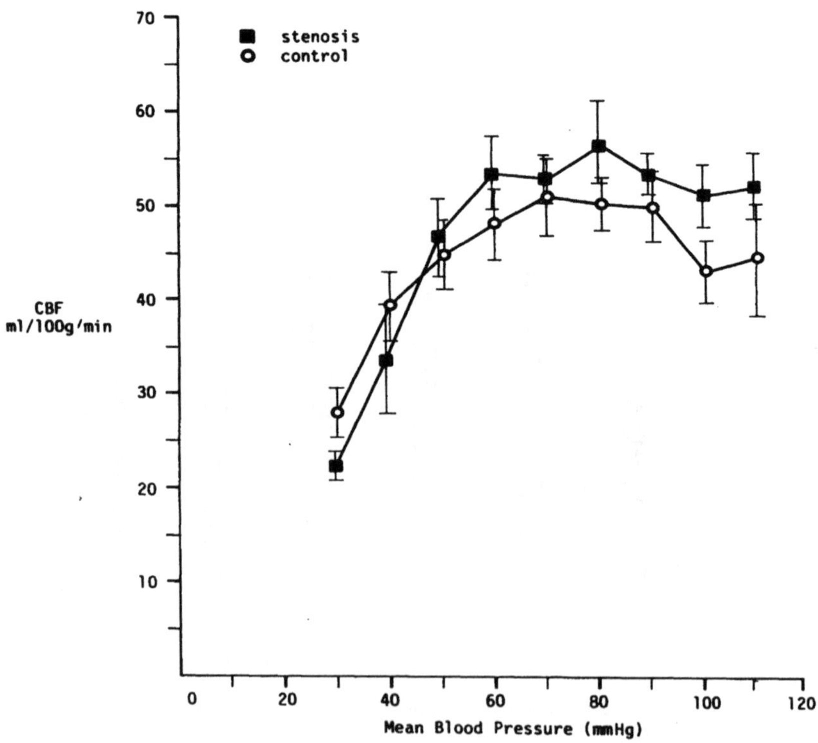

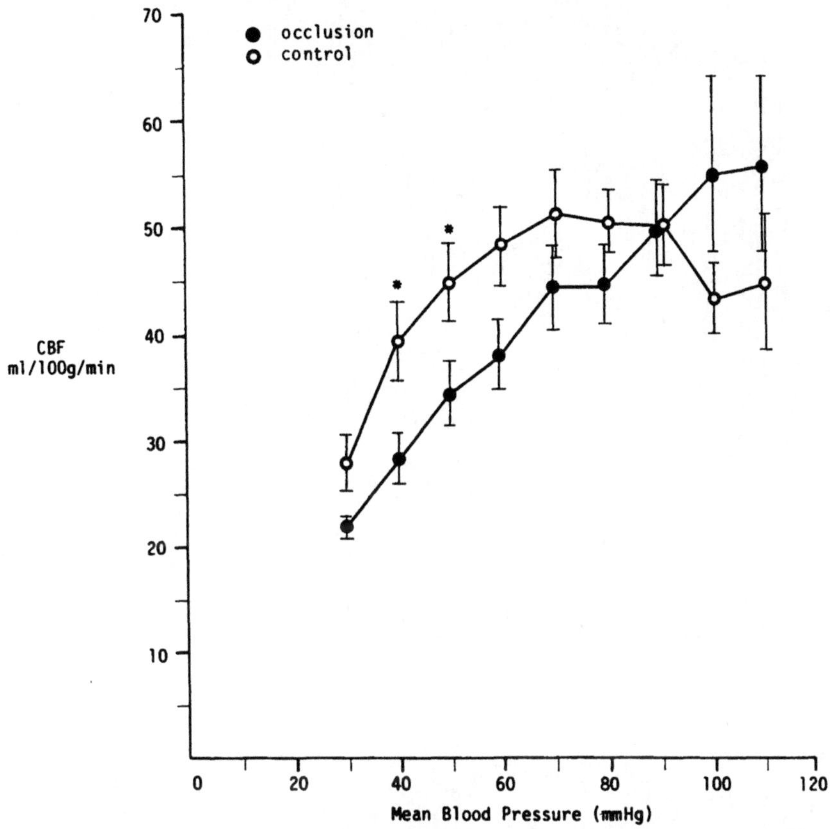

Fig. 6. Cerebral blood flow with xenon-133 at each level of MABP from 30 to 110 mmHg in normal animals and in baboons with ipsilateral internal carotid occlusion. * indicates a significant difference between animals with patent and occluded carotids

◁ **Fig. 5.** Cerebral blood flow with xenon-133 at each level of MABP from 30 to 110 mmHg in normal animals and in baboons with ipsilateral 90% internal carotid stenosis

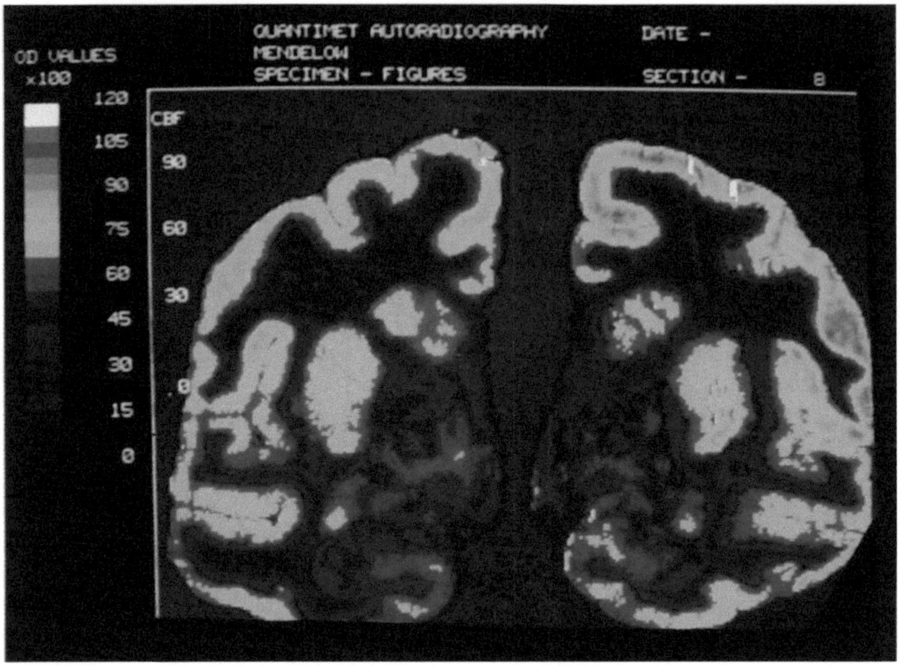

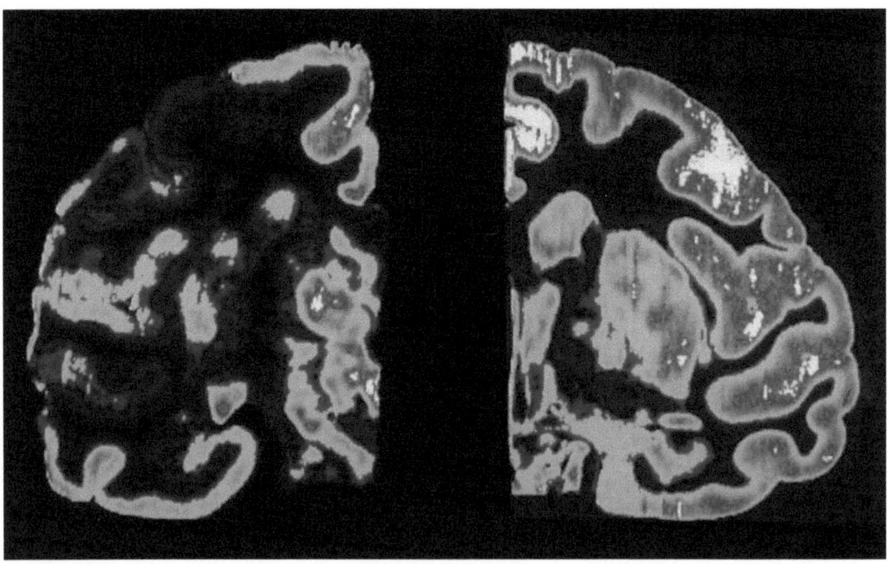

Fig. 7. Cerebral blood flow with carbon-14 autoradiography in baboons with profound hypotension (30 mmHg) with both IC arteries patent (top) and with the right IC artery occluded (bottom).

Discussion

These studies have demonstrated that haemorrhagic hypotension leads to a reduction in CBF which exceeds that seen with vascular occlusion alone. Furthermore, the level of hypotension at which this reduction in CBF takes place is considered to lie within the normal range of autoregulation for intact animals (Harper 1966). In the primate studies haemorrhagic hypotension produced loss of autoregulation with carotid occlusion, but not with the 90% carotid stenosis. In the rat MCA occlusion model, the reduction in CBF was greater with a level of MABP (70 mmHg) still within the accepted range of autoregulation. The area of IBD was larger with haemorrhagic hypotension and, in both the primate and rat ICA occlusion models, it occured within the arterial boundary zones and in the deeper layers of the cortex where the CBF reduction was maximal.

The loss of autoregulation demonstrated here is in agreement with other studies which have also shown a reduction in flow in the penumbral region following MCA occlusion (Dirnagl and Pulsinelli 1990). This consistent finding therefore applies to different species with different types of vascular occlusion from different laboratories. It suggests that maintenance of CPP is important at the time of vascular occlusion and in the subsequent phase during which flow through the collateral circulation may be developing. This has relevance not only to occlusive stroke but also to those clinical conditions in which the mechanism of brain damage is ischaemia as for example in head injury (Graham et al. 1989) and subarachnoid haemorrhage (Crompton 1964).

It is well known that maintenance of CPP is important in head injury and SAH is well known and clinical studies have suggested that CBF is passively dependent upon CPP in SAH (Farrar et al. 1981; Mendelow et al. 1986). In head injury, improvement in CPP with mannitol has also been shown to improve CBF (Mendelow et al. 1985).

This emphasizes that the maintenance of CPP is essential in all these clinical situations: occlusive stroke, head injury and subarachnoid haemorrhage. This is a well-recognized phenomenon but the question arises as to whether increased CPP beyond normal will further improve CBF and limit IBD. Hypertensive and hypervolaemic treatment is well recognized as a form of treatment of delayed cerebral ischaemia in SAH (Kassell et al. 1982). In head injury McGraw (1989) has suggested that a CPP of 80 mmHg or more may be associated with a better outcome than with a CPP of 50 mmHg. Studies in patients with head injury at Newcastle have confirmed this finding (Table 3) (Chambers et al. 1990, unpublished data). Further clinical studies in head injury have indicated that higher levels of CPP (70–80 mmHg) are associated with improved outcome (Rosner and Rosner 1992).

Table 3. Minimum averaged CPP for 1 h in relation to outcome from head injury

	CPP (mmHg)					
	< 40	40–49	50–59	60–69	70–79	80–89
Good recovery	1	1	5	5	4	3
Moderate disability	1	1	1	0	0	0
Severe disability	3	5	2	3	2	0
Vegetative/dead	5	0	2	5	3	1

In occlusive stroke there also may be a place for elevation of CPP, as was originally suggested by Denny-Brown (1951).

In all these situations there is the danger that increased blood pressure may aggravate brain oedema if blood-brain barrier damage has already occurred. This is more likely if hypertensive treatment is delayed. For this reason elevation of CPP is most likely to be beneficial if initiated very early in the development of ischaemia.

In the experimental studies presented here, the reduction in BP occurred at the time of the large vessels occlusion, and it may be that it is only during this early phase that maintenance of BP is important. One implication is that inadvertent reduction of MABP may adversely affect infarct size in stroke, head injury, and SAH. There are many other recognized examples of this phenomenon (Ledingham and Rajagopalan 1979; Graham 1975; Ross Russell and Bharuchia 1978). These findings therefore suggest that the MABP may have profound effects on the pattern and distribution of ischaemia in these clinical situations. Boundary zone regions seem to be the most vulnerable and further clinical studies, which are able to give high-quality images of the distribution of CBF, should be directed toward evaluating the effect of CPP on the distribution of ischaemia.

Acknowledgements. Our thanks go to Miss A. Robinson for her careful preparation of the manuscript. These studies were supported by a grant from the Scottish Home and Health Department in Glasgow and from the Northern Regional Health Authority in Newcastle. Mr. P. Kane was in receipt of a Harker Foundation Fellowship.

References

Chambers IR, Strachan RD, Kane PJ, Clark A, Mendelow AD (1991) Closed loop blood pressure control for cerebral perfusion studies. Clin Phys Physiol Meas 12:171–176

Crompton MR (1964) Infarction following the rupture of cerebral berry aneurysms. Brain 87:263

Denny-Brown D (1951) The treatment of recurrent cerebrovascular symptoms and the question of "vasopasm". Med Clin North Am 35:1457–1474

Dirnagl U, Pulsinelli W (1990) Autoregulation of cerebral blood flow in experimental focal ischaemia. J Cereb Blood Flow Metab 10:327–336

Farrar JK, Gamache FW, Ferguson GG, Barker J, Valkey GP, Drake CG (1981) Effects of profound hypotension on cerebral blood flow during surgery for intracranial aneurysms. J Neurosurg 55:857–864

Fitch W, Jones JV, Graham DI, et al. (1978) Effects of hypotension induced by halothane on the cerebral circulation in baboons with experimental renovascular hypertension. Br J Anaesth 50:119–125

Graham DI (1985) Ischaemic brain damage of cerebral perfusion failure type following treatment for severe hypertension. Br med J 4:737

Graham DI, Ford I, Adams JH, Doyle D, Teasdale GM, Lawrence AE, McLellan DR (1989) Ischaemic brain damage is still common in fatal non-missile head injury. J Neurol Neurosurg Psychiatry 52:346–350

Harper AM (1966) Autoregulation of cerebral blood flow: influence of the arterial blood pressure on the blood flow through the cerebral cortex. J Neurol Neurosurg Psychiatry 29:398–403

Kassell NF, Peerless SJ, Durward QJ, et al. (1982) Treatment of ischaemic deficits from vasospasm with intravascular volume expansion and induced arterial hypertension. Neurosurgery 11:337–343

Ledingham JGG, Rojagopalan B (1979) Cerebral complications in the treatment of accelerated hypertension. Q J Med 48:25

McGraw CP (1989) A cerebral perfusion pressure of greater than 80 mmHg is more beneficial. In: Hoff JT, Betz AL (eds) Intracranial pressure VII. Springer, Berlin Heidelberg New York, pp 839–841

Mendelow AD, Teasdale GM, Russell T, Flood J, Patterson J, Murray GD (1985) Effect of mannitol on cerebral blood flow and cerebral perfusion pressure in human head injury. J Neurosurg 63:43–48

Mendelow AD, Dharker S, Patterson J, Nath F, Teasdale GM (1986) The dopamine withdrawal test following surgery for intracranial aneurysms. J Neurol Neurosurg Psychiatry 49:35–38

Park CK, Mendelow AD, Graham DI, McCulloch J, Teasdale GM (1989) Correlation of triphenyl tetrazolium chloride perfusion staining with conventional neurohistology in the detection of early brain ischaemia. J Neuropathol Appl Neurobiol 14:289–298

Rosner MJ, Rosner SD (1992) Cerebral perfusion pressure management of head injury. In: Avezaat CJJ (ed) ICP and craniospinal dynamics. Springer, Berlin Heidelberg New York (in press)

Ross Russell RWK, Bharuchia N (1978) The recognition and prevention of border zone cerebral ischaemia during carotid surgery. Q J Med 47:303

Sakurada O, Kennedy C, Jehle JW, Brown JD, Carbin JL, Sokoloff L (1978) Measurement of local cerebral blood flow with iodo C-14 antipyrine. Am J Physiol 234:H59–H66

Tamura A, Graham DI, McCulloch J, Teasdale GM (1981) Focal cerebral ischaemia in the rat. I. Description of technique and early neuropathological consequences following middle cerebral artery occlusion. J Cereb Blood Flow Metab 1:53–60

Tuor UI, Fitch W, Graham DI, Mendelow AD (1986) Comparison of quantitative autoradiographic and 133-xenon clearance methods: correlation of grey and white matter cerebral blood flow with compartmental blood flow indices. J Cereb Blood Flow Metab 6:481–485

Wise G, Sutter R, Burkholder J (1972) The treatment of brain ischaemia with vasopressor drugs. Stroke 3:135–140

Young W (1980) H2 clearance measurement of blood flow: a review of technique and polarographic principles. Stroke 11:552–564

Effects of Acetazolamide on EEG and Intracranial Pressure

K. Holl, H. E. Heissler, E. H. Rzesacz, K. Weissenborn, M. N. Nemati,
M. R. Gaab, B. Haubitz, and H. Dietz

Introduction

The investigation of cerebral blood flow (CBF) at rest makes it possible to detect computed tomography (CT)-negative low flow areas (Lassen et al. 1983). Differentiation in areas of lowered metabolism due to incomplete infarction or regions of disturbed blood flow resulting from a diminished cerebrovascular reserve cannot be achieved by CBF studies at rest alone (Holl et al. 1989). Only CBF investigation before and after application of a vasodilator stimulus enables the magnitude of the current reserve in the cerebral vasculature to be estimated.

Various working groups use the intravenous administration of acetazolamide (Diamox) as vasodilator stimulus to determine the cerebrovascular reserve as an alternative to the inhalation of CO_2 or carefully directed variations in blood pressure (Vorstrup et al. 1984; Kreisig et al. 1987; Gaab et al. 1989). For practical reasons, because of its good compliance the unphysiological acetazolamide stimulus is to be preferred to the physiological stimulus. At present there is no agreement about how acetazolamide acts to increase CBF. The majority of authors suppose there is an artificial CO_2 storage caused by a reversible blockade of the carbonic anhydrase (Ehrenreich et al. 1961; Gotoh et al. 1966). In this case after acetazolamide administration the EEG is supposed to alter as it does when inhaling CO_2.

Acetazolamide as an antiepileptic drug was administered orally or intravenously in the past (Woodbury and Kemp 1982). In epileptics with an altered individual EEG a pronounced normalization of the EEG especially an increase in the amplitude and the regularity in the alpha rhythm could be observed (Pateisky and Petsche 1957). Concomitantly, their clinical status improved. After intravenous administration typical EEG alterations occur immediately in epileptic patients (Saldìas et al. 1957).

In spite of this generally known effect of acetazolamide on the EEG in epileptics little is known about potential EEG alterations in normal subjects.

The subject of this study is the EEG response to acetazolamide in nonepileptics. The results will be discussed with respect to the probably different modes of action of acetazolamide and CO_2. Examination of the cerebrovascular reserve by means of a substance resulting in a global and permanent vasodilation affects the cerebrovascular system unphysiologically. A very characteristic side effect of a cerebrovascular vasodilation is elevation of the intracranial pressure (ICP). The present study also aims to describe quantitatively the expected pressure increase, and to define a possibly endangered group of patients.

Materials and Methods

In the past few years use of the Xe-CT technique to examine the CBF was described exhaustively by various working groups (Drayer et al. 1978; Gur et al. 1982; Kohmura et al. 1986). In our clinic 520 Xe-CT-CBF studies were carried out before and after acetazolamide administration to 400 patients during a 42-month period. In some of these patients the EEG and the ICP were monitored before, during, and after acetazolamide administration. The general conditions for these studies were always organized not to interfere with the CBF examination. If scientific and clinical interests collided the relevant clinical CBF studies were always undertaken preferentially. As a principle 1 g acetazolamide was infused into a brachial vein within 5 min with the patient lying in the supine position on the CT table.

EEG Studies

Patients

During a period of 8 months we performed 110 Xe-CT-CBF studies before, and after, acetazolamide administration in 92 patients. In 49 randomly selected patients 55 power EEG investigations were undertaken. For diagnoses refer to Table 1. The protocol and performance of the EEG investigations were arranged following the recommendations for pharmaco-EEG studies (Expert Group 1982).

Preparation of Patients

Patients were interviewed and informed about the intentions underlying the additional EEG investigation, and their agreement was obtained. About 2 h before the Xe-CT study chlorided silver elextrodes were positioned and fixed with collodion on the unshaved scalp of the patient. Optimally, the position of the electrodes should cover the surface of the scalp as well as permit undisturbed CT study. Moreover, the international 10/20 system should be followed. The electrode scheme complying with these requirements was frontal (F3, F4), central (C3, C4), parietal (P3, P4), temporal (T3, T4), and a bipolar star connection against the vertex electrode Cz (Fig. 1). The lead wires were

Table 1. Electroencephalogram sample statistics

	No. of patients	No. of XE-CT studies	Age (years)	Male	Female	Diagnosis		
						Intracranial tumor	Vascular occlusive disease	Other
XE-CT-CBF studies with acetazolamide	92	110	52 ± 14	51	41	40	21	31
EEG sample	49	55	55 ± 12	33	16	24	18	7

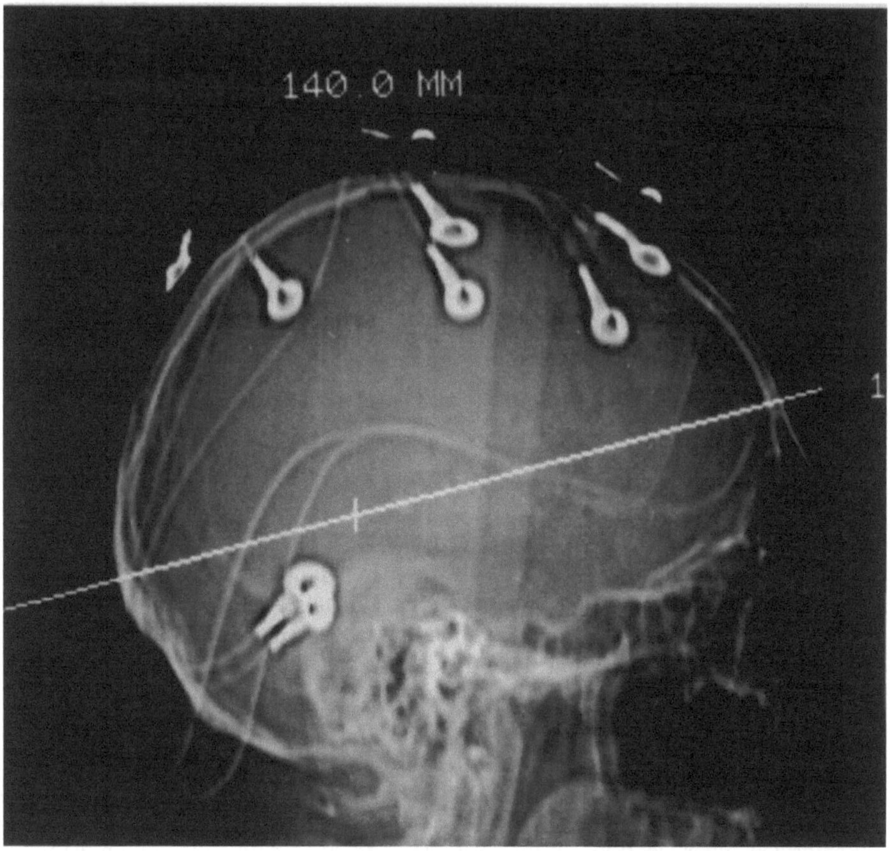

Electrode Connection

channel 1	F3 - Cz	channel 2	Cz - F4
channel 3	C3 - Cz	channel 4	Cz - C4
channel 5	P3 - Cz	channel 6	Cz - P4
channel 7	T3 - Cz	channel 8	Cz - T4

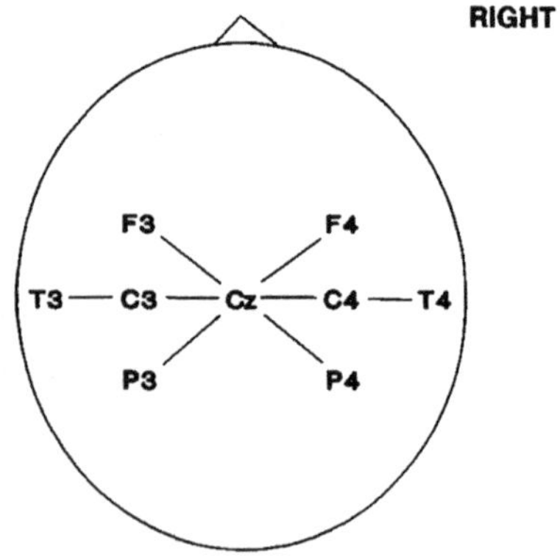

Fig. 1. Electroencephalogram electrodes pictured from scout view, the record diagram, and electrode connections. Placement of electrodes according to the international 10/20 system

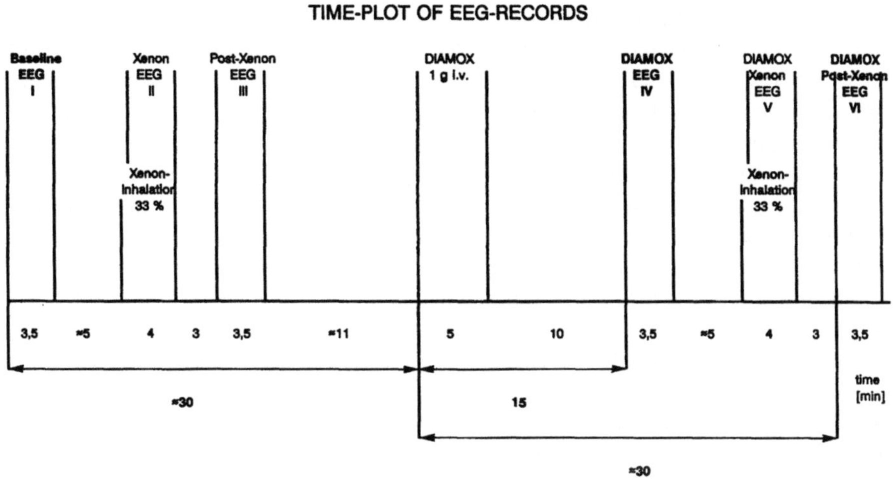

Fig. 2. Survey of the total EEG investigation. In the present study the records of interest were baseline record I (30 min before acetazolamide administration), record IV (at 15 min after acetazolamide administration), and record VI (30 min after acetazolamide administration)

passed through the gantry of the computer tomograph (GE 9800) and connected to eight channels.

EEG Recording

For reasons of data reduction the EEG was not recorded continuously. Therefore, only six EEG records, each of at least 3 min duration, were recorded at fixed times (Fig. 2). Each record consisted of eight channels. In this paper the survey of the EEG response to acetazolamide was compiled from baseline record I and records IV and VI. The baseline record I was 30 min before acetazolamide administration, and records IV and VI 15 and 30 min after administration, respectively. The original EEG was amplified (Mingograph 21, Siemens), filtered (cutoff frequencies at 1.5 and 70 Hz), sampled (sampling frequency 170 Hz), digitized, and stored on computer mass storage (PC-AT 80386/16 MHz, Epson).

Data Analysis

After off-line artifact elimination the EEG time-series were subdivided into blocks of 30 s duration which were subsequently transformed into the frequency domain (Dummermuth 1973). Because of the enormous amount of spectral data the further description was based on adequate spectral parameters being matched to the standard EEG waveforms. Proceeding from the classification into delta (0.5–3.5 Hz), theta (3.5–7.5 Hz), alpha (7.5–12.5 Hz), and beta (>12.5 Hz) frequency bands, the spectral frequency distribution could be described with a relatively small number of parameters. The absolute spectral power of an arbitrary frequency band was the integral of spectral power within the edge frequencies of that band. The median was the frequency at which the integral of the spectral power was 50% of the absolute spectral power, integrating from one edge frequency to the other. The frequency range between 10% and 90% of the absolute spectral power was denoted as the 80% range. It was represented by the difference of the frequency at the 90% and the frequency at the 10% quantile of the absolute power.

For further statistical analysis eight spectral parameters were chosen. A rough estimation of the spectral properties was obtained from median and total power of the spectrum. For detailed assessment of the frequency band between 3.5 and 12.5 Hz the median of the integrated alpha and theta bands was calculated. As a measure of the area under the peak the 80% range was calculated for the alpha band. Additionally, the absolute spectral power in all frequency bands was analyzed. Each of the eight EEG parameters was tested for all eight channels with respect to trends and level.

Trend of EEG parameters

For trend analysis 55 EEG investigations were recorded in 49 patients. In the following, the time courses of the individual EEG parameters of records I, IV, and VI will be designated as the trend. The trend of a parameter is represented by the slope of the linear regression function which obeys the least square error criterion. The recording interval was at least 3 min, which was subdivided into epochs of 30 s duration. Therefore, there were at least six values for any parameter per record and channel in one patient. Subsequently the slope was statistically tested for significance using the Kolmogorov-Smirnov one-sample test.
The trend describes the systematic changes of EEG parameters with time.

Level of EEG parameters

This analysis is based on the data of the previous paragraph. The change in the individual EEG parameters of records IV and VI in relation to the baseline record I will be designated as level. The level of a parameter is caculated from the quotient of parameter mean values for record I and record IV or VI, respectively. The parameter mean values were calculated after a delay of 3 min from the beginning of the record. As the parameters were not distributed in a gaussian fashion, the mean values were compared utilizing the nonparametric paired Wilcoxon test. The level describes the relative parameter changes of records IV or VI, respectively, in relation to baseline record I.

Intracranial Pressure

Patients (Tables 3, 4)

During 26 months an epidural pressure transducer was implanted for further hydrocephalus diagnostics into 16 patients with an average age of 50.5±16 years. Additionally, a Xe-CT-CBF study with acetazolamide was undertaken. The patients showed a variety of diagnoses. In no case were the diagnostic procedures such as long-term pressure monitoring and volume-pressure testing completed at the time of the CBF study. Retrospectively, in half the patients the implantation of a shunt device was indicated on clinical, morphological, and functional criteria. Thus, all patients could be classified into two groups with disturbed (group I) or normal CSF dynamics (group II).

Intracranial Pressure Monitoring

The intracranial pressure was measured with an epidural pressure transducer (Gaeltec ICT/b transducer) in all patients. The transducer was implanted through a frontal burr hole with the patient under local anesthesia. The ICP signal was registered continuously for at least 48 h. During the whole Xe-CT investigation with acetazolamide, the ICP was registered continuously on a chart recorder. To minimize the systematic error of the measuring device, the scale was adapted to its nonlinear static characteristic. For technical reasons the data of patient No. 12 were discarded. In all patients the arterial blood pressure was measured oscillometrically (DINAMAP 1846 SX, Criticon) at time intervals of 2 min.

Statistics

For the evaluation of data, appropriate statistical methods were used. We applied procedures from SAS 6.03 software implemented on a personal computer (HP Vectra Model 60, Hewlett Packard). As a measure of dispersion the single standard deviation was used.

Results

The injection of 1 g acetazolamide dissolved in 10 ml water over 5 min into a brachial vein was tolerated in virtually all 400 patients. Only a few patients felt a short-term tickling in the finger tips or noticed irritations of taste and smell. For instance, one patient complained that mineral water tasted like dung water, and another was worried by persistently smelling gas. In no case were clinically relevant side effects observed.

Acetazolamide: EEG Studies

Visual Inspection

The baseline record I was standardized during the visual artifact rating. In 37 investigations an alpha-type EEG was found, 5 showing beta waveform. Alternating EEG waveforms occured in 13 records. 20 records were characterized by circumscribed focal areas. Due to acetazolamide administration, qualitative changes in the EEG could not be found, nor did the focal activity reveal any changes in activity.

Spectral Analysis: Trend of EEG Parameters (Table 2)

For all parameters and channels the averages were calculated for records I, IV, and VI.

Record I: 30 Min Before Acetazolamide Administration
A positive trend in the integrated alpha and theta frequencies is evident for the median of channel 8 only. All the other parameters show no systematic changes.

Table 2. Survey of EEG results

EEG parameters	record I; Ch1–Ch8[a]	record IV; Ch1–Ch8		Record VI; Ch1–Ch8	
	Trend	Trend	Level	Trend	Level
Median (total power)	ns	Ch1 ↑*, Ch6 ↓*	ns	ns	ns
Median (alpha + theta power)	Ch8 ↑*	ns	ns	ns	ns
Total spectral power	ns	ns	ns	Ch1↓*, Ch2↓**, Ch4↓*	ns
Delta power	ns	ns	ns	Ch1↓*, Ch2↓*	ns
Theta power	ns	ns	ns	Ch1↓*, Ch2↓**, Ch4↓*, Ch7↓*	ns
Alpha power	ns	ns	ns	Ch1↓*, Ch2↓**, Ch4↓*	ns
Beta power	ns	Ch1↑*	ns	Ch1↓*, Ch2↓*, Ch4↓**	ns
80% range (alpha power)	ns	ns	ns	ns	ns

[a] Ch1–Ch8, EEG channels 1–8; ns, $p > 0.05$; *, $p < 0.05$; **, $p < 0.01$
↑↓ denotes direction of trends (slope of trends)

Record IV: 15 Min After Acetazolamide Administration
The median of the total spectrum depicts a positive trend in channel 1 whereas in channel 6 it is negative. The beta power shows a positive trend for channel 1. All the other parameters showed no significant changes.

Record VI: 30 Min After Acetazolamide Administration
A negative trend in both the total spectral power and the power of the individual frequency bands could be found in several channels; however, no changes in the other parameters became evident.

Spectral Analysis: Level of EEG Parameters (Table 2)

For no parameter and channel could significant deviations from record I be proven for either record IV or record VI.

Spectral Analysis: Considering Diagnosis, Individual EEG Pattern, and Side

There were no statistically significant results, neither in the parameter differences between the diagnostic subgroups and the total population, nor among the subgroups themselves. The influence of diagnoses or of individual EEG patterns on the EEG course could not be proven during examination. This holds true for the categorization of data with respect to the side (left and right), and also for the classification into symptomatic and less symptomatic hemispheres.

Table 3. Intracranial pressure sample statistic: group I (disturbed CSF dynamics)

Patient No.	Age (years)	Sex	Diagnosis	ICP[a] before	ICP after
				Acetazolamide administration	
1	20	f	Opticus glioma	24	70
2	49	f	Hydrocephalus	19	33
3	48	m	SAH	4	16
4	38	f	Aqueduct stenosis	5	19
5	69	m	Hydrocephalus	10	24
6	53	m	Tumor third ventricle	9	54
7	40	m	Hydrocephalus	13	20
8	18	f	Porencephalic cyst	25	55

[a] units, mmHg

Acetazolamide: ICP Studies

After acetazolamide administration the intracranial pressure rose in all patients; 23.5±5.6 min after acetazolamide administration the CBF increase was 45% on average ($p<0.05$). The blood pressure showed no statistically significant changes.

Group I: Disturbed CSF Dynamics (Table 3, Fig. 3)

In this group the intracranial mean pressure amounted to 13.6±7.6 mmHg; 13.1±4.5 min after the start of acetazolamide administration a maximum mean pressure of 36.4±19.2 mmHg was reached ($p<0.05$). In patients Nos. 1, 4, 6, and 7 the pressure levels fell to initial levels within the period of investigation after 27, 40, 22 or 32 min respectively. Extreme pressure responses of 70, 54, and 55 mmHg were observed in patients Nos. 1 and 6 suffering from foramen of Monro blockade and in patient No. 8 with a porencephalic cyst, who complained of being sick 12 min after administration of acetazolamide. All the other patients in this group showed no individual responses.

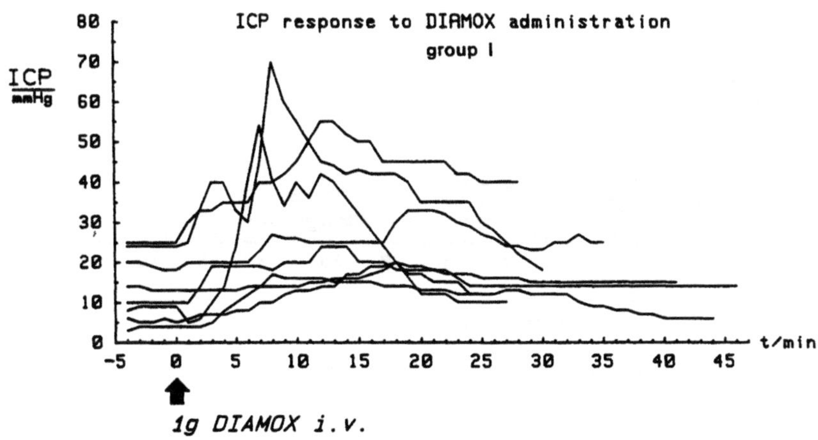

Fig. 3. Group I (disturbed CSF dynamics): plots of individual ICP courses

Table 4. Intracranial pressure sample statistic: group II (normal CSF dynamics)

Patient No.	Age (years)	Sex	Diagnosis	ICP[a] before	ICP after
				Acetazolamide administration	
9	36	f	Atrophy	8	9
10	77	m	Atrophy	7	15
11	65	f	Pineal tumor	4	7
12	51	f	Hemorrhage	_[b]	_[b]
13	43	m	Atrophy	12	20
14	63	f	Atrophy	0	10
15	59	m	Trauma	11	16
16	64	f	Dementia	2	6

[a] Units, mmHg; [b] Missing value

Group II: Normal CSF Dynamics (Table 4, Fig. 4)

The ICP elevations were within clinically unobtrusive ranges. The initial mean pressure was 6.3±4.2 mmHg on average. The maximum pressure was reached at 13.6±1.1 min after starting acetazolamide administration and the peak mean pressure was 11.9±4.8 mmHg ($p<0.01$). There were no individual effects caused by administration of acetazolamide.

Between these two groups under consideration, statistically significant results could only be proven for the intracranial pressure response caused by the acetazolamide stimulus ($p<0.01$): the rise in CBF and the blood pressure showed no systematic differences.

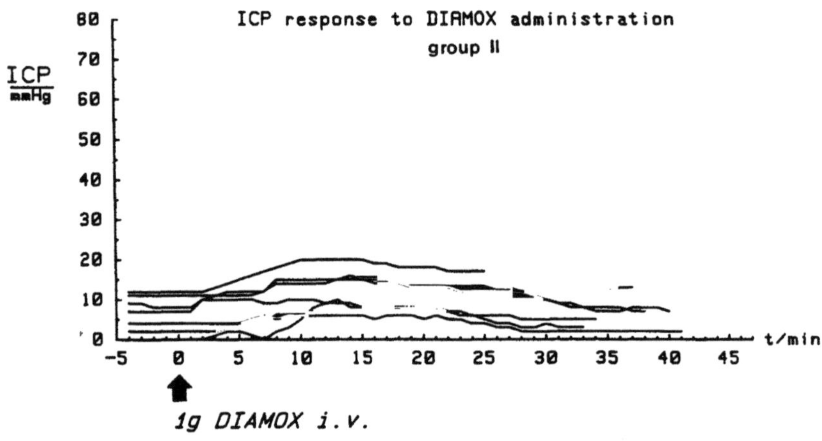

Fig. 4. Group II (normal CSF dynamics): plots of individual ICP courses

Discussion

EEG Studies

In the study under consideration the EEG was recorded in patients who underwent a CBF study with acetazolamide stimulation for clinical reasons. As the clinical management of the patients has always taken priority, only half the patients could be included in the EEG study for a scheduled 8-month period. The selection of patients depended on organizational aspects only, so this population is therefore considered a representative sample.

The EEG was recorded at six fixed times during the CBF study. The results of the records II, III, and V are reported elsewhere. Our experience indicated that the maximum vasodilator response is encountered about 13.5 min after acetazolamide administration (Holl and Heissler, unpublished findings). Thus for evaluation of the acetazolamide effect EEG record IV was used starting 15 min after administration. Record VI starting 15 min later is adequate for observing acetazolamide effects on the EEG. Record VI lies in the 95-min half-life of the acetazolamide effect on the cerebral vessels (Hauge et al. 1983). The occurrence of artifacts decreased toward the end of each record because of adaptation of the patient to the investigation. For the evaluation of parameter levels the EEG of the 3rd min of each record was used exclusively.

The most crucial result of our study is that there are no statistically significant alterations in the mean parameter levels after acetazolamide administration in any EEG channel. The trend of particular parameters was significant in a few channels of records I and IV. Previously, the basline record I showed a significant positive trend in one parameter and channel. Possibly, the sporadic incidence of parameter changes can be attributed to an artificial EEG signal in both records. These artifacts most likely originated from electrodermal and EMG responses which could not have been rejected by previous artifact rating. In opposite order a negative trend was observed throughout in power parameters of several channels in record VI. These parameter variations do not seem to be random or artificial, but rather a result of the preceding xenon inhalation which was terminated 3 min before record VI. At the end of xenon inhalation a positive trend occurs in the power parameters. Concerning the constant parameter level of the 3rd min the negative trend in record VI could therefore be regarded as a decline in parameter values to baseline. This interpretation is more likely because in an earlier report it was found that EEG changes occurred 7 min after inhibition of the xenon inhalation (Holl et al. 1987). Retrospectively, it must be ascertained that the proximity of record VI to the xenon inhalation interfered with the subject of our study.

Considering all the facts, the intravenous administration of 1 g acetazolamide over 5 min cannot be shown to lead to any definite alterations of the EEG, in spite of the application of sophisticated analyses.

In the literature no details were found about EEG responses to acetazolamide in normal subjects. Meyer et al. (1961) reported that there was no immediate effect of acetazolamide (15–25 mg/kg) on the normal EEG in monkeys – but after 10 min slight slowing in the EEG was seen in two experiments. In contrast Falbriard and Gangloff (1955) stated that acetazolamide (100 mg/kg) caused no change in the excitability of cortical cells in rabbits.

Since the study by Ehrenreich et al. (1961), it has been reported repeatedly that the magnitude of the effects on CBF of both 1 g acetazolamide and the inhalation of 5 vol% CO_2 is similar (Fazekas and Alman 1963; Vorstrup et al. 1984). In earlier reports it was supposed that both the quantitative effect and the mode of action were similar. Based on that widespread assumption, acetazolamide blocks the carbonic anhydrase, which results in storage of CO_2 in the brain (Gotoh et al. 1966; Brzezinski et al. 1967; Woodbury and Kemp 1982). Therefore in both CO_2 inhalation and in acetazolamide administration the dilation of the arterioles would be a consequence of an increase in brain tissue CO_2. This concept, however, does not explain the unaltered EEG observed after acetazolamide administration, whereas an equivalent CO_2 stimulus affects the EEG remarkably (Gibbs et al. 1940; Gellhorn 1953; Krnjević et al. 1965). Moreover, the clinical experience that CO_2 but not acetazolamide frequently caused dyspnea would not correspond with the assumption of an uniform mode of action. As the decrease in extracellular pH (pH_e) is well documented for both stimuli, only the use of magnetic resonance imaging (MRI) enabled intracellular pH (pH_i;) to be measured in man. As expected, CO_2 inhalation decreases pH_i, while after acetazolamide administration surprisingly it remains constant (Jensen et al. 1988; Vorstrup et al. 1989). CO_2 inhalation and blockade of carbonic anhydrase commonly increase CBF and reduce the pH_e. This suggests a causal link might be constructed between these effects. In their effects on pH_i acetazolamide and CO_2 are different. Moreover, it is suggested that such side effects as dyspnea, hyperventilation, blood pressure changes, and the EEG alterations which appear using CO_2 stimulus can be traced back to the CO_2-induced decrease in pH_i.

Intracranial Pressure Studies

The effect of acetazolamide on the cerebral vasculature has been investigated by numerous authors using different methods. The increases in blood flow were reported to be 25%–75% (Hauge et al. 1983; Vorstrup et al. 1984; Leinsinger et al. 1988; Sorteberg et al. 1989). In 16 patients with disturbed CSF dynamics an epidural pressure transducer was implanted for further diagnostics and a Xe-CT-CBF study was untertaken. It was found that 23.5±5.6 min after acetazolamide administration CBF increased on average by 45% and lay in the midrange compared with reference values in the literature. The difference in the average CBF increase between groups I and II was not significant. In animal experiments, Knopp et al. (1957) reported a rise in CSF pressure for the first time, which was traced back to an intracranial vascular dilation. Coppen and Russell (1957) also found an increase in CSF pressure in seven epileptic patients after acetazolamide administration (20 mg/kg).

As expected, an endogenous volume load due to acetazolamide administration raised the intracranial pressure in all patients. This transiently induced ICP transient reached its maximum at the same time as the CBF response, which was about 13.5 min after administration. Within the half-life of the acetazolamide effect on CBF, the pressure fell to its initial level again (Holl and Heissler, unpublished findings). Obviously the compensating properties of the CSF compartment restricted the duration of the pressure wave. The differing ICP elevations in group I and II could only be explained by different cerebrospinal compliances. The average increase in CBF and thus the endogenous volume load were equal in both groups. In dogs with artifically reduced intracranial volume reserve a severe rise in ICP to dangerous levels after acetazolamide was noticed by Wilkinson (1989). The present results confirm his observations in principle. However, it is noteworthy that, in spite of considerable ICP rises up to 50–70 mmHg in patients of group I, only in one patient were clinical symptoms encountered. Obviously, pressure elevations caused by an increase in perfusion would be better tolerated than equivalent pressure changes induced by extravascular processes.

However, it cannot be excluded that reactions like vomiting can occur in individual cases depending on cerebrospinal compliance. The application of CBF-measuring methods using tracer inhalation via face mask could result in perilous situations. It should be stated that patients who would normally undergo a CBF study are rather characterized by features of group II than of group I. The ICP increases after acetazolamide administration in group II were clinically still not relevant (Holl et al. 1990).

Conclusion

To determine cerebral vascular reserve, CO_2 and acetazolamide are nowadays available as vasodilator stimuli. The intravenous administration of 1 g acetazolamide or the inhalation of 5–7 vol% CO_2 results in an equivalent response. Therefore, both methods are of equal standing concerning their diagnostic value. While the inhalation of CO_2 causes a severe shortness of breath and distinct alterations in the EEG, the clinical symptoms observed by the use of acetazolamide are comparatively minor and EEG responses can not be shown. This discrepancy could originate from the different effects of CO_2 and acetazolamide on the intracellular pH. It might be stated that, for an equivalent response in CBF, a physiological CO_2 stimulation leads to remarkable cellular alterations in contrast to the unphysiological acetazolamide stimulus. Thus, for intended use of the vasodilator effect acetazolamide should be given preference over CO_2. Basically, it must be supposed that an endogenous volume load caused by vasodilation depending on the cerebrospinal fluid (CSF) volume reserve leads to a rise in intracranial pressure. After acetazolamide administration, ICP in patients with reduced CSF volume reserve reaches values as high as 70 mmHg. This fact does not contraindicate acetazolamide administration, as the magnitude of the pressure response depends on the extent of vasodilation and not on the stimulus. An increase in ICP caused by vasodilation will obviously be better tolerated than ICP elevations originating in other ways, for a CBF increase occurs concomitantly in spite of a reduction of cerebral perfusion pressure. Although the vasodilator effect of acetazolamide has a half-life of 95 min, the ICP reaches its initial level within 20–40 min in four patients.

It should be emphasized that a vasodilation resulting from CO_2 can be better controlled than that induced by acetazolamide. Hence, for determination of the cerebral vascular reserve in patients with increased ICP or reduced CSF volume reserve respectively, CO_2 is to be preferred to acetazolamide for reasons of security. Such an extreme case is an exception in routine CBF studies. Because of the reasons mentioned above, in the majority of cerebrovascular insufficient patients acetazolamide should take precedence as stimulus for the examination of cerebral vascular reserve.

Acknowledgements. We wish to express our gratitude to Frau Swanhild Fischer for computer-assisted preparation of the manuscript and graphic enhancement of this publication. We are also grateful for editorial comments on translation of Dr. Paul Debbage, Anatomische Anstalten, University of Munich.

References

Brzezinski J, Källquist Å, Siesjö BK (1967) Mean carbon dioxide tension in the brain after carbonic anhydrase inhibition. J Physiol (Lond) 188:13–23

Coppen AJ, Russel GFM (1957) Effect of intravenous acetazolamide on cerebrospinal fluid pressure. Lancet 1:926–927

Drayer BP, Wolfson SK Jr, Reinmuth OM (1978) Xenon enhanced CT for analysis of cerebral integrity, perfusion and blood flow. Stroke 9:123–130

Dummermuth G (1973) Numerical spectral analysis of the electroencephalogram. In: Matousek M (ed) Handbook of electroencephalography and clinical neurophysiology, vol 5 A Elsevier, Amsterdam, pp 33–60

Ehrenreich DL, Burns RA, Alman RW, Fazekas JF (1961) Influence of acetazolamide on cerebral blood flow. Arch Neurol 5:125–130

Expert Group of the Federal Health Office, Institute for Drugs (1982) Guidelines for pharmaco-EEG studies in man. Pharmacopsychiatry 15:107–108

Falbriard A, Gangloff H (1955) Action d'un inhibiteur de la carboanhydrase, l'acétazolamide, sur l'excitabilité du cortex, du thalamus et du rhinencéphale. Experientia 11:234–235

Fazekas JF, Alman RW (1983) Vasodilators in cerebral vascular insufficiency. Am J Med Sci 70:68/410–74/416

Gaab MR, Holl K, Nemati MN, Rzesacz E, Becker H, Dietz H (1989) Mapping of rCBF and cerebrovascular reserve capacity by stable Xenon-CT in cerebrovascular disease: pathophysiological aspects and effects of operative therapy. Psychiatry Res 29:309–312

Gellhorn E (1953) On the physiological action of carbon dioxide on cortex and hypothalamus. Electroencephalogr Clin Neurophysiol 5:401–413

Gibbs FA, Williams D, Gibbs EL (1940) Modification of the cortical frequency spectrum by changes in CO_2, blood sugar, and O_2. J Neurophysiol 3:49–58

Gotoh F, Meyer JS, Tomita M (1966) Carbonic anhydrase inhibition and cerebral venous blood gases and ions in man. Arch Intern med 117:39–46

Gur D, Wolfson SK Jr, Yonas H (1982) Progress in cerebrovascular disease: local cerebral blood flow by xenon enhanced CT. Stroke 13:750–758

Hauge A, Nicolaysen G, Thorensen M (1983) Acute effects of acetazolamide on cerebral blood flow in man. Acta Physiol Scand 117:233–239

Holl K, Heissler HE, Nemati N, Gaab MR, Haubitz B, Becker H (1990) Die Wirkung der Acetazolamid-induzierten, endogenen Volumenbelastung des zerebrospinalen Systems auf den intrakraniellen Druck. Neurochirurgia (Stuttg) 33:29–36

Holl K, Nemati N, Heissler HE, Gaab MR, Haubitz B, Becker H, Dietz H (1989) Chronic cerebrovascular insufficiency on the Xenon CT scan. Neurosurg Rev 12:205–210

Holl K, Nemati N, Kohmura E, Gaab MR, Samii M (1987) Stable-xenon-CT: effects of xenon inhalation on EEG and cardio-respiratory parameters in the human. Acta Neurochir (Wien) 87:129–133

Jensen KE, Thomsen C, Henriksen O (1988) In vivo measurement of intracellular pH in human brain during different tensions of carbon dioxide in arterial blood. A ^{31}P-NMR study. Acta Physiol Scand 134:295–298

Knopp LM, Atkinson JR, Ward AA (1957) Effect of Diamox on cerebrospinal fluid pressure of cat and monkey. Neurology (Minneap) 7:119–123

Kohmura E, Gürtner P, Holl K, Nemati N, Stoppe G, Lerch KD, Samii M (1986) Erfahrungen mit der Inhalation eines 33%-igen Xenon (stable)-Sauerstoffgemisches in Zusammenhang mit einer neuen Methode zur lokalen Hirndurchblutungsmessung. Fortschr Geb Röntgenstr 144:531–536

Kreisig T, Schmiedek P, Leinsinger G, Einhäupl K, Moser E (1987) ^{133}Xe-DSPECT: Normalwerte von zerebraler Ruhedurchblutung und Reservekapazität. Nuklear Medizin 26:192–197

Krnjević K, Randić M, Siesjö BK (1965) Cortical CO_2 tension and neuronal excitability. J Physiol (Lond) 176:105–122

Lassen AN, Olsen TS, Hojgaard K, Skriver E (1983) Incomplete infarction: a CT-negative irreversible ischemic brain lesion. J Cereb Blood Flow metab [Suppl 1] 3:602–603

Leinsinger G, Schmiedek P, Kreisig T, Einhäupl K, Bauer W, Moser E (1988) ^{133}Xe-DSPECT: Bedeutung der zerebrovaskulären Reservekapazität für Diagnostik und Therapie der chronischen zerebralen Ischämie. Nuklear Medizin 27:127–134

Meyer JS, Gotoh F, Tazaki Y (1961) Inhibitory action of carbon dioxide and acetazolamide in seizure activity. Electroencephalogr Clin Neurophysiol 13:762–775

Pateisky K, Petsche H (1957) Electroencephalographic and clinical observations concerning the therapeutic effect of DIAMOX® (acetazolamide) in epilepsy and in conditions with increased intracranial pressure. Electroencephalogr Clin Neurophysiol 9:359

Saldías C, Cabieses F, Eidelberg E (1957) Electroencephalographic changes induced by the intravenous administration of acetazolamide (Diamox®) in epileptic patients. Electroencephalogr Clin Neurophysiol 9:333–336

Sorteberg W, Lindegaard KF, Rootwelt K, Dahl A, Nyberg-Hansen R, Russel D, Nornes H (1989) Effect of acetazolamide on cerebral artery blood velocity and regional cerebral blood flow in normal subjects. Acta Neurochir (Wien) 97:139–145

Vorstrup S, Henriksen L, Paulson OB (1984) Effect of acetazolamide on cerebral blood flow and cerebral metabolic rate for oxygen. J Clin Invest 74:1634–1639

Vorstrup S, Jensen KE, Thomsen C, Henriksen O, Lassen NA, Paulson OB (1989) Neuronal pH regulation: constant normal intracellular pH is maintained in brain during low extracellular pH induced by acetazolamide ^{31}P NMR study. J Cereb Blood Flow Metab 9: 417–421

Wilkinson HA (1989) Cerebral blood flow response to acetazolamide. J Neurosurg 70:156

Woodbury DM, Kemp JW (1982) Other antiepileptic drugs: sulfonamides and derivates: acetazolamide. In: Woodbury DM, Penry JK, Pippenger CE (eds) Antiepileptic drugs. Raven, New York, pp 771–789

Mental Activity and Changes in Cerebral Blood Flow Evaluated by Transcranial Doppler Sonography

A. G. Harders, G. Laborde, and D. W. Droste

Introduction

It is well known that brain activity, metabolism, and blood flow are closely related (Bondy 1973; Cooper et al. 1966; Greenberg et al. 1979; Heiss et al. 1979; Raichle 1975). Using the xenon-133 injection technique (Ingvar and Risberg 1965; Ingvar 1975; Lassen et al. 1978; Risberg and Ingvar 1973; Risberg 1986), the xenon-133 inhalation technique (Maximilian 1980; Obrist et al. 1967; Prohovnik 1980; Risberg 1980, 1986), single photon emission computed tomography (SPECT) (Sokoloff et al. 1977), and positron emission tomography (PET) (Heiss et al. 1986; Mazziotta et al. 1981, 1982; Raichle et al. 1981), the dependency of brain activity on the increase in cerebral blood flow (CBF) and metabolism can be clearly demonstrated. These techniques have the advantage of a high spatial resolution, but the disadvantage of a low temporal resolution.

Using transcranial Doppler sonography (TCD), blood flow velocities can be measured atraumatically and continuously through the intact skull (Aaslid 1986; Harders 1986). During the performance of tasks which activate the right and/or left hemisphere, we measured the blood flow velocities in both middle cerebral arteries (MCA_s). The velocities in the postcommunicating segment of the posterior cerebral artery (P_2) were recorded while the left and/or right visual field was being activated.

Assuming that the diameter of the large cerebral arteries in the circle of Willis (measuring points) does not change markedly, velocity changes are necessarily related to volume flow changes. Hence diameter changes in the small-resistance vessels caused by metabolic changes should result in corresponding velocity changes.

The objective of this study was primarily to evaluate the time course of velocity changes during mental activities. Further questions we investigated were whether there is a difference according to side in the MCA blood flow velocity with regard to handedness and what effect selective activation of the visual field has on the velocities in the posterior cerebral arteries.

Mental Activities and TCD

Subjects and Methods

Sixty-eight subjects with no clinical signs of cerebrovascular disease were entered in the study. Thirty-seven were right handed (RH) with no familial sinistrality (FS), 9 were RH with FS, 16 were LH with no FS, and 8 were LH with FS. Age ranged from

Table 1. Task order during blood flow measurement in the right and left MCA

Task
1. Reading aloud (90 s), rest (42 s)
2. Dot/distance estimation silently (90 s), rest (42 s)
3. Finding nouns aloud (90 s), rest (42 s)
4. Spatial imagination silently (90 s), rest (42 s)
5. Multiplication aloud (90 s), rest (42 s)
6. Face recognition silently (90 s), rest (42 s)

16 to 63 years; 37 persons were under and 33 patients were over 30 years of age. There were 29 women and 41 men. Twenty-nine were in academic and 41 in nonacademic professions.

We used the TC2-64 transcranial Doppler device (EME GmbH, Überlingen, FRG). The highest velocity in the MCA was searched for at a depth of about 45 or 50 mm. The ultrasound intensity was 100 mW/cm^2. The time-averaged peak frequencies (mean) calculated by the machine every 3 s (cm/s) were recorded by hand. Continuous measurements were possible by securing the probe in a headband.

The subjects performed six tasks according to the schedule shown in Table 1. Three right-hemispheric tasks were performed silently and three left-hemispheric mispheric tasks were performed aloud. The subjects were instructed to sit comfortably and in a relaxed manner throughout the entire procedure. Eyes were kept closed during the rest periods. Each person had to perform the task twice (once on the left side and once on the right side).

In 36 subjects the right side was measured first and in 34 subjects the left side was measured first.

Results

As we found a steady state within the rest values after 33 s, we used the last 9 s as a reference value and set the mean of the six rest phases at 1.00. The typical time courses of the velocity changes are shown in Figs. 1–4.

In all the tasks a maximum velocity is reached about 8 s after the task is begun, which is followed by a decrease, resulting in a steady state. When the tasks were stopped the velocities continued to be in the steady state for about 9 s, after which there was a decrease with an "undershoot" (below 1.00), followed by normalization within at least 33 s. No obvious differences in the time courses could be observed in subgroups such as handedness, familial handedness, profession, order, sex, and age.

The steady state began after about 24–42 s. The calculations of relative increase were performed using the values of the last 48 s in the task phase. None of the values measured during mental activities was 1.00. During performance of the three left hemispheric tasks there was a statistically significant difference in favor of the left hemisphere in contrast to the right hemispheric tasks. Statistically, there was no difference between the left MCA and the right MCA, the left-right difference for each task between the two subgroups as left-handers (n=23) and right-handers (n=23).

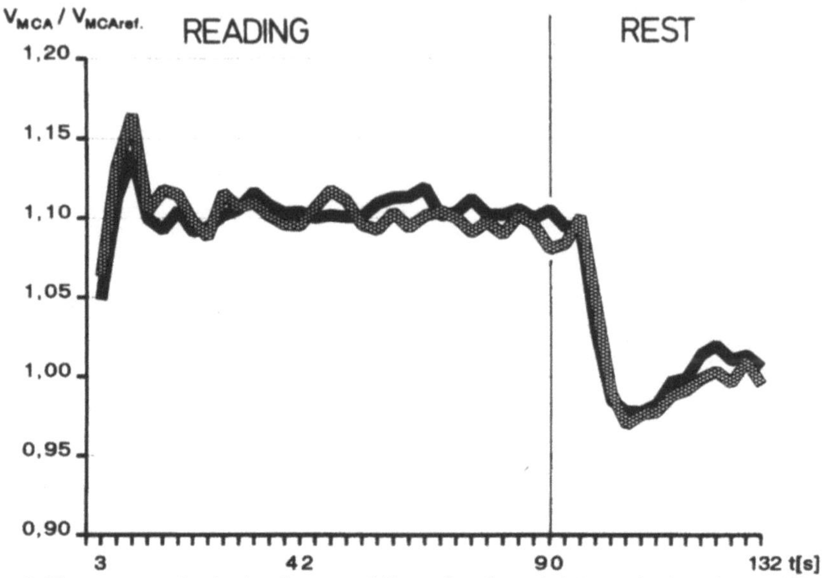

Fig. 1. Time course of velocity changes while performing a left hemspheric task. no differences between sides and a velocity increase of about 10% were seen during the task.

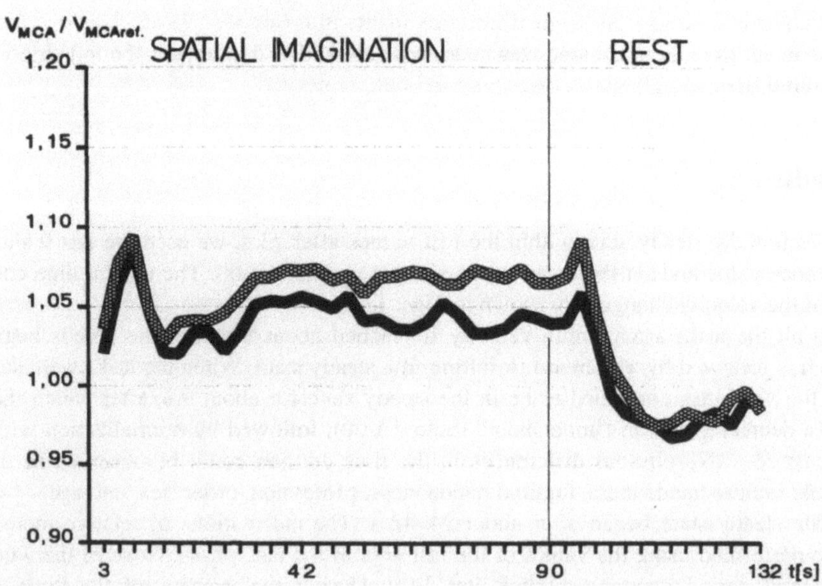

Fig. 2. In this "right hemispheric" task there is a statistically higher velocity increase in the right MCA than in the left.

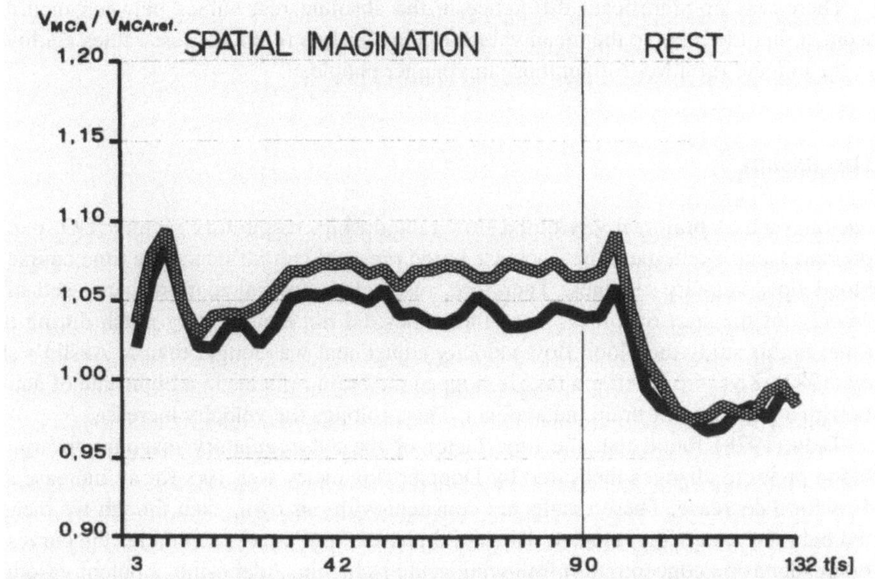

Fig. 3. Time course of velocity changes during a spatial imagination task; right-left difference is statistically significant

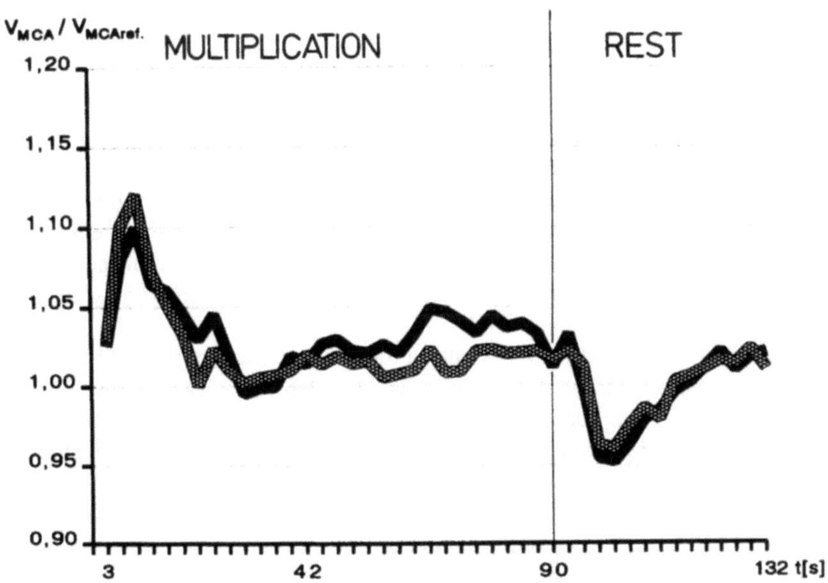

Fig. 4. Only slight velocity changes during multiplication tasks. No difference between sides

There was no significant difference in the absolute rest values between men and women. In older people the mean values of the absolute reference rest values are lower in the left and right MCA than those in younger people.

Discussion

Factors such as brain activity/blood flow relationship, respiratory factors (CO_2 partial pressure), and excitement that increase blood pressure can influence the time course of blood flow velocity changes. Therefore, rest values for calculation were used after 24–42 s of the start of a task, since the values did not change very much during this time. In this study the blood flow velocity adjustment was longer than in Aaslid's study (1987), 8 vs. 4.6 s. After a task is stopped the brain remains in a high state of activity with a high state of brain metabolism. This prolongs the velocity increase.

Tada (1978) found that the time factor of the autoregulatory response to arterial blood pressure changes measured by Doppler flowmetry was 10 s for an increase and 16 s for a decrease. These results are consitent with our own, even though we measured only the parameter velocity. The initial phase of our curves resembles the curves of brain adenosine concentration following acute ischemia. Adenosine, a potent vasodilatator, is claimed to play a role in autoregulation (Winn et al. 1985).

All of the six tasks increased the MCA blood flow velocity on both sides, which indicated the participation of both hemispheres in cognitive activities, although 133-xenon inhalation studies showed that the regional CBF during rest and the performance of verbal and spatial tasks showed higher regional CBF on the left side during the verbal task and on the right side for the spatial task (Gur et al. 1982, 1987; Risberg et al. 1975).

The three "right-hemispheric" tasks were accompanied by a significantly higher blood flow velocity in the right MCA. The three "left-hemispheric" tasks did not show corresponding results. This may be due to the influence of bilateral motor cortex activity, habituation, motivation, excitement, and respiratory factors in the three tasks performed aloud. It is also possible, however, that these tasks require more participation of both hemispheres. Handedness failed to show a significant influence on hemispheric specialization. This is consistent with two EEG studies reported by Jung et al. (1984; Jung and Landwehrmeyer 1987).

We found that the blood flow velocity in the MCA increased bilaterally in women more than in men during the dot/distance task and that there was a higher right>left difference in men for this task.

We found no differences in all of the five other tasks. It is remarkable that habituation takes place *between* the tasks, but not during the tasks.

With transcranial Doppler sonography, changes in the brain activity in the area supplied by the MCA can be measured indirectly with a high temporal resolution, allowing the speed and the extent of blood flow changes to be determined. Perhaps this reflects the very rapid onset of autoregulation.

Table 2. Task order during activation of the visual cortex task

Task
1. Illumination of the left visual field (90 s), rest
2. Illumination of the right visual field, rest
3. Illumination of both visual field, rest
4. Looking at six pictures (different contrast and interest, (6x45 s), rest (45 s)
5. Reading silently at 100 W illumination, rest
6. Fixing a point on a white sheet of paper, rest
7. Fixing a point in darkness (as dark as possible), rest

Rest, 45 s with closed eyes

Visual Cortex Activity and Blood Flow in the Posterior Cerebral Artery

Subjects and Methods

The objective of this investigation was to detect blood flow velocity changes in the posterior cerebral artery during activation of the right and/or left visual field. Stimulated by the investigations of Aaslid (1987), we examined 76 persons with no clinical signs of cerebral vascular disease, 40 women and 36 men, 24 between 20 and 30 years of age, and 32 between 31 and 49 years of age. The visual cortex was activated by looking at pictures of different interests. We tried to identify the response in the P_2 segment of the posterior cerebral artery while measuring the blood flow velocities with the TCD method. The P_2 segment of the posterior cerebral artery was insonated at depths between 5 and 6 cm from the skull surface, and the time-averaged peak frequencies (mean) were recorded.

The subjects performed seven tasks, as shown in Table 2. In 24 persons (12 women, 12 men) the velocities in the P_2 segment were measured; in 12 persons the investigation was started on the left side and in the other 12 on the right side. All of the persons were right handed.

Results

During activation of the left visual field the increased velocities in the corresponding P_2 segment of the posterior cerebral artery were significantly higher than velocities in the left P_2 segment during activation of the right visual field. During all of the tasks, the velocities on the right side were higher than those on the left side, except for when the right visual field was stimulated (Fig. 5).

The time course of velocity changes showed that the maximum was reached after about 18 s; this value was set as a maximum when it was followed by three lower values. Then there was more or less a decrease until a "steady state" of activated velocities set in. Five seconds after the tasks had been stopped there was a rapid decrease of the velocities with an "undershoot" and then normalization within 33 s. Activation of both visual fields resulted in an increase in both P_2 segments, showing no statistical difference between sides (Fig. 6). Task 4 illustrates the repeated velocity increase in

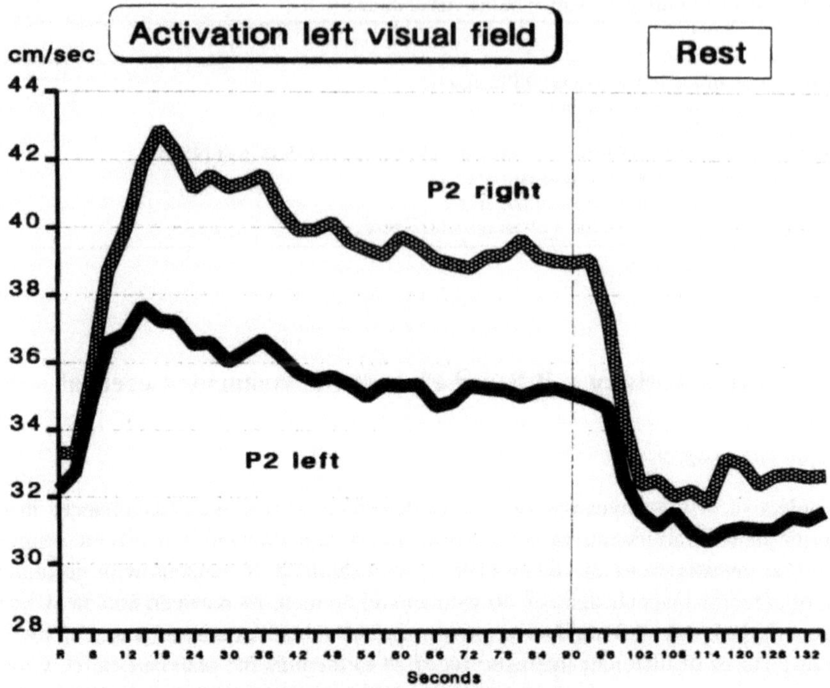

Fig. 5. Corresponding to the activation of the left visual field, there is a statistically significantly higher velocity increase in the right P_2 segment than in the left

close relation to new states of occipital lobe activation by six consecutive, highly complex pictures (Fig. 7). The velocity in the right P_2 segment was always higher than that in the left P_2 segment. Looking at a white sheet of paper produced no statistically significant velocity changes compared with task seven, where the persons had to look at a point in a dark room (Fig. 8). Sex and age of the volunteers had no influence on the results, nor did the order in which the tasks were performed. All the "working values" were statistically different from the rest value.

Fig. 6. Activation of both visual fields results in a velocity increase in both P_2 segments with no ▷ difference between sides

Fig. 7. Six pictures of different complexity. At the beginning there is always an overshoot of velocity increase, with no sign of habituation during the task. The right P_2 segment always showed higher velocities than the left, even though both visual fields were activated

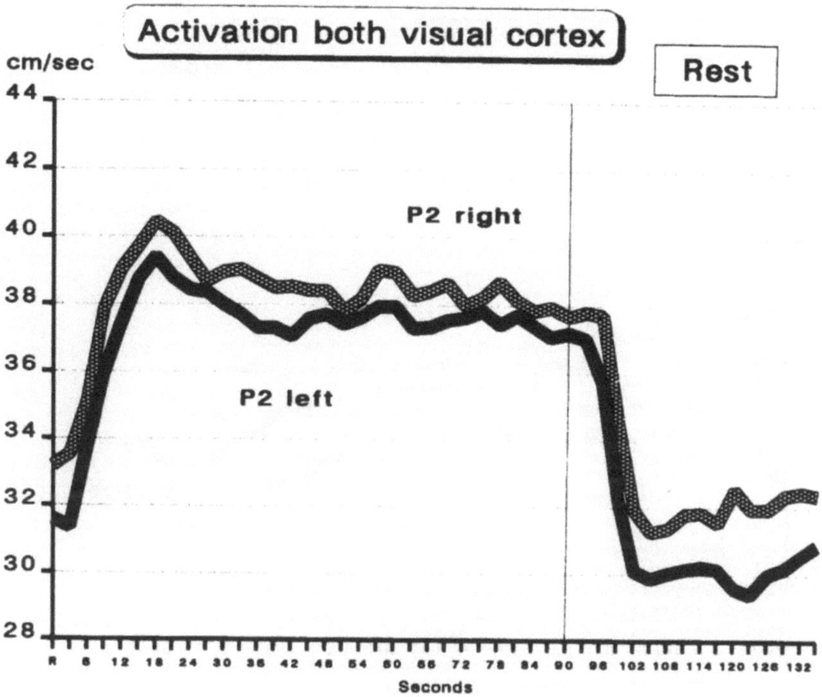
Activation both visual cortex
Rest
cm/sec
44
42
40
38
36
34
32
30
28
P2 right
P2 left
R 6 12 18 24 30 36 42 48 54 60 66 72 78 84 90 96 102 108 114 120 126 132
Seconds

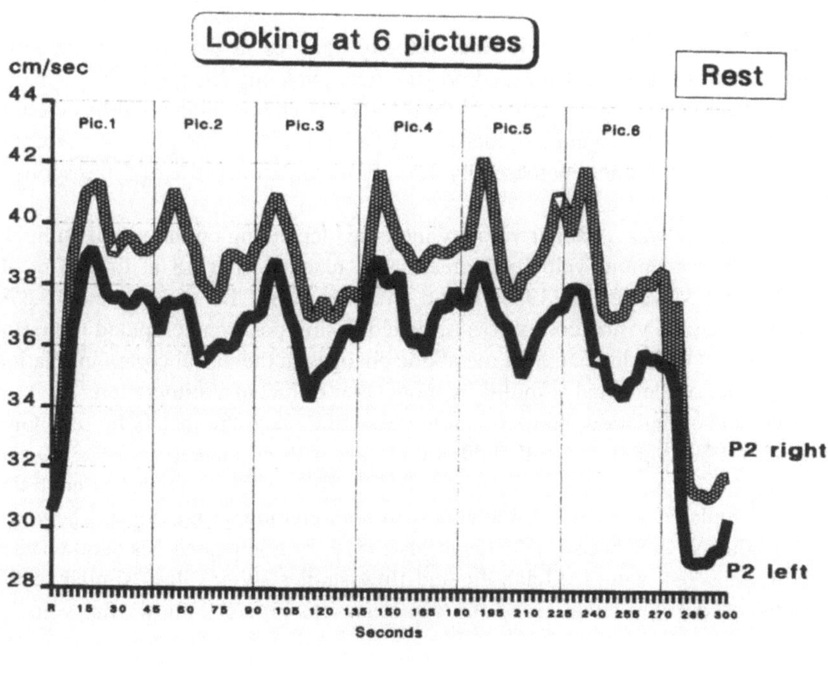
Looking at 6 pictures
Rest
cm/sec
44
42
40
38
36
34
32
30
28
Pic.1
Pic.2
Pic.3
Pic.4
Pic.5
Pic.6
P2 right
P2 left
R 15 30 45 60 75 90 105 120 135 150 165 180 195 210 225 240 255 270 285 300
Seconds

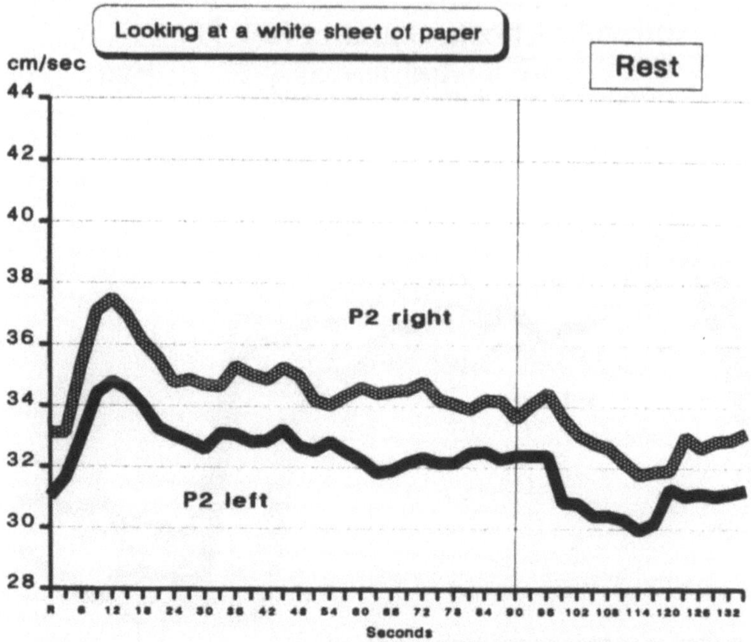

Fig. 8. Looking at a white sheet of paper, the increase in velocity was only about 4%

Discussion

Aaslid (1987) was the first to show that velocity changes in the posterior cerebral artery under mild stimulation. He found no significant velocity change in the supracerebellar artery and only a very small arrhythmic velocity change in the middle cerebral artery in 3% of cases. He found a velocity increase of 16.4% in the posterior cerebral artery, while the flow volume increased by 22%. Full regulation (90% of full response) took 46 s.

In our study there was a similar velocity increase, depending on the visual stimulus (Figs. 5–8). The maximum velocity increase was reached after 18 s. Lassen et al. (1977, 1978) and Meyer et al. (1981) found an increase in CBF of 20% and 16.8%, respectively, when the visual cortex was activated. Using positron computed tomography, Phelps et al. (1979) investigated metabolic changes in the visual cortex in relation to the complexity of the visual stimulus by monocular or biocular stimulation.

With full field stimulation, he found an increase of 23% in the metabolic rate. Greenberg et al. (1979) reported a half-field stimulation with an increase of 8%±3% and Reivich et al. (1979) also found an increase of 15%–20% in the visual cortex contralateral to the stimulated visual field. Patients with homonymous hemianopsia showed a decrease in glucose metabolism (Phelps et al. 1981a, b; Phelps and Mazziotta 1983) under the normal rest values. Metabolic and flow studies show values similar to the values obtained during activation of the visual cortex. Figure 9 shows the velocity

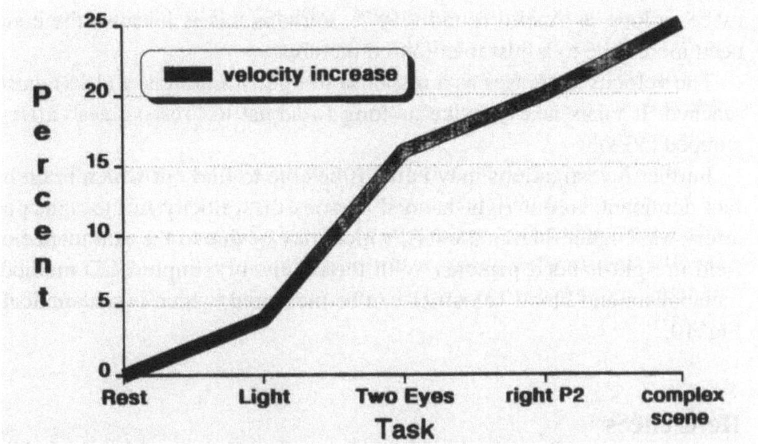

Fig. 9. Increasing the complexity of visual stimuli velocity increases by 25% (*rest,* closed eyes, relaxed; *light,* looking at a white sheet of pater; *two eyes,* looking at a colored picture straight ahead; *right* P_2, stimulation of the left visual field with the same picture as in the last task; *complex scene,* picture with high colored contrast resulting in emotional reactions

increase in relation to the tasks with increasing complexity. This relationship is understandable, since the diameter of the large cerebral arteries does not change during brain activity changes, although volume flow changes cause the same amount of velocity changes.

Due to the high temporal resolution of the TCD method, it is now possible to obtain information on the very rapid adjustment of the brain to a higher state of activity. With our stimuli the maximum of velocity increase was reached after 18 s, which is about

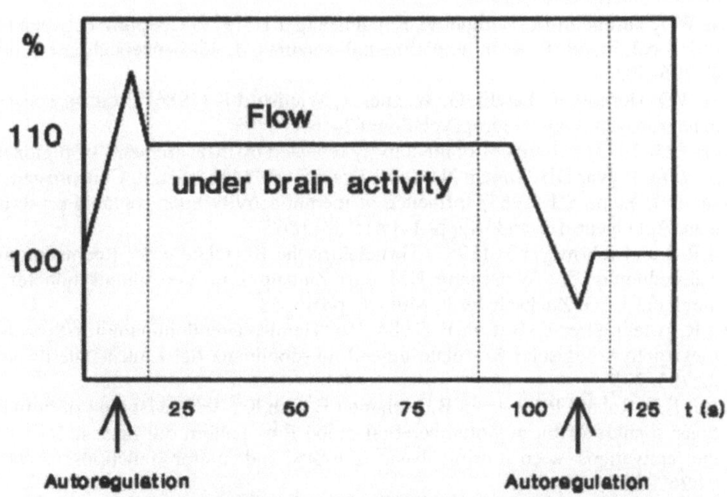

Fig. 10. This typical time course of velocity changes represents the high temporal resolution of TCD measurements under brain activation

twice as long as Aaslid found (1987). Perhaps this is because the cones of the retina need more time to adjust to coloured pictures.

The velocity increases as a response to light stimuli tasks (18 s) until a maximum is reached. It takes nearly twice as long to adjust to "rest values" after the stimuli are stopped (33 s).

Further investigations may perhaps be able to find out which brain hemisphere is in fact dominant. In our right-handed persons the velocity in the right posterior cerebral artery was higher than in the left, which may be due to the dominance of the left visual field in right-handed persons. With the relatively simple TCD method, brain activity metabolism and blood velocities can be measured, which is schematically illustrated in Fig. 10.

References

Aaslid R (1986) Transcranial Doppler sonography. Springer, Berlin Heidelberg New York

Aaslid R (1987) Visually evoked dynamic blood flow response of the human cerebral circulation. Stroke 18:771–775

Bondy SC (1973) The regulation of regional blood flow in the brain by visual input. J Neurol Sci 19:425–432

Cooper R, Crow HJ, Grey Walter W, Winter AL (1966) Regional control of cerebral vascular reactivity and oxygen supply in man. Brain Res 3:174–191

Greenberg J, Hand P, Sylvestro A, Reivich M (1979) Localized metabolic-flow couple during functional activity. Acta Neurol Scand [Suppl 72] 60:12–13

Gur RC, Gur RE, Obrist WD, Hungerbuhler JP, Younkin D, Rosen AD, Sholnick BE, Reivich M (1982) Sex and handedness differences in cerebral blood flow during cognitive activity. Science 217:659–661

Gur RC, Gur RE, Obrist WD, Skolnick BE, Reivich M (1987) Age and regional cerebral blood flow at rest and during cognitive activity. Arch Gen Psychiatry 44:617–621

Harders A (1986) Neurosurgical applications of transcranial Doppler sonography. Springer, Berlin Heidelberg New York

Heiss WD, Turnheim M, Vollmer R, Rappelsberger P (1979) Coupling between neuronal activity and focal blood flow in experimental seizures. Electroencephalogr Clin Neurophysiol 47:396–403

Heiss WD, Herholz K, Pawlik G, Wagner R, Wienhard K (1986) Positron emission tomography in neuropsychology. Neuropsychologia 24:141–149

Ingvar DH (1975) Patterns of brain activity revealed by measurements of regional cerebral blood flow. In: Ingvar DH, Lassen NA (eds) Brain work. Munksgaard, Copenhagen, pp 397–413

Ingvar DH, Risberg J (1965) Influence of mental activity upon regional cerebral blood flow in man. Acta Neurol Scand [Suppl 14] 41:183–186

Jung R, Landwehrmeyer B (1987) Hirnelektrische Korrelate einer Rechtsdominanz der Raumwahrnehmung. In: Weinmann HM (ed) Zugang zum Verständnis höherer Hirnfunktionen durch das EEG. Zuckschwerdt, Munich, pp 46–58

Jung R, Altenmüller E, Natsch B (1984) Zur Hemisphärendominanz für Sprache und Rechnen: Elektrophysiologische Korrelate einer Linksdominanz bei Linkshändern. Neuropsychologia 22:755–775

Lassen NA, Roland PE, Larsen B, Melamed E, Soh K (1977) Mapping of human cerebral functions: a study of the regional cerebral blood flow pattern during rest, its reproducibility and the activations seen during basic sensory and motor functions. Acta Neurol Scand 64:262–263

Lassen NA, Ingvar DH, Skinhj E (1978) Brain function and blood flow. Sci Am 239:62–71

Maximilian VA (1980) Funtional changes in the cortex Curing mental activation. Applications of regional cerebral blood flow measurements in neuropsychological research. Gleerup, Malmö

Mazziotta JC, Phelps ME (1985) Human neuropsychological imaging studies of local brain metabolism: strategies and results. In: Sokoloff L (ed) Brain imaging and brain function. Raven, New York, pp121–137

Mazziotta JC, Phelps ME, Miller J, Kuhl DE (1981) Tomographic mapping of human cerebral metabolsim: normal unstimulated state. Neurology (NY) 31:503–516

Maziotta JC, Phelps ME, Carson RE, Kuhl DE (1982) Tomographic mapping of human cerebral metabolism: sensory deprivation. Ann neurol 12:435–444

Meyer JS, Hayman LA, Amano T, Nakajima S, Shaw T, Lauzon P, Derman S, Karacan I, Harati Y (1981) Mapping local blood flow of humans brain by CT scanning during stable xenon inhalation. Stroke 12:426–436

Obrist WD, Thompson PhD, King CH, Shan Wang H (1967) Determination of regional cerebral blood flow by inhalation of 133-xenon. Circ Res 20:124–135

Phelps ME, Mazziotta JC (1983) Human sensory stimulation and deprivation as demonstrated by positron computed tomography. In: Heiss WD, Phelps ME (eds) Positron emission tomography of the brain. Springer, Berlin Heidelberg New York, pp 139–152

Phelps ME, Huang C, Hoffmann EJ, Selin C, Sokoloff L, Kuhl DE (1979) Tomographic measurement of local cerebral glucose metabolic rate in humans with /F–18)2-fluoro-2-deoxy-D-glucose: validation of method. Ann Neurol 6:371–388

Phelps ME, Mazziotta JC, Kuhl DE, Nuwer M, Packwood J, Metter J, Engel J (1981a) Tomographic mapping of human cerebral metabolism: visual stimulation and deprivation. Neurology (NY) 31:517–529

Phelps ME, Kuhl DE, Mazziotta JC (1981b) Metabolic mapping of the brain's response to visual stimulation: studies in humans. Science 211:1445–1448

Prohovnik I (1980) Mapping brainwork: theoretical and methodological considerations in applying the regional cerebral blood flow method to neuropsychology. Gleerup, Malmö

Raichle M (1975) Sensori-motor area increase of oxygen uptake and blood flow in the human brain during contralateral hand exercise; preliminary observations by the 0–15 method. In: Ingvar DH, Lassen NA (eds) brain work. Munksgaard, Copenhagen, pp 372–377

Raichle ME, Markham J, Larson K, Grubb RL Jr, Welch MJ (1981) Measurement of local cerebral blood flow in man with positron emission tomography. J Cereb Blood Flow Metab [Suppl 1] 1:19–20

Reivich M, Kuhl D, Wolf W, Greenberg J, Phelps M, Ido T, Casella V, Fowler J, Hoffmann E, Alavi A, Som P, Sokoloff L (1979) The [^{1}8F]fluorodeoxyglucose method for the measurement of local cerebral glucose utilization in man. Circ Res 44:127–137

Risberg J (1980) Regional cerebral blood flow measurements by 133-Xe inhalation: methodology and applications in neuropsychology and psychiatry. Brain Lang 9:9–34

Risberg J (1986) Regional cerebral blood flow in neuropsychology. Neuropsychologia 24:135–140

Risberg J, Ingvar DH (1973) Patterns of activation in the grey matter of the dominant hemisphere during memorizing and reading. Brain 96:737–756

Risberg J, Halsey JH, Wills EL, Wilson EM (1975) Hemispheric specialization in normal man studied by bilateral measurements of the regional cerebral blood flow: a study with the 133 Xe-inhalation technique. Brain 98:511–524

Sokoloff L, Reivich M, Kennedy C, Des Rosiers MH, Patlak CS, Pettigrew KD, Sakurada O, Shinohara M (1977) The [14C] deoxyglucose method for the measurement of local cerebral glucose utilization: theory, procedure, and normal values in the conscious and anesthetized albino rat. J Neurochem 28:897–916

Tada K (1978) A study on cerebral blood flow autoregulation. Osaka Daigaku 28:321–337

Wallesch CW, Henriksen L, Kornhuber HH, Paulson OB (1985) Observations on regional cerebral blood flow in cortical and subcortical structures during language production in normal man. Brain Lang 25:224–233

Winn HR, Morii S, Berne RM (1985) The role of adenosine in autoregulation of cerebral blood flow. Ann Biomed Eng 13:321–328

Chapter 4
Clinical Application of Stimulated Cerebral Blood Flow Studies

Natural History of Patients Defined by Assessment of Cerebral Blood Flow Reserves

H. Yonas, S.R. Durham, and H.A. Smith

History

Xenon has proven to be a useful tracer in the measurement of cerebral blood flow (CBF). While radioactive xenon has been extensively utilized for the measurement of CBF since the 1950s, the first reports of using stable xenon as a flow indicator appeared in 1977 (Haughton et al. 1976; Winkler et al. 1977). The following year, Kelcz et al. (1978) defined the blood-brain partition coefficient for xenon and Drayer et al. (1978) reported the first CBF measurements using the stable xenon technique. In 1983 General Electric, with other manufacturers following soon, incorporated this technique within a CT scanning system. In subsequent years, the xenon/CT (Xe/CT) technique has been validated as a quantitative CBF method in animal studies (Gur et al. 1985; Faturos et al. 1987; DeWitt et al. 1989; Wolfson et al. 1990; Yonas et al. 1988, 1990), and is currently used clinically in the diagnosis and management of patients with acute stroke (Drayer et al. 1980; Hughes et al. 1989; Yonas et al. 1989), occlusive vascular disorders (DeVries et al. 1990), vasospasm (Yonas et al. 1989; Yonas 1990), arteriovenous malformation (Okabe et al. 1983; Marks et al. 1988), and head trauma (Wozney et al. 1985; Darby et al. 1988; Marion et al. 1991) at over 40 institutions worldwide.
In this report we will focus attention on our experience since 1987 in over 350 patients with occlusive vascular disorders who have undergone Xe/CT CBF studies before and after "acetazolamide challenge." While numerous reports suggest that hemodynamically different groups can be defined by the measurement of the CBF combined with a "stress test" of cerebral flow reserves, the prognostic significance of these findings remains undefined. We have, therefore, sought to define the natural history of these individuals and retrospectively correlate this information with baseline Xe/CT CBF values and hemodynamic reserve status.

Methods

Flow studies were performed on the Xe/CT CBF system adapted to the GE 9800 CT scanner (General Electric Medical System Division, Milwaukee, Wisconsin) and used medical-grade xenon/oxygen (Linde XeScan, USP mixture, Union Carbide Rare Gases, Somerset, NJ).

Xenon/CT CBF with acetazolamide challenge has been used primarily as a routine outpatient study. The average time to complete a double study is 60–90 min with a 20 min break between studies during which 1 g acetazolamide is injected intravenously. Details of the Xe/CT method of mapping CBF have been recently reviewed (Gur et al.

1989). In brief the method involves indirectly characterizing the arterial xenon buildup curve by recording the end-tidal xenon curve. The tissue buildup curve is obtained through the analysis of two baseline and six sequential CT scans performed while the patient inhales 33% xenon /67% oxygen for 4.3 min. A blood flow measurement for each of the 20000–30000 CT voxels is then calculated to create a high-resolution map of blood flow. Flow data are currently displayed on a CT console on a gray scale which is arbitrarily set at 0–100 with units in millimeters per 100 g per minute.

We compared pre- and postacetazolamide CBF studies by placing regions of interest (ROIs) consistent with vascular territories reported by Damasio (1983). Pre- and postacetazolamide blood flow maps were then compared for evidence or flow change in corresponding vascular territories. Based on normative data from 67 patients ranging in age from 20 to 67 years, we have established that normal blood flow is 53±10 ml/100 g per minute with a slight decrease of mean cortical blood flow through the decades (Yonas et al. 1991).

In this paper we present our initial observations of the first 68 individuals we have followed for a mean of 18 months, none of whom underwent surgical intervention during the follow-up period. All subjects had a history consistent with symptomatic occlusive vascular disease.

Results

On initial review, 45% of the patients had normal flow and flow activation (an increase of 10%–40%), 31% had low flows which augmented normally following acetazolamide challenge, and 24% had an abnormal response as defined by either no activation or regional decrease of CBF. Regional flow compromises tended to be consistent with major vascular territories. In this study, individuals in a group that either did not increase or actually decreased flow following acetazolamide challenge appear to have a significantly elevated incidence of subsequent transient ischemic attacks (TIAs) and strokes (55% and 23%, respectively) (Rutigliano et al. 1989).

In an effort to better define the clinical significance of compromised flow reserves, we separated our study population into group 1, those individuals whose regional flow was augmented by greater than 5% in all vascular territories, group 2, those whose flow did not vary greater than 5%, and group 3, those whose flows decreased more than 5% in one or more vascular territory. If 50% of a vascular territory was atrophic by reference to the CT image, presumably due to prior infarction, then that territory was eliminated from analysis. We observed that group 3 patients had the greatest number of occluded and/or stenotic vessels, but that a history of past stroke and TIA was evenly distributed among the three groups.

The incidence of subsequent stroke was, however, significantly different between groups, with a 38% incidence of subsequent stroke in group 3 patients. Seven of the nine ischemic events in group 3 occured ipsilateral to the vascular territory with compromised reserves (Fig. 1). In one individual the region of stroke was contralateral to the low reserve region and in the other we were unable to determine the site of injury although the patient was said to have died of a stroke (Durham et al. 1991). Patients in groups 1 and 2 had no significant incidence of stroke during the follow-up period.

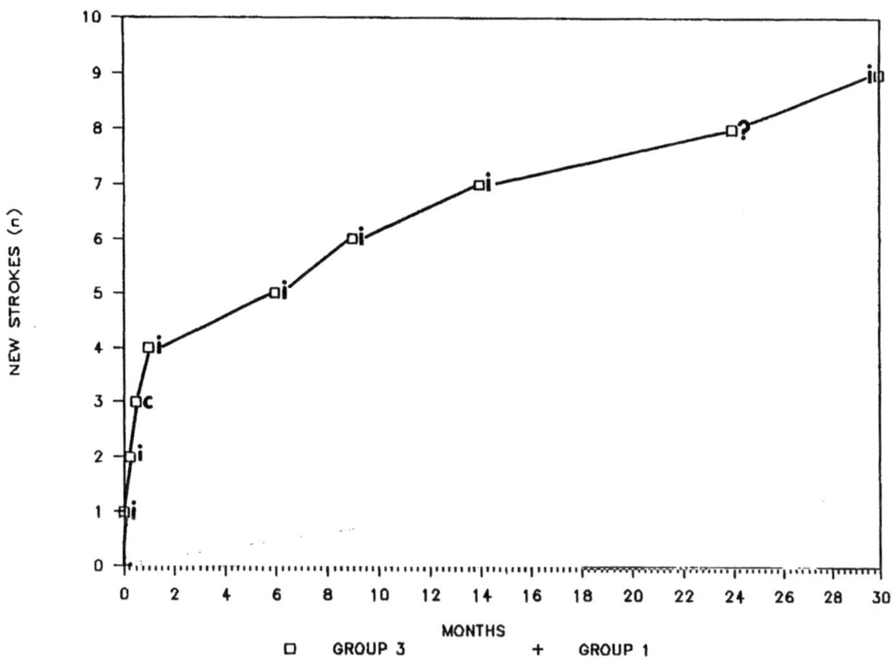

Fig. 1. Cumulative incidence of new stroke

Discussion

A number of reports have identified a subgroup in which blood flow is not activated after a vasodilatory challenge with acetazolamide. These individuals presumably have a severe degree of hemodynamic compromise and are in a chronic state of maximal vasodilation. Studies with positron emission tomography have also shown that patients with decreased reserves meet the criteria for "misery perfusion" as defined by Baron et al. (1981; Kanno et al. 1988). Studies are currently underway to observe whether clinical outcome in patients with severely compromised hemodynamics can be improved by flow augmentation surgery.

Our studies, although still preliminary, support the premise that a group of individuals with severe hemodynamic compromise are at increased risk for subsequent stroke and can be identified by relatively simple studies of CBF reserve. Our observation of an increased incidence of stroke in only those individuals with decreased flows following introduction of acetazolamide suggests that those at increased risk of subsequent stroke are those who are not only maximally vasodilated but also dependent on leptomeningeal collaterals for the maintenance of regional CBF. Although we have only examined hemodynamic parameters in this study, we postulate that this group may be at increased risk for infarction due not only to small decreases in perfusion pressure, but also to relatively small, soft, and otherwise insignificant intraluminal thrombi. Because of the indirect route of blood delivery in group 3 patients, severe dampening of intraluminal pulsatility would be expected. Thus even small clots would be likely to lodge and permanently occlude vessels.

Quantitative technologies, which use xenon as a diffusible tracer and directly measure blood flow by solving the Kety-Schmidt equation, have been able to define a group at risk because of the ability to define the full spectrum of both positive and negative regional CBF responses that can accompany a stress test of cerebral hemodynamics. Both radioactive and stable Xe/CT CBF studies can be repeated within 20–30 min, which corresponds to the peak effectiveness of acetazolamide. Xe/CT CBF also provides coupled anatomical CT data, which is important because, without the ability to identify and eliminate vascular regions with significant (<50%) prior infarctions from analysis, our flow data yield little predictability. Xe/CT CBF also has the potential for wide availability because of its capacity for integration within existing modern CT scanners. New systems, which recycle xenon, are also making Xe/CT CBF less expensive, and advancements in computer applications are making access to quantitative CBF analyses easier at more brain levels per study.

Conclusion

Acetazolamide challenge studies obtained with the stable Xe/CT method appear to identify a subgroup of individuals with occlusive vascular disease who are at significantly increased risk of subsequent infarction. The greatest risk appears to be within a relatively short time frame from the onset of symptoms in those individuals who demonstrated a greater than 5% "steal phenomenon." These results suggest that strategies for the prevention of stroke focused upon the subgroup of patients identified to be at greatest risk may be warranted based on preliminary studies of cerebral hemodynamic reserves.

References

Baron JC, Bousser MG, Comar D et al. (1981) Noninvasive tomographic study of cerebral blood flow and oxygen metabolism in vivo. Potentials, limitations, and clinical applications in cerebral ischemic disorders. Eur neurol 20:273–284

Darby JM, Yonas H, Marion DW, Latchaw RE (1988) Local "inverse steal" induced by hyperventialtion in head injury. Neurosurgery 23:84–88

Demasio H (1983) A computed tomographic guide to the identification of cerebral vascular territories. Arch Neurol 40:138–142

DeVries EJ, Sekhar LN, Horton JA et al. (1990) A new method to predict safe resection of the internal carotid artery. Laryngoscope 100:85–88

DeWitt DS, Fatouros PP, Wist AO et al. (1989) Stable xenon versus radiolabeled microsphere cerebral blood flow measurements in baboons. Stroke 20:1716–1723

Drayer BP, Wolfson SK Jr, Reinmuth OM et al. (1978) Xenon enhanced computed tomography for the analysis of cerebral integrity, perfusion, and blood flow. Stroke 9:123–130

Drayer BP, Gur D, Yonas H et al. (1980) Abnormality of the xenon brain:blood partition coefficient and blood flow in cerebral infarction: an in vivo assessment using transmission computed tomography. Radiology 135:349–354

Durham SR, Smith HA, Rutigliano MJ, Jonasa H (1991) Assessment of cerebral vasoreactivity and stroke risk using Xe/CT acetazolamide challenge. Stroke 22:138

Faturos PP, Wist AO, Kishore PRS (1987) Xenon/computed tomography cerebral blood flow measurements: methods and accuracy. Invest Radiol 20:705–712

Gur D, Yonas H, Jackson DL et al. (1985) Simultaneous measurements of cerebral blood flow by the xenon/CT method and the microsphere method: a comparison. Invest Radiol 20:672–677
Gur D, Yonas H, Good WF (1989) Local cerebral blood flow by xenon-enhanced CT: current status, potential improvements, and future directions. Cerebrovasc Brain Metab Rev 1:68–86
Haughton V, Harrington G, Schmidt J et al. (1976) Xenon inhalation enhancement for computed tomography scanning in multiple sclerosis. International Symposium on Computer Assisted Tomography in Nontumoral Diseases of the Brain, Spinal Cord and Eye, Oct 11–15, National Institute of Health, Bethesda
Hughes RL, Yonas H, Gur D, latchaw RE (1989) Cerebral blood flow determination within the first 8 hours of cerebral infarction using stable xenon-enhanced computed tomography. Stroke 20:754–760
Kanno I, Uemura K, Higano S et al. (1988) Oxygen extraction fraction a maximally vasodilated tissue in the ischemic brain estimated from the regional CO_2 responsiveness measured by positron emission tomography. J Cereb Blood Flow Metab 8:22–235
Kelcz F, Hilal SK, Hartwell P, Joseph PM (1978) Computed tomographic measurement of the xenon brain-blood partition coefficient and implications for regional blood flow: a preliminary report. Radiology 127:383–392
Marion DW, Darby J, Yonas H (1991) Acute regional cerebral blood flow changes caused by severe head injuries. J Neurosurg 74: 407–414
Marks MP, O'Donahue J, Fabricant JI et al. (1988) Cerebral blood flow evaluation of arteriovenous malformations with stable xenon CT. AJNR 9:1169–1175
Okabe T, Meyer JS, Okayasu H (1983) Xenon-enhanced CT CBF measurements in cerebral AVMs before and after excision. J Neurosurg 59:2121–31
Rutigliano MJ, Yonas H, Johnson DW (1989) Natural history of patients with compromised cerebral reserves. J Cereb Blood Flow Metab 9:S609
Winkler SS, Sacket JF, Holden JE et al. (1977) Xenon inhalation as an adjunct to computerized tomography of the brain: preliminary study. Invest Radiol 12:15–18
Wolfson SK Jr, Clark J, Greenberg JH et al. (1990) Xenon-enhanced computed tomography compared with [^{14}C]iodoantipyrine for normal and low cerebral blood flow states in baboons. Stroke 21:751–757
Wozney P, Yonas H, Latchaw RE et al. (1985) Central herniation revealed by focal decrease in blood flow without elevation of intracranial pressure: a case report. Neurosurgery 17:641–644
Yonas H (1990) Cerebral blood measurements in vasospasm. In: Winn R, Mayber M (eds) Neurosurgery clinics of North America, vol 1, no 2. Saunders, Philadelphia, pp 307–317
Yonas H, Gur D, Claasen D et al. (1988) Stable xenon enhanced computed tomography in the study of clinical and pathologic correlates of focal ischemia in baboons. Stroke 19:228–238
Yonas H, Sekhar L, Johnson DW, Gur D (1989) Determination of irreversible ischemia by xenon-enhanced computed tomographic monitoring of cerebral blood flow in patients with symptomatic vasospasm. Neurosurgery 24:368–372
Yonas H, gur D, Claasen D et al. (1990) Stable xenon-enhanced CT measuurement of cerebral blood flow in reversible focal ischemia in baboons. J Neurosurg 73:266–273
Yonas H, Darby JM, Marks EC et al. (1991) CBF measured by Xe/CT: approach to analysis and normal values. J Cereb Blood Flow Metab 11:716–725

Aspects of Cerebrovascular Autoregulation Following Subarachnoid Haemorrhage

J. D. Pickard, R. J. Nelson, A. H. J. Lovick, R. W. B. Coull, J. C. Stanley, D. H. Read, J. Herbetko, and M. Campbell

Scientific Background

Delayed cerebral ischaemia remains a major cause of morbidity and mortality in those patients with subarachnoid haemorrhage (SAH) who survive the initial catastrophe. A recent study of 3521 SAH patients from 68 neurosurgical units found no difference in outcome between early surgery (0–3 days) and late surgery (11–14 days) (Kassell et al. 1990), and so the neurosurgeon is presented with the task of weighing up the possible relative risk of precipitating cerebral ischaemia by early surgery to clip the aneurysm against those of delaying surgery and increasing the chances of a second haemorrhage for each individual patient.

The aetiology of delayed ischaemic deficit (DID) has not been fully elucidated. The appearance of angiographic vasospasm has been thought to correlate with the development of DID by several workers (Allcock and Drake 1965; Fisher et al. 1977; Weir et al. 1978). However, Millikan (1975) in a series of 198 consecutive SAH patients found no such relationship. Forty-one percent of his patients had angiographic vasospasm and 45.7% of these had apparent ischaemic deficit, whereas, of the 59% of patients with no vasospasm, 52.2% had abnormal neurological signs. The incidence of angiographic vasospasm is generally thought to peak around the 7th day after the haemorrhage (Kassell et al. 1985; Weir et al. 1978), although a large series of 797 cases suggests that vasospasm is most commonly seen on angiography between the 10th and 17th day (Kwak et al. 1979). Pickard et al. (1989) in a recent study found that the peak incidence of DID is at the end of the 1st week (Data on file, Brant Study).

Several studies have demonstrated a fall in cerebral blood flow (CBF) following SAH, and some have suggested that low flows and large falls in CBF are related to poor outcome (Meyer et al. 1983). There may be some correlation between vasospasm and regional CBF (Geraud et al. 1984), although experimental work in the monkey indicates that a decrease in vessel calibre of at least 50% is needed to decrease CBF by 60% of the control value (Simeone et al. 1972). This is presumably due to vasodilation of the parenchymal arterioles distal to the stenosis. In healthy man, normal baseline CBFs fall within a wide range, and so a baseline CBF study has little predictive value for the individual patient. In health CBF is maintained at normal values until mean arterial systemic blood pressure falls to 60 mmHg. It has been noted that SAH patients may develop a neurological deficit in association with an episode of hypotension, and that the induction of relative hypertension may improve the clinical state of some patients with an ischaemic deficit (Kosnik and Hunt 1970). As might be expected from these observations, work in both primates and man demonstrates that autoregulation of

CBF to changes in systemic blood pressure and reactivity of CBF to arterial CO_2 concentration is impaired following SAH, and such impairment correlates with poor prognosis (Mendelow et al. 1981; Boisvert et al. 1979; Messeter et al. 1987; Voldby et al. 1985; Dernbach et al. 1988; Pickard et al. 1980; Ishii 1979; Heilbrun et al. 1972). Pickard et al. (1980) used the intravenous xenon-133 technique intraoperatively to study the CBF response in SAH patients to the controlled hypotension, then used to assist dissection and clipping of aneurysms. Fifteen of the 20 patients studied demonstrated a rise in CBF during the halothane-induced hypotension, whereas in 5 of the 20 CBF fell. These 5 were deemed to have impaired autoregulation and, of these 5, 4 went on to develop DID as compared with only 1 of the 15 with a normal CBF response ($p<0.001$, chi-square test). In these 20 patients impairment of autoregulation appeared to be an excellent predictor of the development of DID.

It is likely that DID is multifactorial in aetiology, and a combination of a fall in baseline CBF and impairment of autoregulation of CBF renders the cerebral circulation vulnerable to further insults, for example vasospasm, hypotension, hyponatraemia, hypovolaemia, or the development of hydrocephalus that may complicate SAH. To further evaluate the predictive value of impairment of autoregulation in the preoperative patient with SAH in the Wessex Neurological Centre, Southampton General Hospital, we have developed a technique for the assessment of autoregulation of CBF following SAH in man (Lovick et al. 1982).

Methods of Assessment of the Cerebral Circulation Following SAH

Wessex CBF Trolley

The Wessex CBF Trolley is robust and portable and may be readily used both in and out of theatre. A quantity of 60 MBq xenon-133 is injected intravenously, and the subsequent cerebral clearance of xenon-133 measured by scintillation counters. Initially only global CBF was measured using a single probe, but more recently two probes have been used to record hemispherical values. Analysis of the clearance curve is restricted to a period of 1–3 min after the injection, and the initial slope index used for CBF computation. End-tidal PCO_2 is measured via a catheter in the postnasal space, and a chest probe is used to estimate arterial xenon concentration. This technique may be repeated every 10 min and the results are available within 6 min after the injection of xenon. The need for a face mask is obviated, facilitating use in theatre and minimizing the cooperation required from the patient.

Preoperative Assessment of CBF Autoregulation in SAH Patients: The "Stress Test"

In the awake, preoperative SAH patient, hypotension is induced by infusion of trimetaphan, a short-acting ganglion blocker, until mean arterial blood pressure falls to 70% of its baseline value. Patients are sedated with diazepam during the procedure and tilted to 30° whilst hypotension is induced. CBF is recorded both before and during hypotension. If global CBF (or hemispherical CBF in later studies) falls by more than 30% from baseline values, the patient is deemed to have significantly impaired autoregulation.

Studies Involving the "Stress Test" in Preoperative Assessment of Cerebrovascular Autoregulation in SAH Patients in the Wessex Neurological Centre

Correlation of Preoperative Cerebrovascular Autoregulation with Delayed Postoperative Cerebral Ischaemia and Outcome Following SAH

Methods

One hundred and three patients with proven SAH were studied. The "stress test" was performed prior to clipping of the aneurysm once the surgeon had made the decision to operate on the usual clinical and radiological grounds. The results of the test were withheld from the neurosurgeons.

There were three end points to the trial; immediate ischaemic deficit (present immediately on reversal of anaesthesia), delayed ischaemic deficit, and clinical outcome at 3 months. A bad outcome was defined as severe disability or death.

Results

Two groups of patients, A or B, were defined on the basis of whether CBF fell by more than 30% (group B) during the period of hypotension. Patients in group B were considered to have significantly impaired autoregulation. The incidence of immediate deficit was the same in the two groups, but the risk of progression or failure to improve was increased from 10.5% in group A to 50% in group B. The incidence of DID was 9% in group A, but 37% in group B. Similarly the risks of a bad outcome were higher in group B at 28% as opposed to 12% in group A. Preliminary analysis of the data demonstrates that the presence of substantial cisternal blood on the CT scan in conjunction with impaired autoregulation significantly increases the risk of DID. Five out of six (83%) patients with both these risk factors developed cerebral ischaemica (Table 1).

Table 1. Preoperative assessment of SAH patients using the Stress Test

	Postoperative ischaemic deficit		Poor outcome
	Immediate	Delayed	
Group A $n = 74$	31%	9%	12%
Group B $n = 29$	23%	37%	28%

Group A, patients without significantly impaired autoregulation; group B, patients with significantly impaired autoregulation

Preliminary Results of a Retrospective Study of the Correlation Between Impairment of Autoregulation of CBF and Other Factors Following SAH

Methods

Between 1982 and 1990, 165 patients with SAH have had a total of 196 stress tests and we have recently finished a retrospective analysis of our preoperative "Stress Test" data to determine any relationship between impairment of CBF autoregulation and other factors following SAH. After the analysis of the previous study in 1985, the Stress Test has been part of the routine clinical management SAH patients in the Wessex Neurological Centre. Data have been collected retrospectively on all the patients who have undergone Stress Tests under the following categories:

Stress Test Result. Percentage fall in hemispherical or global CBF from baseline during hypotension.

Clinical Data. These were obtained from the patient's case notes, and included age, sex, hypotension, smoking, family history of subarachnoid haemorrhage, diastolic blood pressure on admission, World Federation of Neurological Societies grade on admission, duration of coma following haemorrhage and drugs administered.

Radiological Data. Two independent reports were made on each CT scan and cerebral angiogram, by a neurosurgeon and by a neuroradiologist. The reports were compared and a consensus reached. The amount of subarachnoid blood in the basal cisterns was determined from the CT scan and substantial cisternal blood was defined as either a clot of greater than 2 mm or blood diffusely dispersed throughout the basal cisterns. Previous studies suggest that the amount of cisternal blood is an accurate predictor of subsequent vasospasm and DID (Bell et al. 1980; Fisher et al. 1980). The degree of arterial narrowing of the circle of Willis was determined from the angiogram.

Statistics.
Multiple regression analysis was used to determine the relationship between the clinical and radiological variables, and the percentage fall in CBF during the Stress Test.

Results

Patient studies were aged 16–70 years with a mean age of 47 years. Fifty-seven percent were female. Preoperative Stress Tests were carried out between 1 and 95 days following SAH (median 9 days). During the Stress Test two patients developed transient deficits that had been present earlier during their admission. There were no permanent sequelae.

Time Course of Impaired Autoregulation.
There was a significant relationship between the fall in CBF during the Stress Test and the time after SAH. We found that autoregulation is impaired immediately following

SAH, and remains impaired for 2–3 weeks before starting to return towards normal (multiple regression analysis, $p<0.05$).

Other Factors Associated with Impaired Autoregulation.
The only other factor significantly related to the percentage fall in CBF during hypotension was age ($p<0.05$, multiple regression analysis). Elderly patients had greater degrees of impairment of autoregulation. There were no other factors significantly associated with impaired autoregulation.

Discussion

We have shown that even in this group of relatively well patients autoregulation of CBF may be impaired immediately following SAH, and impairment may last for 2–3 weeks. Impaired autoregulation was associated with an increase in DID and a poorer outcome at 3 months. There was also an association with increasing age of the patient. Our results are in agreement with those of other workers. Messeter et al. (1987) in a small series of patients found that diminished reactivity to controlled hyperventilation correlated with an increased incidence of DID compared with patients with intact reactivity. Also in a small series of patients, Heilbrun et al. (1972) noted poorer postoperative results in patients with global lack of autoregulation. Interestingly, Voldby et al. (1985) noted a clear association between the presence of vasospasm and impaired autoregulation, and also that the severity of the vasospasm was related to the degree of impairment of autoregulation, although the resting CBF and neurological condition of the patient may have been normal. They also found that CBF reactivity to hyperventilation was impaired, though these changes were less marked, and a preserved CO_2 response was seen in some patients with impaired autoregulation and also slight vasospasm.

Impaired autoregulation or reactivity to hypercapnia is not the sole cause of postoperative DID and subsequent poor outcome, but it will put the patient at increased risk of cerebral ischaemia, should the circulation be subjected to further insults, e.g., vasospasm, hypotension, hyponatraemia, hypovolaemia or hydrocephalus. Such a hypothesis would explain why patients with substantial cisternal blood (and thus increased risk of vasospasm) had such a high risk of developing delayed ischaemia in our study.
The Stress Test is now part of the routine preoperative assessment of SAH patients in the Wessex Neurological Centre, and provides valuable data for the neurosurgical management of these patients.

Acknowledgements. The early part of this work was supported by the Chest Heart and Stroke Association.

References

Allcock JM, Drake CG (1965) Ruptured intracranial aneurysms – the role of arterial spasm. J Neurosurg 22:21–29
Bell B, Kendall B, Symon L (1980) Computed tomography in aneurysmal subarachnoid haemorrhage. J Neurol Neurosurg Psychiatry 43:522–524

Boisvert DPJ, Pickard JD, Graham DI (1979) Delayed effect of subarachnoid haemorrhage on cerebral metabolism and the cerebrovascular response to hypercapnia in the primate. J Neurol Neurosurg Psychiatry 42:892–898
Dernbach P, Little JR, Jones SC, Ebrahim Z (1988) Altered cerebral autoregulation and CO_2 reactivity after aneurysmal subarachnoid haemorrhage. Neurosurgery 22:822–826
Fisher CM, Roberson GH, Ojemann RG (1977) Cerebral vasospasm with ruptered saccular aneurysm – the clinical manifestations. Neurosurgery 1:245–248
Fisher CM, Kistler JP, Davis JM (1980) Relationship of cerebral vasospasm to subarachnoid haemorrhage visualised by computerised tomographic scanning. Neurosurgery 6:1–9
Geraud G, Tremaulet M, Gueii A, Beo A (1984) The prognostic value of non-invasive cerebral blood flow measurement in subarachnoid haemorrhage. Stroke 15:301–305
Heilbrun MP, Olesen J, Lassen N (1972) Regional cerebral blood flow studies in subarachnoid haemorrhage. J Neurosurg 37:36–44
Ishii R (1979) Regional cerebral blood flows in patients with ruptured intracranial aneurysms. J Neurosurg 50:587–594
Kassell NF, Sasaki T, Colohan ART, Nazar G (1985) Cerebral vasospasm following aneurysmal subarachnoid haemorrhage. Stroke 16:562–572
Kassell NF, Torner JC, Haley EC, Jane JA, Adams HP, Kongable GL et al. (1990) The International Cooperative Study on the Timing of Aneurysm Surgery. I. Overall management results. J Neurosurg 73:18–36
Kosnik E, Hunt W (1970) Postoperative hypertension in the management of intracranial arterial aneurysms. J Neurosurg 45:148–154
Kwak R, Niizum H, Takatsugu O, Suzuki J (1979) Angiographic study of cerebral vasospasm following rupture of intracranial aneurysms. I. Time of the appearance. Surg Neurol 11:257–267
Lovick AJ, Pickard JD, Goddard BA (1982) Prediction of late ischaemic complications after cerebral aneurysm surgery – use of a mobile microcomputer system for the measurement of pre-, intra- and post-operative cerebral blood flow. Acta Neurochir (Wien) 63:37–49
Mendelow AD, McCalden TA, Hattingly J, Coull A, Rosendorff C, Eidelman BH (1981) Cerebrovascular reactivity and metabolism after subarachnoid haemorrhage in baboons. Stroke 12:58–65
Messeter K, Brandt L, Ljunggren B, Svendgaard NA, Algotsson L, Romner B, Ryding E (1987) Prediction and prevention of delayed ischaemic dysfunction after aneurysmal subarachnoid haemorrhage and early operation. Neurosurgery 20:548–553
Meyer CHA, Lowe D, Meyer M, Richardson PL, Neil-Dwyer G (1983) Progressive change in cerebral blood flow during the first three weeks after subarachnoid haemorrhage. Neurosurgery 12:58–76
Millikan CH (1975) Cerebral vasospasm and ruptured intracranial aneurysm. Arch Neurol 32:433–449
Pickard JD, Mathieson M, Pattersen J, Wyper D (1980) Prediction of late ischaemic complications after cerebral aneurysm surgery by the intraoperative measurement of CBF. J Neurosurg 53:305–308
Pickard JD, Murray GD, Illingworth R, Shaw MDM, Teasedale GM, Foy PM, Humphrey PRD, Lang DA, Nelson R, Sinar J, Bailey S, Skene A (1989) Effect of nimodipine on cerebral infarction and outcome after aneurysmal subarachnoid haemorrhage: British Aneurysm Nimodipine Trial. BMJ 298:636–642
Simeone FA, Trepper PJ, Brown DJ (1972) Cerebral blood flow evaluation of prolonged experimental vasospasm. J Neurosurg 37:302–311
Voldby B, Enevoldsen EM, Jensen FT (1985) Cerebrovascular reactivity in patients with ruptured intracranial aneurysms. J Neurosurg 62:59–67
Weir B, Grace M, Hansen J, Rothberg C (1978) Time course of vasospasm in man. J Neurosurg 48:173–178

Doppler CO_2 Test in Interal Carotid Artery Occlusions: Prospective and Retrospective Results

B. Kleiser and B. Widder

Introduction

The transcranial Doppler CO_2 test is a simple method of investigating the cerebral reserve capacity in internal carotid artery (ICA) occlusion, giving quantitative information about the efficiency of the collaterals. To prove the clinical value of the technique, we investigated patients with ICA occlusions retro- and prospectively.

Methods

To evaluate the cerebrovascular reserve capacity, time averaged middle cerebral artery (MCA) blood flow velocity was monitored continuously by transcranial Doppler sonography together with end-tidal PCO_2 measured by an infrared analyzer. Measurements were performed during at least four steady states of different PCO_2 values (Widder et al. 1986):

1. Normoventilation by breathing ambient air
2. Hypercapnia by breathing a fixed mixture of 5% CO_2 in 95% O_2 ("carbogene")
3. Hyperventilation in ambient air
4. Normoventilation giving feedback about position artifacts of the probe during the investigation

To assess MCA blood flow velocity changes using a standardized method, a blood PCO_2 of 40 mmHg was taken as a reference point and the increase/decrease in flow during hyper- and hypocapnia of 1 vol%. CO_2 was calculated as the "normalized CO_2

Table 1. Interpretation of the Doppler CO_2 test. (After Widder 1989)

		Change in MCA velocity in relation to baseline values at 40 mmHg PCO_2	
Type	Auto-regulatory capacity	Increase during hypercapnia (+1 vol. % CO_2)	Decrease during hypocapnia (–1 vol. % CO_2)
A	Normal	$\geq$ 10%	$\geq$ 10%
B	Diminished	–	$\geq$ 10%
C	Exhausted	–	–

reactivity" (NCR). Based on standard values obtained from former investigations in normal subjects and patients with various degrees of carotid artery stenosis (Widder et al. 1986; Widder 1989), three categories of NCR were distinguished (Table 1).

Results

Between 1985 and 1989, 293 patients with ICA occlusions were investigated. The retrospective evaluation of clinical symptoms and the comparison with the CO_2 reactivity is shown in Fig. 1. The neurological symptoms were subdivided into recent attacks and those where the time interval between the (last) onset of symptoms and the Doppler CO_2 test was more than 3 months. In all cases, the neurological attacks were due to ischemia. Other causes such as cerebral hemorrhage were excluded by cranial computed tomography (CCT). Of 49 patients with nearly or completely absent CO_2 reactivity 31 (63%) had developed at least one stroke or transient ischemic attack (TIA) during the previous 3 months. Of 92 with a markedly diminished CO_2 reactivity

Fig. 1. Correlation between the "normalized CO_2 reactivity" *(NCR) and ipsilateral clinical findings in 293 ICA occlusions*

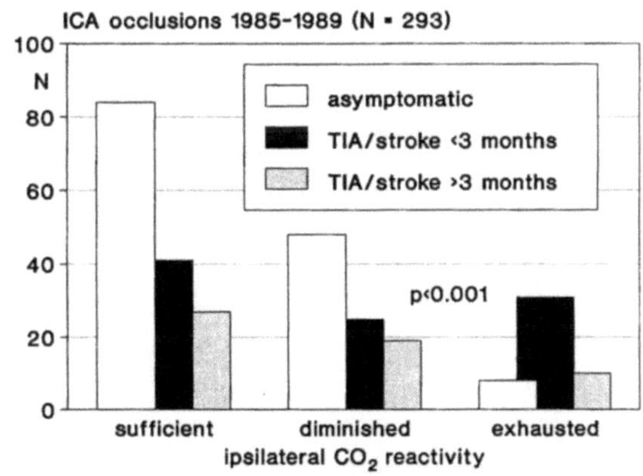

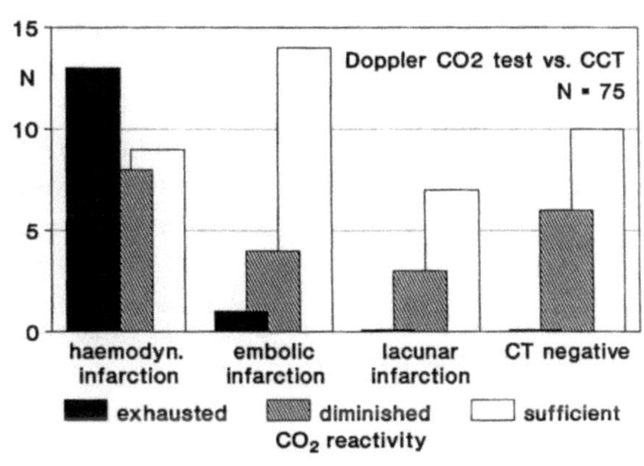

Fig. 2. Correlation between the "normalized CO_2 reactivity" *(NCR) and ipsilateral CCT lesions in 75 ICA occlusions*

25 (27%) had recently suffered symptoms, and in 41 out of 152 (27%) with higher CO_2 reactivity acute cerebral ischemia occurred. The correlation between low CO_2 reactivity and recent cerebral ischemia was highly significant ($p<0.001$).

In 75 patients with ICA occlusions, CCT images were available. The patterns of infarction were evaluated without knowledge of the CO_2 reactivity. Thirteen out of 30 cases with hemodynamic infarctions had an exhausted cerebrovascular reserve capacity, compared with only 1 out of 19 with territorial infarctions. None of the ten in the group with lacunar lesions and none of the CT-negative patients showed an exhausted CO_2 reactivity. Though the number of cases evaluated was not very large, the difference was significant with $p<0.01$ (Fig. 2).

One hundred and three patients with 100 uni- and 3 bilateral occlusions of the ICA were followed for an average time of 27 months. Sixteen suffered an ipsilateral ischemic deficit (eight TIAs or PRINDs, eight strokes) corresponding to an annual stroke rate of 3.5%. Seven died from noncerebral causes. In the group with sufficient autoregulatory reserve, 3 out of 43 (7%) developed a TIA or prolonged reversible ischemic neurological deficit (PRIND), none a stroke, and 3 patients died from other causes. In the group with diminished CO_2 reactivity, 7 out of 26 (27%) suffered an ipsilateral ischemic attack (3 TIAs, 4 strokes), and 2 patients died from other causes. The annual stroke rate in this group was 7.4%. Of the patients with exhausted autoregulatory reserve, 5/15 (33%) developed an ipsilateral neurological deficit (1 TIAs, 4 strokes). Three attacks occurred in the first 3 months after the measurement of the CO_2 reactivity. The annual stroke rate in this group was 14.5%. The difference between the patients with sufficient and those with diminished or exhausted CO_2 reactivity was significant ($p<0.01$) (Fig. 3a–c).

Nineteen patients were submitted for extra-intracranial bypass surgery prior to the development of the Doppler CO_2 test. Only one patient developed a PRIND in the follow-up period of 29 months (Fig. 3d).

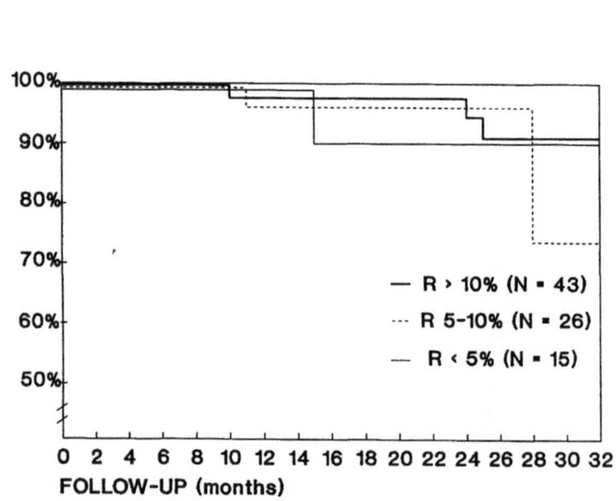

Fig. 3a. Lifetime analysis for ipsilateral TIA/PRIND in 84 patients with ICA occlusions.

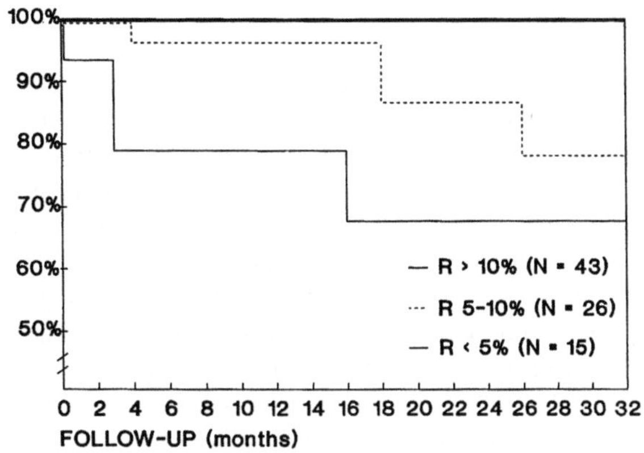

Fig. 3b. Lifetime analysis for ipsilateral stroke in 84 patients with ICA occlusions.

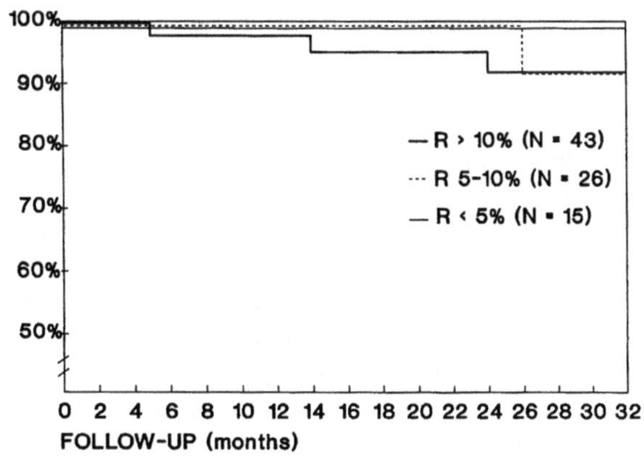

Fig. 3c. Lifetime analysis for noncerebral causes of death in 84 patients with ICA occlusions.

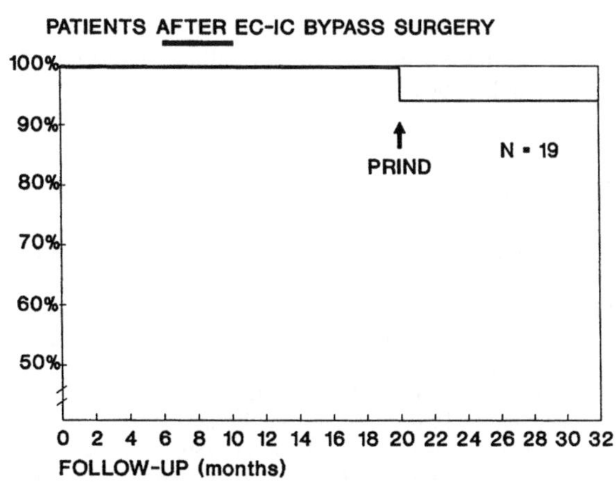

Fig. 3d. Lifetime analysis for the incidence of ipsilateral neurological symptoms in 19 patients with extraintracranial bypass

Discussion

The retrospective investigation of patients with ICA occlusions showed a highly significant correlation between an exhausted autoregulatory reserve and the incidence of ipsilateral neurological deficits such as TIA or stroke in the last 3 months. This corresponds to earlier published data about carotid artery stenosis (Widder et al. 1986).
The evaluation of the CCT scans revealed a significant correlation between an exhausted CO_2 reactivity and hemodynamic infarctions. Thromboembolic and lacunar lesions did not influence the CO_2 reactivity, indicating that the cerebrovascular reserve capacity is not dependent upon structural brain damage itself, but on the pathogenetic mechanism causing the lesion. This corresponds to a retrospective study by Ringelstein et al. (1988), who found an association of low-flow infarctions, ischemic ophthalmopathy, and hypostatic ischemic attacks with reduced vasomotor reactivities.
In the follow-up study, the overall rate for ipsilateral ischemic attacks was similar to the prognosis in other investigations (Cote et al. 1983; Hennerici et al. 1986; EC/IC Bypass Study Group 1985). But these studies did not consider the intracranial collateralization. The classification into three groups according to CO_2 reactivity resulted in different outcomes. The patients with an exhausted reserve capacity had a significantly higher rate of ipsilateral strokes than those with a sufficient reserve capacity. In a study using positron emission tomography, Powers et al. (1989) found no influence of cerebral hemodynamics on stroke risk. But his group was limited to 30 patients, and the follow-up time was only 1 year.

The patients with an extra-intracranial bypass showed a risk of ipsilateral neurological symptoms similar to that of patients with a sufficient cerebrovascular reserve capacity. But this study only recorded the follow-up after successful extra-intracranial bypass surgery, not the perioperative risk.

In conclusion, these results support the hypothesis that the Doppler CO_2 test may be a suitable method for the evaluation of the cerebrovascular reserve capacity. Patients with an exhausted CO_2 reactivity have a significantly higher risk of developing ischemic neurological symptoms than patients with a sufficient reserve capacity. This test could exclude patients who are not in need of EC/IC bypass surgery. On the other hand, the Doppler CO_2 test helps to identify a subgroup of patients who may benefit from EC/IC bypass surgery. To compare the use of operative and conservative treatment in patients with insufficient collateralization, a prospective study is in preparation (Schmiedek 1990).

References

Cote R, Barnett HJM, Taylor DW (1983) Internal carotid occlusion: a prospective study. Stroke 14:898–902

EC/IC Bypass Study Group (1985) Failure of extracranial intracranial arterial bypass to reduce the risk of ischemic stroke. Results of an international randomized trial. N Engl J Med 313:1191–1200

Hennerici M, Hülsbömer H-B, Rautenberg W, Hefter H (1986) Spontaneous history of asymptomatic internal carotid occlusion. Stroke 17:718–722

Powers WJ, Tempel LW, Grubb RL (1989) Influence of cerebral hemodynamics on stroke risk: one year follow-up of 30 medically treated patients. Ann Neurol 25:325–330

Ringelstein EB, Sievers C, Ecker S, Schneider PA, Otis SM (1988) Noninvasive assessment of CO_2-induced cerebral vasomotor response in normal individuals and patients with internal carotid artery occlusion. Stroke 19:963–969

Schmiedek P (1990) Zerebrale Ischämie: Neuansatz für die mikrochirurgische Behandlung. Dtsch Aerztebl 87:1518–1523

Widder B, Paulat K, Hackspacher J, Mayr E (1986) Transcranial Doppler CO_2-test for the detection of hemodynamically critical carotid artery stenosis and occlusions. Eur Arch Psychiatry Neurol Sci 236:162–168

Widder B (1989) The Doppler CO_2 test to exclude patients not in need of extracranial/intracranial bypass surgery. J Neurol Neurosurg Psychiatry 52:38–42

Changes in CBF After Carotid Endarterectomy: Follow-up in Neurologically Asymptomatic Patients

J. A. REM, O. GRATZL, H. R. MÜLLER, J. MÜLLER-BRAND, and E. W. RADÜ

Introduction

According to a previous report (EC/IC Bypass Study Group 1985), patients with high-grade stenoses or occlusions of cerebral arteries, who were expected to benefit from surgical procedures, did not actually benefit clinically. We tried to define a subgroup in neurologically asymptomatic patients by two quantiative methods, namely regional cerebral blood flow (CBF) and ultrasonic common carotid flow (CCF) measurements. Mean hemispheric CBF was measured at rest and after administration of 1 g acetazolamide (Diamox). Several authors demonstrated that the acetazolamide test is a reliable indicator of critically reduced cerebral perfusion pressure (Schroeder 1986; Sillesen et al. 1988) and may unmask perfusion deficits even in patients with normal baseline values (Vorstrup et al. 1986; Sullivan et al. 1987). In this report we compare the preoperative and postoperative CBF and CCF values and discuss the significance of prophylactic carotid endarterectomy.

Material and Methods

Ultrasonic CCF was measured with the Hayashi Denki VFM 1000 instrument, which measures mean spatial velocity, using an angle-independent double-beam technique, and internal vessel diameter by means of a high-resolution one-dimensional impulse echo technique (Furuhata et al. 1978). CCF was measured in patients with a Doppler flowmeter (Müller et al. 1984) pre- and postoperatively. CBF and CCF in a test group were significantly correlated (Müller et al. 1985). Only patients with hemodynamically significant carotid stenosis (Doppler sonography showing a peak systolic frequency shift greater than 8 kHz using a transmitted frequency of 4 MHz) were considered for inclusion in this study.

For CBF studies we used the intravenous xenon-133 technique (Novo Cerebrograph; Schroeder 1986). Data were analyzed according to the bicompartmental model yielding fast (gray matter) blood flow values (F1), initial slope index (ISI), and initial slope (IS). CBF was measured during rest and 10–15 min after administration of 1 g acetazolamide to obtain global cerebral vasodilatation (Vorstrup et al. 1986). According to Schroeder (1986) and Schroeder et al. (1987), the increase following acetazolamide was expressed as a percentage of baseline flow. CBF baseline asymmetry (BA) and acetazolamide asymmetry (AA) were calculated as:

$$\frac{\text{CBF contralateral} - \text{CBF ipsilateral} \times 100}{\text{mean CBF}} \%$$

Acetazolamide asymmetry enhancement (AAE) was calculated as acetazolamide CBF asymmetry (AA) minus CBF baseline asymmetry. Studies by Schroeder (1986) and Schroeder et al. (1987) have shown BA exceeding ±5% and AAE exceeding ±7% to be significant. CBF was measured within 6 weeks preoperatively and 1–3 weeks, 6 weeks, 3 months, and 1 year postoperatively.

Computed tomography scan and four-vessel angiography were carried out in the patients considered for carotid endarterectomy. Postoperative Doppler sonography and digital subtraction angiography were performed to confirm patency.

Results

Sixty neurologically asymptomatic patients were seen over a 5-year period. Some of them had, however, suffered from previous attacks of amaurosis fugax bruits. Data from these patients are shown in Table 1. In all patients CBF was measured because of the presence of a peak Doppler frequency shift exceeding 8 kHz. Forty-two patients had normal cerebral perfusion (group I) and 18 patients underwent carotid endarterectomy because of amaurosis fugax (10 patients), significant CBF baseline asymmetry, and/or AAE (seven patients) and a severe, disturbing carotid bruit (one patient) (group II).

Table 1. Patient data

	Group I (conservative)	Group II (surgical)
Number of patients	42	18
Male	30	16
Female	12	2
Amaurosis fugax	20	10
Carotid bruits	22	8
Mean age (years)	64.3	63.9
Age range (years)	58–81	53–77

Table 2. Cerebral blood flow ipsilateral to the carotid stenosis and side-to-side CBF asymmetry

	Group I (conservative)	Group II (surgical)
Number of patients	42	18
Baseline CBF (ml 100 g^{-1} min^{-1})	37.10 [6.7]	37.32 [6.42]
Acetazolamide CBF (ml 100 g^{-1} min^{-1})	50.46 [10.0]	51.05 [8.36]
Baseline CBF asymmetry (%)	2.55 [6.61]	3.73 [7.64]
Acetazolamide CBF asymmetry (%)	2.86 [6.02]	0.51 [3.71]
Acetazolamide asymmetry enhancement (%)	0.32 [5.28]	–3.22 [6.89]

[], ± SD

Preoperative CBF values ipsilateral to the carotid stenosis and side-to-side CBF asymmetry are listed in Table 2; there is no statistically significant difference between these two groups. None of the surgically treated patients showed a cerebral infarction in the respective arterial distribution in CT scans. Doppler sonography and angiography demonstrated carotid stenosis of >60%. The BAs and AAEs (15 postoperative

Table 3. Baseline asymmetry and acetazolamide asymmetry enhancement

	Preoperative	Postoperative
No. patients	18	15
Baseline CBF asymmetry (%)	3.73 [7.64]	0.14 [5.27]
Acetazolamide asymmetry enhancement (%)	–3.22 [6.89]	–0.17 [4.11]

[], ± SD

Table 4. Side-to-side CBF asymmetry in seven patients exceeding a baseline asymmetry of ± 5% and/or acetazolamide asymmetry enhancement of ± 7%

	Preoperative	Postoperative
Baseline CBF asymmetry (%)	7.63 [11.14]	0.56 [7.35]
Acetazolamide asymmetry enhancement (%)	–6.61 [10.14]	–0.19 [5.04]

[], ± SD

Table 5. Cerebral blood flow results of group II over a 1-year period

	Baseline CBF (ml 100 g^{-1} min^{-1})	Acetazolamide CBF (ml 100 g^{-1} min^{-1})	BA (%)	AA (%)	AAE (%)	No. patients
Preoperative	37.32 [6.47]	51.05 [8.36]	3.73 [7.64]	0.51 [3.71]	–3.22 [6.89]	18
Postoperative						
1–3 weeks	34.02 [3.83]	46.91 [4.24]	0.14 [5.27]	0.03 [2.70]	–0.17 [4.11]	15
6 weeks	36.79 [6.27]	50.71 [6.60]	0.65 [2.83]	0.37 [1.99]	–0.28 [1.64]	10
3 months	36.05 [4.03]	49.60 [3.20]	–0.54 [1.02]	–0.11 [2.56]	0.43 [2.38]	6
1 year	35.11 [4.26]	50.24 [6.97]	0.09 [3.90]	1.86 [2.10]	1.77 [3.67]	7

[], ± SD

Table 6. Ultrasonic common carotid flow measurement pre- and postoperatively, ipsilateral and contralateral to stenosis of the internal carotid artery

	Preoperative values	Postoperative values
No. patients	11	9
Ipsilateral (ml/s) [± SD]	5.11 [1.5]*/**	6.93 [2.16]*
Contralateral (ml/s) [± SD]	7.74 [1.9]**	7.47 [2.53]

* $p < 0.05$; ** $p < 0.01$

values) of 18 surgically treated patients are listed in Table 3. In Table 4 pre- and postoperative side-to-side CBF asymmetry of the seven patients exceeding a BA of ±5% and/or AAE of ±7% is presented; there is a marked but statistically insignificant difference. Table 5 summarizes the CBF values of group II over a 1-year period. The results of ultrasonic CCF measurement pre- and postoperatively are shown in Table 6. Preoperative measurements demonstrated a statistically significant lower flow ipsilateral rate (p<0.01) and postoperatively there was a significant increase (p<0.05) in the ipsilateral flow rate.

Discussion

Cerebral blood flow studies and Doppler CCF measurements appear to provide an adequate basis for defining criteria for subgroups of cerebral vascular disease (Schroeder 1986; Vorstrup et al. 1986; Sullivan et al. 1987; Müller et al. 1985). In the determination of CBF parameters, the presence of hemispheric asymmetry has the greatest relevance and is the most sensitive parameter (Schroeder 1986; Schroeder et al. 1987). In addition, tests of cerebrovascular reactivity with acetazolamide can disclose perfusion deficits (Schroeder 1986; Schroeder et al. 1987; Sillesen et al. 1988; Sullivan et al. 1987).

Our data show CBF parameters tend to improve after surgical procedures, but this improvement is not statistically significant. Sullivan et al. (1987) observed a postoperative improvement in CBF after endarterectomy in five patients. Fourteen patients were investigated by Russell et al. (1990) before and 3 months after endarterectomy. These authors found a normalization of the vasoreactivity 3 months after the operation. Our failure to find a statistically significant difference can be explained by (a) the small number of patients and (b) calculating the hemispheric asymmetry as the sole parameter and not focusing on the region of interest.

Ultrasonic CCF measurements demonstrated a significant postoperative improvement in the flow on the operated side.

The pathophysiological significance of an asymmetry of CBF for cerebral perfusion is known, especially under acetazolamide exposure, but the question is not settled as to whether the disturbed cerebrovascular reactivity also entails a higher risk of stroke (Clifton et al. 1988). Considering as many parameters as in our study, and a follow-up to compare the group treated surgically and the group treated conservatively, surgery will probably clarify questions regarding the significance of prophylactic carotid endarterectomy.

So far, it appears that long-term survival after prophylactic endarterectomy is comparable with that of a corresponding age group of the population, i.e., premature deaths caused by stroke can probably be reduced by the operation (Rosenthal et al. 1987). However, without a favorable perioperative course there are no prospects for a significant effect of the operation on long-term outcome. Since a combined surgical morbidity and mortality rate of 2.1% can be attained for carotid endarterectomy even in symptomatic cases (Zeiger et al. 1987), we expect that the surgical procedure will be able to compete with the conservative management of asymptomatic carotid atherosclerosis.

References

Clifton GL, Haden HT, Taylor JR, Sobel M (1988) Cerebrovascular CO_2 reactivity after carotid artery occlusion. J Neurosurg 69:24–28

EC/IC Bypass Study Group (1985) Failure of extra-/intracranial arterial bypass to reduce the risk of ischemic stroke: results of an international randomized trial. N Engl J Med 313:1191–1200

Furuhata H, Kanno R, Kodaira K, Aoyagi T, Hayashi J, Matsumodo H, Joshimura S (1978) An ultrasonic blood flow measuring system to detect absolute volume flow. Iyodenshi To Seitai Kogaku [Suppl] 16:334

Müller HR, Radü EW, Gratzl O (1984) Common carotid cw Doppler flow measurement in neurovascular surgery. In: Kurjak A, Kossoff G (eds) Recent advances in ultrasound diagnosis, vol 4. Elsevier, Amsterdam, pp 17–36

Müller HR, Buser M, Müller J, Schneider T (1985) Correlation of mean hemispheric blood flow by Xenon 133 clearance to common carotid flow by QFM Doppler in 100 patients. Ultrasound Med Biol [Suppl] 1:442

Rosenthal D, Ruddermann R, Borrero E, Hafner DH, Perdue GD, Lamis PA, Clark MD, Daniel WW (1987) Carotid endarterectomy to correct asymptomatic carotid stenosis: ten years later. J Vasc Surg 6:226–230

Russel D, Dybevold S, Kjartansson O, Nyberg-Hansen R, Rootwelt K, Wiberg J (1990) Cerebral vasoreactivity and blood flow before and 3 months after carotid endarterectomy. Stroke 21:1029–1032

Schroeder T (1986) Cerebrovascular reactivity to acetazolamide in carotid artery disease. Neurol Res 8:231–236

Schroeder T, Sillesen H, Sorènsen O, Engell HC (1987) Cerebral hyperperfusion following carotid endarterectomy. J Neurosurg 66:824–829

Sillesen H, Schroeder T, Buchardt Hansen HJ (1988) Haemodynamic evaluation of the cerebral circùlation by periorbital Doppler examination and cerebral blood flow (CBF) measurement in carotid artery disease. Neurol Res 10:57–60

Sullivan HG, Kingsbury TB, Morgan ME, Jeffcoat RD, Allison JD, Goode JJ, McDonnel DE (1987) The rCBF response to Diamox in normal subjects and cerebrovascular disease patients. J Neurosurg 67:525–534

Vorstrup S, Brun B, Lassen NA (1986) Evaluation of the cerebral vasodilatory capacity by the acetazolamide test before EC-IC bypass surgery in patients with occlusion of the internal carotid artery. Stroke 17:1291–1298

Zeiger HE, Zampella EJ, Naftel DC, McKay RD, Varner PD, Morawetz RB (1987) A prospective analysis of 142 carotid endarterectomies for occlusive vascular disease. J Neurosurg 67:540–544

Effect of Stenosis and Endarterectomy on Internal Carotid Artery Blood Flow

C. R. Bishop

Patients

A total of 122 patients were studied (84 men, 38 women) of mean age 59 years (range, 38–76 years). These patients were all referred to the Department of Surgery for assessment of their carotid arteries by duplex ultrasound scanning and agreed to undergo a hypercapnia stress test as part of their investigation. Reasons for referral included detection of asymptomatic neck bruits on routine examination, symptoms suggestive of amaurosis fugax, transient ischaemic attacks (TIAs), or referral for consideration of carotid endarterectomy following investigation elsewhere. In order to investigate the effect of disease of the opposite internal carotid artery (ICA) on the response of blood flow velocity to hypercapnia in the ICA under study, these 122 patients were divided into two groups.

Group 1: 79 Patients (54 Men, 25 Women)

This group of patients either had minimal bilateral ICA stenosis or if a stenosis was present had less than 50% diameter reduction of the opposite ICA. On the basis of duplex ultrasound scanning, confirmed where clinically indicated by angiography, each ICA was found to be widely patent (<20%) diameter reduction), moderately stenosed (20%–49% diameter reduction), or severely stenosed (50%–99% diameter reduction). On this basis, these patients could be subdivided as follows:

Both ICAs widely patent	13 patients
One ICA moderately stenosed and the other ICA widely patent	13 patients
One ICA severely stenosed and the other ICA widely patent	19 patients
Both ICAs moderately stenosed	7 patients
One ICA severely stenosed and the other ICA moderately stenosed	27 patients

Forty-nine of these patients subsequently underwent carotid endarterectomy.

Group 2: 43 Patients (30 Men, 13 Women)

This group of patients were found on Duplex ultrasound scanning, and in the majority confirmed by angiography, to have severe bilateral ICA stenoses or a totally occluded ICA in combination with a contralateral ICA stenosis:

Both ICAs severely stenosed	18 patients
One ICA moderately stenosed and the other ICA occluded	10 patients
One ICA severely stenosed and the other ICA occluded	15 patients

Twenty-three of these patients subsequently underwent carotid endarterectomy.

Methods

All patients underwent duplex ultrasound scanning of both carotid bifurcations using the Philips SDU 3000 real-time B scanner and the Philips SDD 500 continuous-wave Doppler scanner. The ICA was scanned from the bifurcation to the angle of the jaw. The maximum peak frequency (PF) found was recorded and taken to present the stenosis. A PF of less than 4 KHz represents a widely patent artery; in other words either a normal ICA or one with a reduction in diameter of 1%–19%. A PF of between 4 and 6 KHz represents a moderately stenosed ICA with a diameter reduction of between 20% and 49% and a PF of greater than 6 KHz represents a severely stenosed ICA which has a diameter reduction of between 50% and 99%.

The vertebral arteries were also scanned in the majority of patients to establish the patency of these vessels. The vertebral artery was insonated just inferior to the mastoid process, where it winds around the lateral mass of the atlas bone.

Following the completion of the duplex ultrasound scan, the response of ICA blood flow velocity to hypercapnia (5% CO_2 in air) was measured and expressed as a reactivity index. The measurement was performed above, i.e., distal, to any stenosis that was present.

Angiography (IV digital subtraction angiography, DSA,in the majority) was performed at the discretion of the referring clinician. The results reported in this chapter are based on the duplex ultrasound findings rather than being specifically compared with angiographic findings as not all patients underwent angiography. On the rare occassion where there was difficulty in interpreting between occlusion and patency of the ICA, the angiogram (if it had been performed) was referred to.

In group 1, 28 of the 32 patients with reactivities to CO_2 in the ICA of less than 10 underwent carotid endarterectomy. Twenty-five of these 28 patients had the study repeated between 6 weeks and 3 months following surgery to assess whether removal of the stenotic plaque had resulted in the restoration of normal reactivity to CO_2. Of the remaining four patients with reactivities less than 10, two had occluded their ICAs by the time they were admitted for surgery and two did not undergo operation as they were asymptomatic.

In group 2, there were 39 patients with ICAs which demonstrated a reactivity to CO_2 of less than 10, 20 of which subsequently underwent carotid endarterectomy. Of these 20, 18 were restudied between 6 weeks and 3 months following surgery. The remaining 19 patients with ICAs with a reactivity below 10 were not restudied, in 10 because no operation was performed and in 9 because they were on the contralateral side to one of the 20 operated arteries, although 4 of these did subsequently undergo contralateral carotid endarterectomy. These results are only based on the side on which the first operation was performed.

Statistical analysis was performed by linear regression analysis and Student's *t* test using the Litton Monroe 1930 calculator. *P* values derived from regression coefficients (*r* values) were obtained from tables in *Documenta Geigy* (Anonymous 1970).

Results

Group 1

Results of Doppler scanning of the 158 ICAs were as follows:

PF	<4 KHz	59 (No. of ICAs)
	4–6 KHz	53
	6–8 KHz	5
	8–10 KHz	10
	10–12 KHz	9
	12–14 KHz	8
	14–16 KHz	6
	16–18 KHz	0
	18–20 KHz	0
	20–22 KZz	8

Both vertebral arteries were patent in 63 patients. Only one vertebral artery was patent in eight patients and in eight patients the status of the vertebral arteries was unknown because it was not recorded.

For each ICA, reactivity to CO_2 was plotted against peak frequency (Fig. 1) to assess the effect of stenosis on the response. This demonstrated that, if the ICA stenosis was less than 10 KHz, reactivity to CO_2 was preserved. Two patients had unexpected results, one had a reactivity of 5 in an ICA of PF 4.5 KHz, and one had a reactivity of 0 in an ICA of PF 8 KHz.

Figure 2 illustrates the mean reactivity of all ICAs falling into each of the following ranges of PF:

PF	<4 KHz	Reactivity 14.7 (±1.9) (SD)
	4– 6 KHz	14.7 (±2.7)
	6– 8 KHz	14.4 (±1.5)
	8–10 KHz	11.6 (±4.8)
	10–12 KHz	4.3 (±3.4)
	12–14 KHz	1.7 (±1.4)
	14–16 KHz	1.6 (±1.9)
	16–18 KHz	–
	18–20 KHz	–
	20–22 KZz	0.7 (±0.60)

The first column of Fig. 2 represents the mean ICA reactivity of 25 normal subjects.

Reactivity was normal if the ICA stenosis PF was less than 8 KHz. With a stenosis PF between 8 and 10 KHz, mean reactivity was reduced compared with the widely patent ICAs (PF<4 KHz) and this was statistically significant ($p<0.01$, Student's *t* test). If the stenosis was greater than 10 KHz, then the reduction in mean reactivity compared with the widely patent ICAs was highly statistically significant (Student's *t* test); PF 10–12 KHz, $p<0.001$; PF 12–14 KHz, $p<0.001$; PF 14–16 KHz, $p<0.001$; PF 20–22 KHz, $p<0.001$.

For each of the 79 patients, reactivity of the right ICA was plotted against reactivity of the left ICA (Fig. 3).

Closed circles refer to those patients where both ICAs had a PF of less than 10 KHz and therefore both ICAs would be expected to have normal reactivity. Correlation between left and right ICA reactivity in these patients was good ($r=0.531$, $p<0.001$), despite the fact that two patients, as mentioned earlier, had wayward results. The open circles refer to those patients where one ICA had a PF of more than 10 KHz and therefore that ICA would be expected to have reduced reactivity as previously demonstrated (Figs. 1, 2). Obviously no correlation could be expected in those patients between the right ICA and the left ICA.

The mean increase in end expiratory CO_2 was 1.31 (vol%)±0.3 SD. Mean increase in systolic blood pressure was 5 mmHg and in diastolic pressure 3 mmHg.

Group 2

Results of Doppler scanning of the 86 ICAs were as follows:

PF	4– 6 KHz	10 (No. of ICAs)
	6– 8 KHz	16
	8–10 KHz	10
	10–12 KHz	7
	12–14 KHz	6
	14–16 KHz	4
	16–18 KHz	5
	18–20 KHz	1
	20–22 KZz	2
	Occluded	25

Both vertebral arteries were patent in 34 patients. Only one vertebral artery was patent in two patients and the status of the vertebral arteries was unknown in seven patients because it was not recorded.

Obviously it was not possible to measure reactivity in a totally occluded ICA. For the 61 nonoccluded ICAs, reactivity to CO_2 was plotted against peak frequency (Fig. 4), demonstrating that ICA reactivity to CO_2 was reduced in some patients when the contralateral ICA was severely diseased. With a stenosis PF of less than 6 KHz, reactivity was preserved above 10 in all but one ICA, but with a stenosis PF of greater than 6 KHz many patients demonstrated an ICA reactivity of below 10.

Figure 5 illustrates the mean reactivity of all ICAs falling into each of the following ranges of PF. The mean (±SD) values are also as follows:

PF	4– 6 KHz	Reactivity 13.4 (±3.5) (SD)
	6– 8 KHz	10.0 (±5.6)
	8–10 KHz	10.3 (±5.4)
	10–12 KHz	5.0 (±3.9)

Table 1. Comparison of patients with severe contralateral ICA disease with PF greater than 6 with groups with PF between 4 and 6 KHz and normals

		Compared with normals	Compared with ICAs of PF 4–6 KHz
PF	4– 6 KHz	$p<0.01$	–
	6– 8 KHz	$p<0.001$	$p<0.2$
	8–10 KHz	$p<0.001$	$p<0.2$
	10–12 KHz	$p<0.001$	$p<0.001$
	12–14 KHz	$p<0.001$	$p<0.001$
	14–16 KHz	$p<0.001$	$p<0.001$
	16–18 KHz	$p<0.001$	$p<0.001$
	18–20 KHz	–	–
	20–22 KHz	–	–

12–14 KHz	1.4 (±1.3)
14–16 KHz	0.4 (±0.5)
16–18 KHz	0.4 (±1.6)
18–20 KHz	0
20–22 KZz	0

The first column of Fig. 5 represents the mean ICA reactivity (15.4±1.4 SD) of 25 normal subjects. These mean values illustrate that in this group of patients with severe contralateral ICA disease there is a reduction in ICA reactivity in every range of PF. When those subgroups were compared (Student's *t* Test) with the 25 normal subjects and when stenoses of PF greater than 6 KHz were compared (Student's *t* test) with those between 4 and 6 KHz, the *p* values shown in Table 1 were obtained.

Referring back to Fig. 4, it can be seen that, if the ICA stenosis PF was less than 6 KHz, reactivity to CO_2 was preserved. If the ICA stenosis PF was greater than 10 KHz, reactivity to CO_2 was lost. This loss of reactivity is similar to the findings in group 1 patients. i.e., those without severe contralateral disease. In order to elucidate the effect of contralateral ICA disease on the reactivity of ICAs with a stenosis PF of between 6 and 10 KHz, patients with such a stenosis were divided into the following three groups according to the status of the contralateral ICA:

PF of contralateral ICA	Mean reactivity ± SD
<6 KHz	12.5±4.1
6–10 KHz	12.4±5.5
>10 KHz or occluded	7.8±4.9

Figure 6 illustrates the mean reactivities (±SD) for these three groups of patients. This shows that, even with a contralateral stenosis PF of 6–10 KHz, reactivity was preserved. When the opposite ICA was unable itself to increase flow in response to CO_2 (i.e., PF>10 KHz or occluded), then this reduced the reactivity in contralateral ICAs with a stenosis PF of between 6 and 10 KHz. This reduction was statistically significant ($p<0.01$, Student's *t* test).

Figure 7 shows the individual reactivities according to the status of the contralateral ICA.

The mean increase in end expiratory CO_2 was 1.33 (vol%)±0.3 SD. Mean increase in systolic blood pressure was 1 mmHg and in diastolic pressure 3 mmHg.

Effect of Carotid Endarterectomy

The effect of carotid endarterectomy on those ICAs which had a reactivity preoperatively of less than 10 was investigated by repeating the study between 6 weeks and 3 months following surgery. Figure 8 illustrates the individual and mean results for the 25 patients in group 1. Mean reactivity increased from 1.9 (±2.2 SD) to 12.3 (±2.4 SD), which was highly significant ($p<0.001$, paired *t* test).

In the 18 patients from group 2 which were restudied postoperatively, mean reactivity increased from 2.1 (±2.6 SD) to 11.7 (±2.4 SD), which was highly significant ($p<0.001$, paired *t* test). Figure 9 illustrates the individual changes and increase in mean reactivity for these 18 patients.

Discussion

Patients with a tightly stenotic lesion at the origin of the internal carotid artery have the highest incidence of subsequent stroke (Ziegler and Hassanein 1973) and this has been further confirmed in patients with a haemodynamically significant carotid stenosis (Busuttil et al. 1981). Early studies suggested that arterial stenosis caused by atherosclerotic plaques led to cerebral infarction by simply decreasing cerebral blood flow (CBF) (Schwartz and Mitchell 1961; Hutchinson and Yates 1957). More recently it has been demonstrated experimentally that the haemodynamic changes associated with critical stenoses result in endothelial cell injury and thrombus formation (Blaumanis and Grady 1981; Grady and Blaumanis 1983). Such stenoses therefore appear to predispose to embolic cerebral infarction as well as causing a reduction in CBF.

The aims of these studies was to develop a test using hypercapnia which would identify those stenoses which were physiologically flow limiting and to assess the effect of carotid endarterectomy on the blood flow in these vessels. Experimental evidence suggests that increasing the flow through a stenosis "unmasks" the haemodynamic consequenes of such stenoses, and stenoses which are not flow limiting at normal flow rates may become so at elevated rates of flow (May et al. 1963; Young et al. 1977). This is of particular relevance in the ICA as cerebral autoregulation in response to reduced systemic pressure will increase CBF and hence increase flow through the ICA. If an ICA stenosis prevents the required increase in flow, then cerebral ischaemia may result.

Several studies have investigated the effect of ICA stenosis on flow through the vessels. Tindall et al. (1962) demonstrated that lumen reduction of the order of 90% is required before ICA flow is reduced, which was of a similar magnitude as had previously been shown experimentally in dogs– 94.5% (Cannon et al. 1960). Brice et al. (1964a, b) argued that absolute lumen area was important but their studies suggested that a lumen reduction of 84%–93% was necessary for reduction of ICA flow. De Weese et al. (1970) in an angiographic and anatomical dissection study of the ICA also came to the same conclusions – showing that lumen reduction of the order of 87% always produced a significant pressure drop distal to the stenosis.

There are two factors which would be expected to influence the increase in flow with hypercapnia through an internal carotid artery stenosis: firstly the severity of the stenosis itself and secondly the degree of contralateral disease. In order to assess the effect of the stenosis itself, only patients with minimal contralateral disease should be considered. For this reason the patients studied were divided into the two groups described. In group 1 patients any stenosis present was associated with a peak frequency of less than 6 KHz of the opposite ICA. This has been shown by angiographic studies to represent a stenosis of 50% lumen reduction (Zwiebel et al. 1982; Thomas et al. 1985) and therefore well below the sort of lumen reduction which would reduce flow through the vessel even at the elevated flow rates caused by hypercapnia.

Figure 1 illustrates that in those patients with unilateral disease the increase of ICA flow secondary to hypercapnia is not markedly impaired until the stenosis reaches a peak frequency of 10 KHz. This is equivalent to a lumen reduction of approximately 80% (Zwiebel et al. 1982), which is slightly lower than the lumen reductions which reduced flow in the reported studies discussed above. However, all of those studies were performed with patients under general anaesthesia and therefore may not have represented true resting flow rates.

Spencer and Reid (1979) in a theoretical study comparing angiography with Doppler suggested that a lumen reduction of the order of 90% was required for ICA flow reduction. Therefore the results reported here have shown that increasing ICA flow with hypercapnia reduces the stenosis required for flow reduction down to 80%.

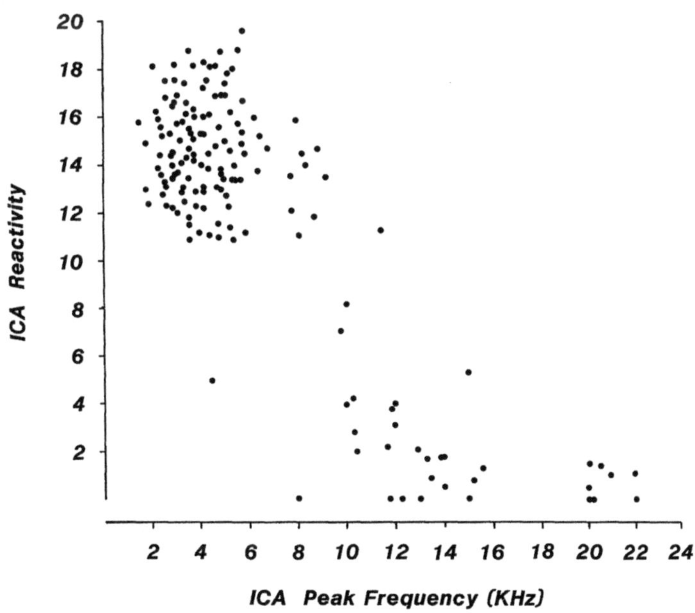

Fig. 1. Effect of ICA stenosis (expressed as peak frequency in kilohertz) on the ICA reactivity to CO_2 in 79 patients with minor contralateral ICA desease

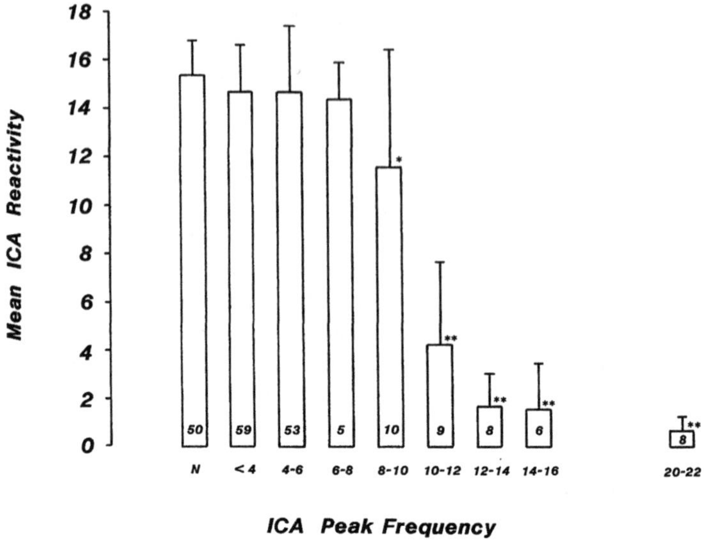

Fig. 2. Effect of ICA stenosis (expressed as peak frequency in kilohertz) on the mean (±SD) ICA reactivity to CO_2 in 79 patients with minor contralateral disease. The first column *(N)* represents the mean ICA reactivity of 25 normal subjects. *Numbers inside the columns* represent the number of ICAs with a peak frequency in that particular range. * $p<0.01$ compared with column <4 KHz; ** $p<0.001$ compared with column <4 KHz

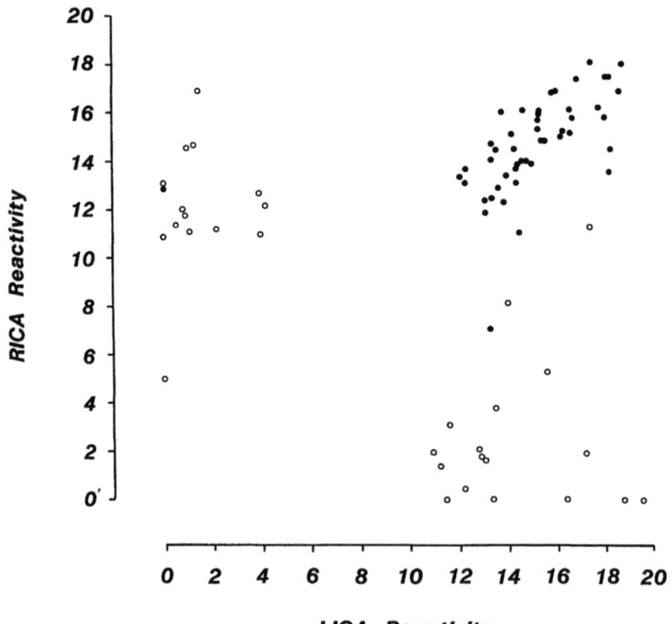

Fig. 3. Correlation between right and left ICA reactivity to CO_2 in 79 patients with minor contralateral disease. *Closed circles,* PF of both ICAs <10 KHz (r=0.531); *open circles,* PF of one ICA >10 KHz

The two patients who showed unexpectedly low reactivities may possibly be explained by the presence of an undetected stenosis in the ICA above the angle of the jaw (which would have been missed on the Duplex scan). Disease in the distal ICA is unusual without coexisting disease at the bifurcation but its existence in these two patients would suffice to explain the reduced reactivity found. Unfortunately it was not possible to confirm this by referral to angiograms, because the DSA was of insufficient quality in one patient and angiography was not performed in the other patient.

With a stenosis of PF greater than 10 KHz, there is a highly significant ($p<0.001$) reduction in ICA reactivity to CO_2 as shown in Fig. 2, which also shows that patients with a stenosis of 8–10 KHz (70%–80% lumen reduction) had a mean reactivity that was significantly lower ($p<0.01$) than those ICAs which were widely patent. Therefore it can be concluded that in some patients with unilateral disease a reduction of lumen to 70% becomes haemodynamically significant at the elevated flow rates induced by hypercapnia.

In those patients where both ICAs would be expected to have normal reactivity, the correlation between left and right ICA reactivity was good (Fig. 3), which is in agreement with the findings on normal subjects.

Considering now the effect of severe contralateral disease on ICA reactivity to CO_2 (group 2 patients), it can be seen that contralateral disease reduces reactivity in some stenoses which might be expected to respond normally, i.e., those between 6 and 10 KHz (50%–80% lumen reduction) (Fig. 4). The mean values (Fig. 5) show a significant reduction of reactivity in stenoses of PF greater than 6 KHz (50% lumen reduction) when compared with both normal subjects and those ICAs in this group of pati-

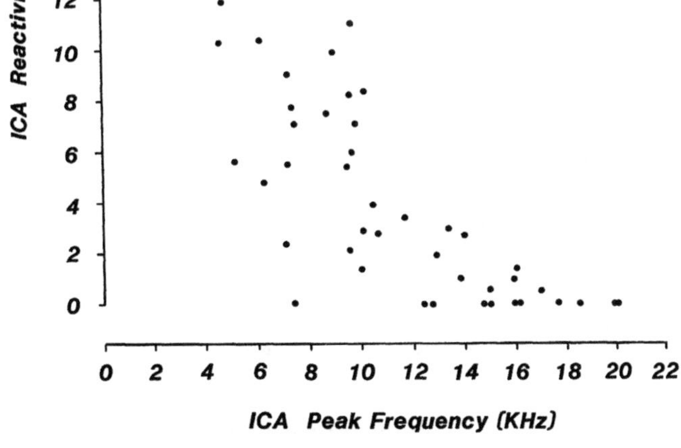

Fig. 4. Effect of ICA stenosis (expressed as peak frequency in kilohertz) on the ICA reactivity to CO_2 in 43 patients with severe contralateral ICA disease

ents with stenoses of PF between 4 and 6 KHz (20–50% lumen reduction). Somewhat surprisingly there was no ICA in this group which had a PF of less than 4 KHz in association with a contralateral occlusions. Patients with an ICA PF of less than 4 KHz with a contralateral stenosis of any degree would obviously have been included in the group 1 patients for analysis.

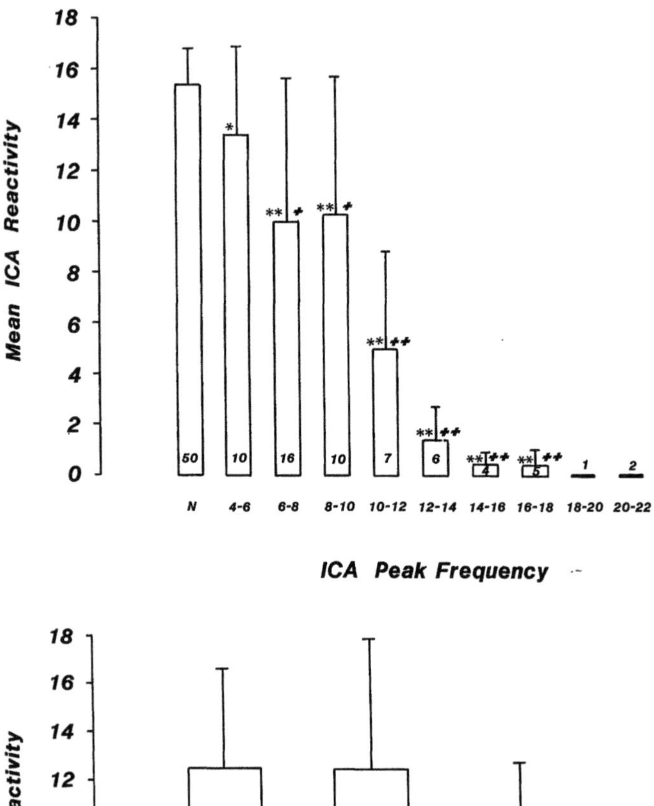

Fig. 5. Effect of ICA stenosis (expressed as peak frequency in kilohertz) on the mean (±SD) ICA reactivity to CO_2 in 43 patients with severe contralateral ICA disease. The first column *(N)* represents the mean ICA reactivity of 25 normal subjects. *Numbers* inside the columns represent the number of ICAs with a peak frequency in that particular range. * $p<0.01$ compared with normals *(N)*; ** $p<0.001$ compared with normals *(N)*; # $p<0.2$ compared with column 4–6 KHz; ## $p<0.001$ compared with column 4–6 KHz

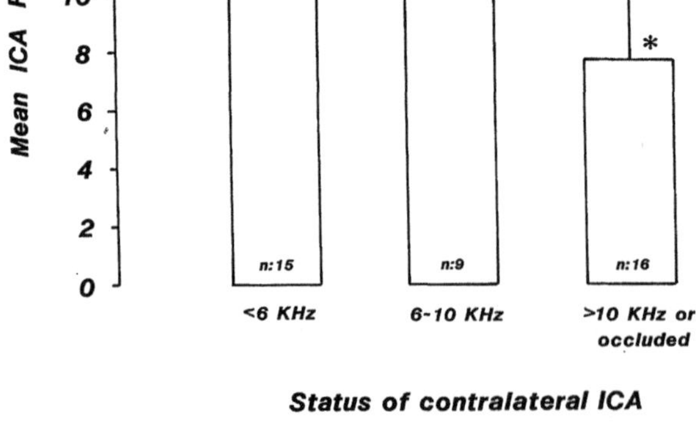

Fig. 6. Effect of contralateral ICA disease (expressed as peak frequency in kilohertz or total occlusion) on the mean (±SD) reactivity to CO_2 of ICAs with a stenosis peak frequency between 6 and 10 KHz (*n*, number of patients). * $p<0.01$

Therefore these results show that severe contralateral disease renders some ICA stenoses haemodynamically significant at elevated flows when the stenosis represents only a 50% reduction in lumen diameter. However, the contralateral ICA disease must itself show reduced reactivity (i.e., PF>10 KHz or occluded) before the effect on the opposite ICA becomes statistically significant (Fig. 6). Even when the contralateral

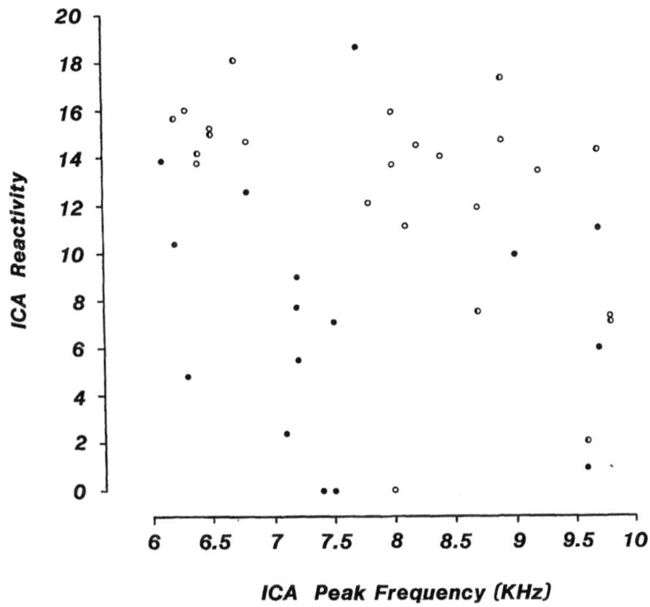

Fig. 7. Effect of ICA stenosis (peak frequency between 6 and 10 KHz) on ICA reactivity to CO_2 related to state of contralateral ICA. *Open circles,* contralateral ICA PF<6 KHz; *half-open circles,* contralateral ICA PF 6–10 KHz; *closed circles,* contralateral ICA PF>10 KHz or occluded

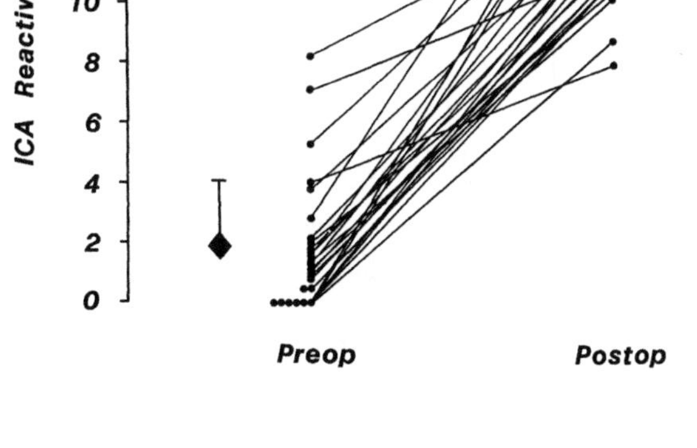

Fig. 8. Effect of carotid endarterectomy on ICA reactivity to CO_2 in 25 patients with minor contralateral ICA disease. *Diamonds,* means ± SD; * $p<0.001$

ICA PF was between 6 and 10 KHz (50%–80% lumen reduction), this did not statistically affect ICA mean reactivity in the equivocal vessels (i.e., those with PF between 6 and 10 KHz) on the opposite side.

Carotid endarterectomy restored ICA reactivity (Figs. 8, 9) and this provides further evidence that the reduced reactivity to CO_2 preoperatively is secondary to the haemodynamic effects of the ICA stenosis. Not all patients had a reactivity greater than 10 following surgery. This can be explained by residual stenosis in group 1 patients (Fig. 8) and by either residual stenosis or severe contralateral disease in group 2 patients (Fig. 9). Crawford et al. in 1960 first reported the effects of carotid endarterectomy on ICA blood flow using intraoperative pressure measurements and found an improvement only in those vessels with severe stenoses and this was more recently confirmed in studies using electromagnetic flowmeters (Boysen 1973).

One further point requires comment. The length of the ICA stenosis was not evaluated in these studies with respect to the reactivity to CO_2. However, it is generally agreed that the length of the constriction has only a small haemodynamic effect (von Ruden et al. 1964; Kindt and Youmans 1969).

In conclusion, these studies have demonstrated that unilateral carotid stenosis is always haemodynamically significant if the stenosis is greater than 80% lumen reduction and may be significant below this. Furthermore in patients with severe bilateral disease, a stenosis of 50% and greater lumen reduction may be haemodynamically significant, especially if the contralateral ICA is totally occluded. In the present climate of debate concerning carotid endarterectomy (Strother and Crummy 1982; Barnett et al. 1984), it may become necessary to restrict the use of carotid endarterectomy for stenoses which are shown to be flow reducing by a test such as developed in this work. In this situation, endarterectomy would remove lesions which may not only produce cerebral ischaemia by reducing CBF but would also remove sources of emboli which themselves are more likely to develop if the lesion is haemodynamically significant.

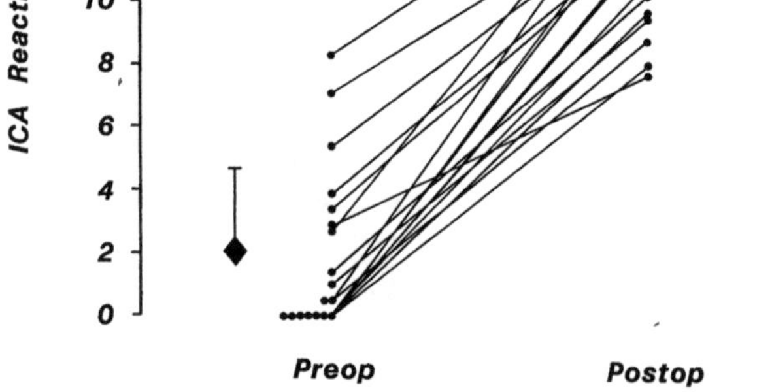

Fig. 9. Effect of carotid endarterectomy on ICA reactivity to CO_2 in 18 patients with severe contralateral ICA disease. *Diamonds,* means ± SD; * $p<0.001$

References

Anonymous (1970) Documenta Geigy scientific tables, 7th edn., Basel
Barnett HJM, Plum F, Walton JN (1984) Carotid endarterectomy – an expression of concern. Stroke 15:941–943
Blaumanis OR, Grady PA (1981) Shear stress injury to arterial walls. Adv Neurol 30:167–174
Boysen G (1973) Cerebral haemodynamics in carotid surgery. Acta Neurol Scand 52:1–84
Brice JG, Dowsett DJ, Lowe RD (1964a) The effect of constriction on carotid blood flow and pressure gradient. Lancet 1:84–85
Brice JG, Dowsett DJ, Lowe RD (1964b) Haemodynamic effects of carotid artery stenosis. Br Med J 2:1363–1366
Busuttil RW, Baker JD, Davidson RK, Machleder HI (1981) Carotid artery stenosis – haemodynamic significance and clinical course. JAMA 245:1438–1441
Cannon JA, Lobpreis EL, Herrold G, Frankenberg HL (1960) Experience with a new electromagnetic flow-meter for use in blood-flow determinations. Ann Surg 152:635–646
Crawford ES, Bakey ME, Blaisdell FW, Morris GC, Fields WS (1960) Haemodynamic alterations in patients with cerebral arterial insufficiency before and after operation. Surgery 48:76–94
DeWeese JA, May AG, Lipchik EO, Ob CG (1970) Anatomic and haemodynamic correlations in carotid artery stenosis. Stroke 1:149–157
Grady PA, Blaumanis OR (1983) Arterial wall changes in experimental stenosis. In: Reitich M, Hurtig H (eds) Cerebrovascular diseases. Raven, New York, pp 347–362 (13th Princeton Conference)
Hutchinson EC, Yates PO (1957) Carotico-vertebral stenosis. Lancet 1:2–8
Kindt GW, Youmans JR (1969) The effect of stricture length on critical arterial stenosis. Surg Gynecol Obstet 128:729–734
May AG, DeWeese JA, Rob CG (1963) Haemodynamic effects of arterial stenosis. Surgery 53:513–524
Schwartz CJ, Mitchell JRA (1961) Atheroma of the carotid and vertebral arterial systems. Br Med J 2:1057–1063
Spencer MP, Reid JM (1979) Quantitation of carotid stenosis with continuous-wave Doppler ultrasound. Stroke 10:326–330
Strother CM, Crummy AB (1982) Cervical arteriosclerosis – diagnostic advances in need of a clinical answer. Stroke 13:551–556
Thomas MH, Otis SM, Rush MM, Zygroff J, Dilley RB, Bernstein EF (1985) The contribution of spectral analysis to the diagnosis of carotid artery disease. J Vasc Surg 2:270–277
Tindall GT, Odom GL, Cupp HB, Dillon ML (1962) Studies on carotid artery flow and pressure. Observations in 18 patients during graded occlusion of proximal carotid artery. J Neurosurg 19:917–923
Von Ruden WJ, Blaisdell FW, Hall AD, Thomas AN (1964) Multiple arterial stenoses: effect on blood flow. Arch Surg 89:307–315
Young DF, Cholvin NR, Kirkeeide RL, Roth AC (1977) Haemodynamics of arterial stenoses at elevated flow rates. Circ Res 41:99–107
Ziegler DK, Hassanein RS (1973) Prognosis in patients with transient ischaemic attacks. Stroke 4:666–673
Zwiebel WJ, Zagzebski JA, Crummy AB, Hirscher M (1982) Correlation of peak Doppler frequency with lumen narrowing in carotid stenosis. Stroke 13:386–39

Cerebrovascular Reserve Capacity Measured with 133-Xenon Dynamic SPECT Before and After Carotid Endarterectomy

G. LEINSINGER, H. FÜRST, P. SCHMIEDEK, K. EINHÄUPL, and C. M. KIRSCH

Introduction

The role of surgery in patients with carotid artery disease remains controversial. Whereas it is generally agreed that endarterectomy is beneficial in patients with symptomatic conditions and ulcerative arteriosclerotic lesions, the optimal management of patients with stenotic lesions of the carotid artery has not been established yet. Previous randomized studies document that the spontaneous rate of stroke in patients with carotid artery stenoses is below 20% over a follow-up period of 2 years (Fields et al. 1970). The aim of the present study was to establish a functional test in order to identify patients with cerebral ischemia due to hemodynamic failure. Therefore, regional cerebral blood flow (rCBF; ml/100 g per minute) was measured at resting conditions and after stimulation with acetazolamide (Diamox) using the 133-xenon inhalation technique. Serial rCBF measurements were performed in a consecutive and unselected group of patients in order to study the effect of carotid endarterectomy on CBF and cerebrovascular reserve capacity.

Patients

The study includes 61 patients (46 men and 15 women, mean age 66±9 years, range 38–82 years). The indication for carotid endarterectomy was based on findings from

Table 1. Findings from Doppler ultrasound examination in 61 Patients before carotid endarterectomy

Ipsilateral	Contralateral	*n*	Surgery
ICA stenosis 80%–90%	No stenosis	10	Unilateral
ICA stenosis >90%	No stenosis	25	Unilateral
ICA stenosis 80%–90%	ICA stenosis 80%–90%	3	Unilateral (1) Bilateral (2)
ICA stenosis >90%	ICA stenosis 80%–90%	4	Unilateral (3) Bilateral (2)
ICA stenosis >90%	ICA stenosis >90%	7	Unilateral (4) Bilateral (3)
ICA stenosis 80%–90%	ICA occlusion	3	Unilateral
ICA stenosis >90%	ICA occlusion	9	Unilateral

ICA, internal carotid artery

Doppler studies of the extracranial brain-supplying arteries (Table 1). Surgery was performed in 61 patients on 19 high grade stenoses (80%–90%) and 48 filiform stenoses (>90%). Neurologically, 20 patients were asymptomatic for the operated hemisphere; 3 patients presented with contralateral transitory ischemic attacks (TIA) because of internal carotid occlusion. Thirty-seven patients had a history of unilateral and four patients of bilateral TIA. Patients with extensive cerebral infarctions or a history of stroke were excluded from the study. Measurements of rCBF were performed before surgery and in the early (6 days; n=24) and later postoperative period (3 months; n=36). Carotid endarterectomy was performed in all patients irrespective of rCBF findings.

Control rCBF data were obtained from 41 patients (33 males, 8 females; mean age 45±13 years with a range from 19 to 77 years). From the history and a neurologic examination the presence of cerebrovascular disease could be excluded in all cases. This was further established by normal findings of Doppler studies.

Methods

The rCBF was measured using the 133-xenon inhalation technique and dynamic SPECT (Tomomatic 64; Medimatic, Copenhagen, Denmark). After inhalation of 133-xenon gas (approximately 400 MBq/l) for 1 min and exhalation for 3 min, rCBF values were calculated using a special algorithm developed by Kanno and Lassen (1979). The flow maps (2, 6 and 10 cm above the orbitomeatal line) were evaluated by standardized regions of interest. For the present study only regions over the middle cerebral artery territory in slice 2 were assessed. All measurements were first performed at resting conditions. After a period of 30 min 1 g Diamox was injected intravenously. Fifteen minutes after the administration of Diamox rCBF measurements were repeated. Cerebrovascular reserve capacity was calculated from the difference between the Diamox-activated flow and the resting flow in the middle cerebral artery territory and expressed in ml/100 g per minute.

Table 2. Regional cerebral blood flow (ml/100 g per minute) before and after intravenous injection of 1 g Diamox in 41 normal subjects

	rCBF (range)	
Before Diamox		
MCA left	64±11	(45– 87)
MCA right	66±11	(46– 90)
After Diamox		
MCA left	81±10	(62–103)
MCA right	82± 9	(60–101)
Increase		
MCA left	17±11	(9– 29)
MCA right	16± 6	(4– 29)

rCBF, regional cerebral blood flow; MCA, middle cerebral artery

Results

Control

After administration of 1 g Diamox in normal subjects a significant increase of rCBF was noted in the middle cerebral artery territory, as indicated in Table 2.

The stimulated flow values were compared with their respective baseline values. A linear dependency was found which can be expressed in the following equation:

$rCBF_{stim} = 0.75\ rCBF_{rest} + 33$ (ml/100 g per minute); $r = 0.87$ (Fig. 1)

Therefore, individuals with low baseline flow values reach lower values following stimulation with Diamox when compared with subjects exhibiting high baseline flow values. The increase in rCBF, however, was more pronounced in subjects with low baseline values than in those with high baseline flow values.

In order to allow a more sensitive evaluation of the cerebrovascular reserve capacity of patients with cerebrovascular disease the flow increase following Diamox administration is shown with its corresponding dependency on resting flow value (Fig. 2). The 95% tolerance limits for this regression show the upper and lower limits of normal

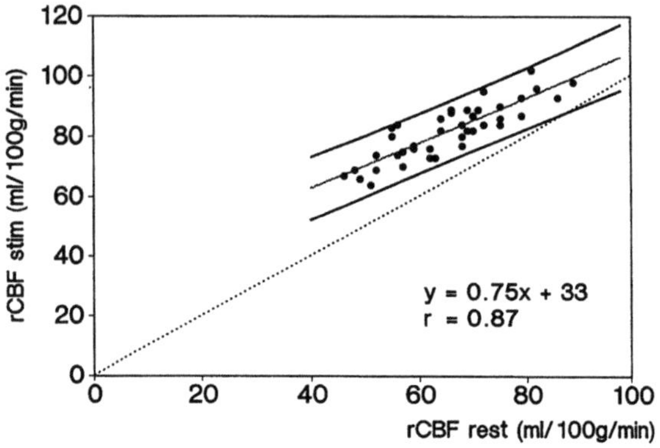

Fig. 1. Stimulated flow values in comparison with the respective baseline values in 41 normal subjects

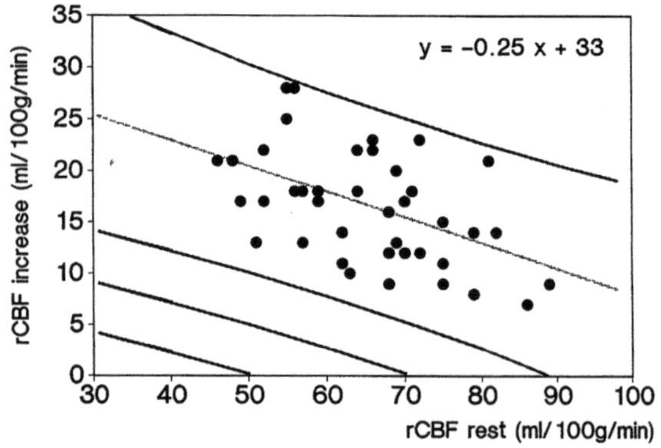

Fig. 2. Tolerance limits of cerebrovascular reserve capacity in terms of regional cerebral blood flow (rCBF)

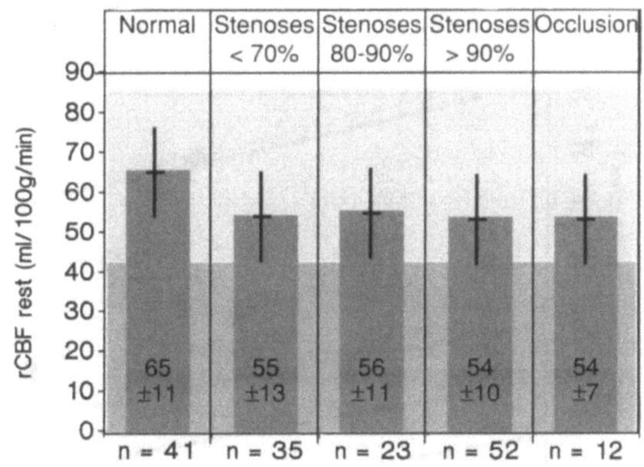

Fig. 3. Resting regional cerebral blood flow ($rCBF_{REST}$) in comparison with the degree of stenosis

values. Flow values below the lower tolerance limit represent a decreased cerebrovascular reserve capacity. Equidistant curves (5 ml/100 g per minute) to the lower tolerance limit define ranges of slight, moderate or severe reduction of cerebrovascular reserve capacity.

Preoperative rCBF Measurements in Carotid Artery Disease

Preoperative mean resting flow over the middle cerebral artery territory of the operated hemispheres was 54±10 ml/100 g per minute. However, there was no correlation of $rCBF_{rest}$ and the degree of stenosis (Fig. 3).

Normal cerebrovascular reserve capacity was found in 33 of 35 carotid arteries which were normal or showed stenoses under 70% at ultrasound examination. Cerebrovascular reserve capacity was reduced in 2 of 23 (9%) of the high grade stenoses, in 20 of 52 (38%) of the filiform stenoses and in 9 of 12 (75%) of the internal carotid artery occlusions (Fig. 4). Severe reduction of cerebrovascular reserve capacity or even a decrease of rCBF after administration of Diamox ("steal phenomenon") was found in 2 of 52 (4%) of the filiform stenoses and in 3 of 12 (25%) of the occlusions. All patients with steal phenomenon had a history of TIA.

Measurements of rCBF After Carotid Endarterectomy

In the follow-up after carotid endarterectomy patients were divided into three groups according to their preoperative cerebrovascular reserve capacity. The results of the postoperative rCBF measurements are given in Fig. 5.

Group 1 represented those patients with preoperatively normal reserve capacity. In this group, postoperative studies failed to show any change of resting flow or Diamox-stimulated flow in the middle cerebral artery territory of the hemispheres operated on. In group 2 preoperative reserve capacity was slightly reduced. In these patients resting flow values remained unchanged in the follow-up after carotid endarterectomy. Diamox-stimulated flow values, however, increased in the early postoperative period but 3 months later almost decreased to the level measured preoperatively.

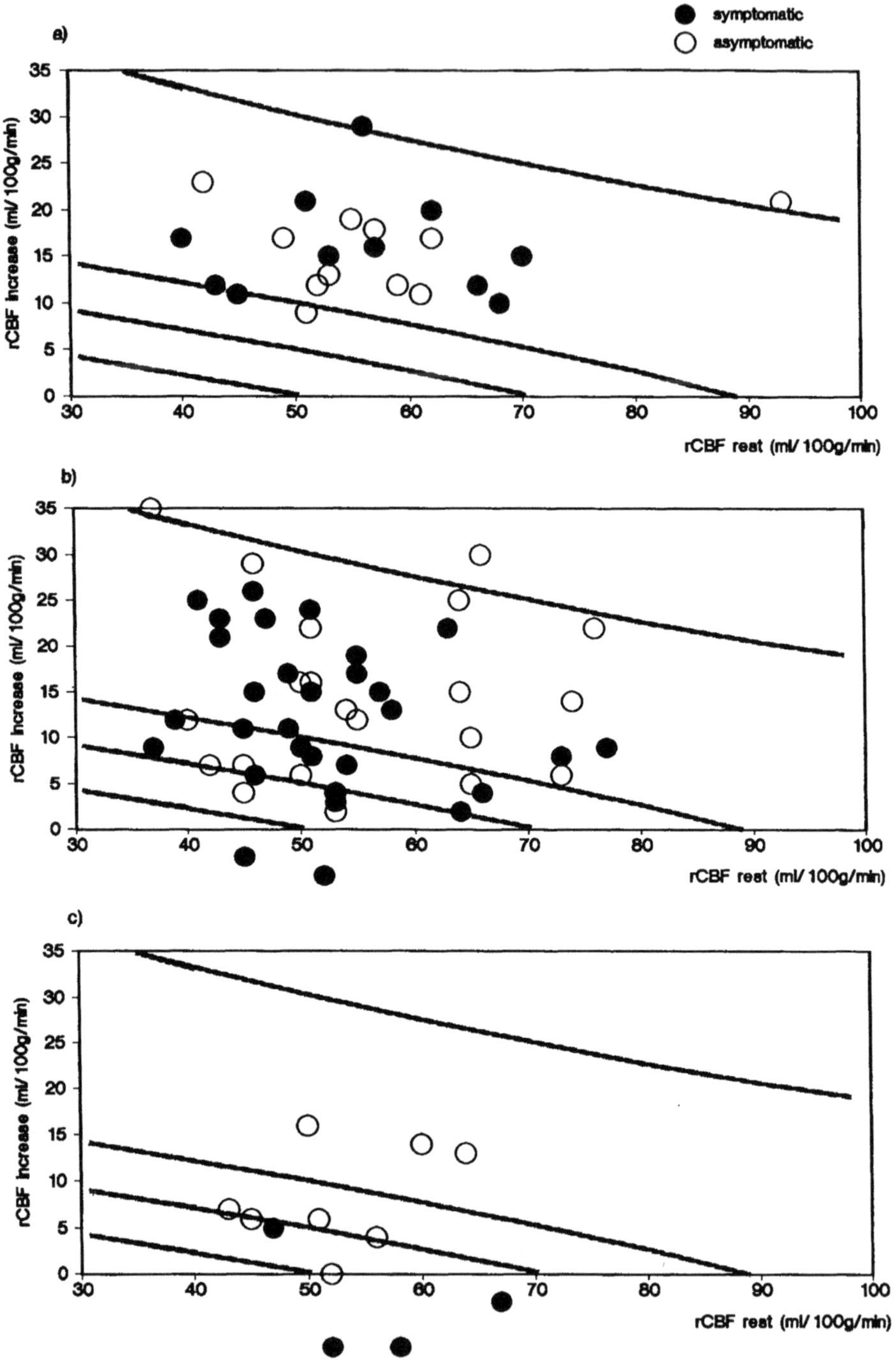

Fig. 4a–c. Cerebrovascular reserve capacity in symptomatic *(closed circles)* or asymptomatic *(open circles)* internal carotid artery stenosis or occlusion. **a** Stenosis of 80%–90%, **b** stenosis of over 90, and **c** occlusion

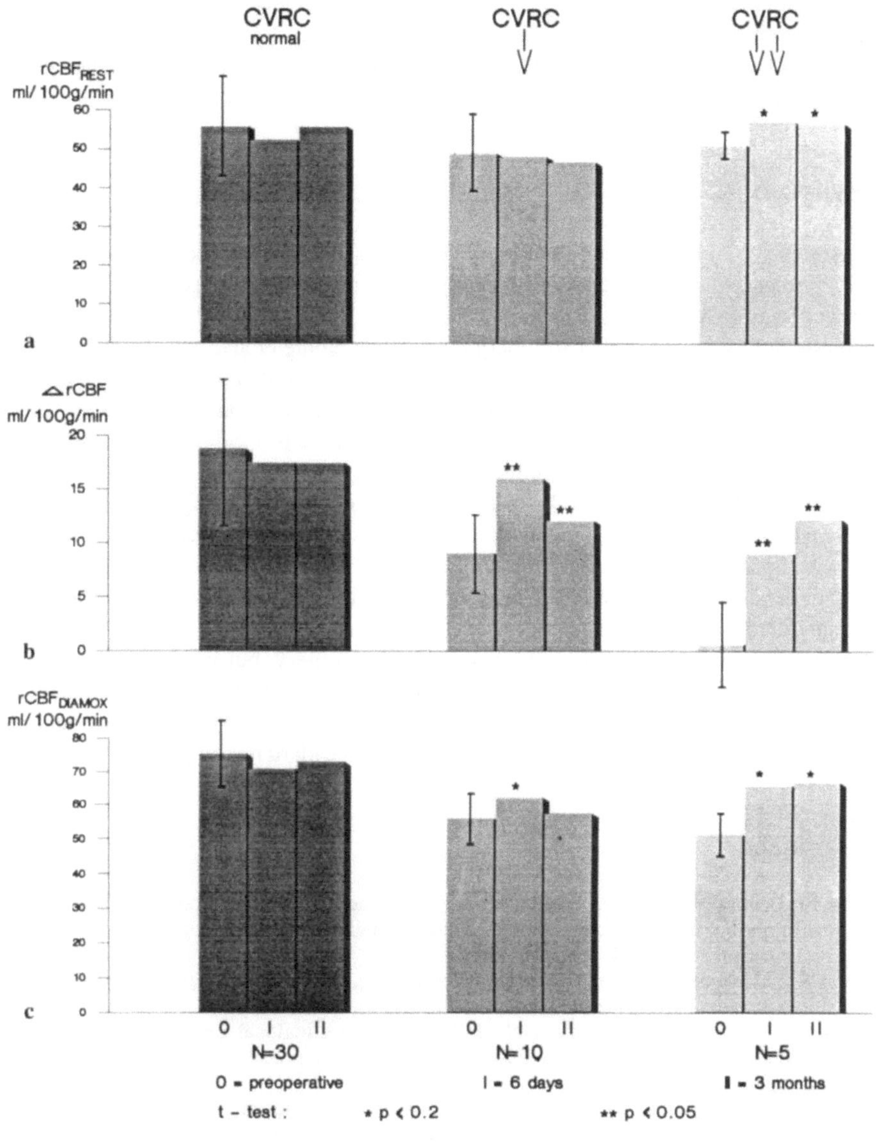

Fig. 5a–c. Regional cerebral blood flow (rCBF) at follow-up after carotid endarterectomy. **a** $rCBF_{REST}$; **b** △rCBF; **c** rCBF after administration of Diamox. *CVRC*, cerebrovascular reserve capacity; *0*, preoperative; *I*, 6 days; *II*, 3 months. According to *t*-test * $p<0.02$; ** $p<0.05$

Group 3 included those patients with preoperatively moderate or severe reduction of cerebrovascular reserve capacity. In this group a significant improvement of resting flow and Diamox-stimulated flow was noted in the early as well as in the later postoperative studies.

Discussion

Measurements of cerebrovascular reserve capacity using the Diamox test were performed in order to estimate the risk of hemodynamic insufficiency in patients with carotid artery disease. After administration of Diamox cerebral blood flow significantly increased in normal subjects (Sorteberg et al. 1989; Bonte et al.1988). In patients with internal carotid artery occlusion previous studies demonstrated a severely reduced response to stimulation with Diamox especially when insufficient arterial collateralization was documented by panangiography (Leinsinger et al. 1988). Some authors reported a high risk of stroke in those patients with severely impaired cerebrovascular reserve capacity (Rutigliano et al. 1989). In the present study, however, most of the patients with high grade or filiform stenosis of the internal carotid artery preoperatively presented with normal cerebrovascular reserve capacity. Only in a small group of patients with moderate or severe reduction of reserve capacity was an improvement after carotid endarterectomy noted. These data are supported by the results of Vorstrup et al. (1987), who used the Diamox test during vascular surgery, but who also found perioperative risks were highest in the group with an abnormal Diamox test. Therefore, cerebrovascular reserve capacity should be an essential parameter in further randomized studies in order to evaluate the benefit of carotid endarterectomy.

References

Bonte FJ, Devous MD, Reisch JS (1988) The effect of acetazolamide on regional cerebral blood flow in normal human subjects as measured by single-photon emission computed tomography. Invest Radiol 23:564–568

Fields WS, Maslenikow V, Meyer JS, Hass WK, Remington RD, Macdonald M (1970) Joint study of extracranial arterial occlusion. JAMA 211:1993–2003

Kanno I, Lassen NA (1979) Two methods for calculating regional cerebral blood flow from emission computed tomography of inert gas concentrations. J Comput Assist Tomogr 3:71–76

Leinsinger G, Schmiedek P, Kreisig T, Einhäupl K, Bauer W, Moser E (1988) 133-Xe-DSPECT: Bedeutung der zerebrovaskulären Reservekapazität für Diagnostik und Therapeutik der chronischen zerebralen Ischämie. Nucl Med 27:127–134

Rutigliano MJ, Yonas H, Johnson DW (1989) Natural history of patients with compromised cerebral reserves. J Cereb Blood Flow Metab 9:S609

Sorteberg W, Lindegaard K-F, Rootwelt K, Dahl A, Nyberg-Hansen R, Russell D, Nornes H (1989) Effect of acetazolamide on cerebral artery blood velocity and regional cerebral blood flow in normal subjects. Acta Neurochir (Wien) 97:139–145

Vorstrup S, Boysen G, Brun B, Engell HC (1987) Evaluation of the regional cerebral vasodilatory capacity before carotid endarterectomy by the acetazolamide test. Neurol Res 9:10–18

Extra-Intracranial Bypass Surgery in Patients with Hemodynamic Cerebral Ischemia

P. Schmiedek, A. Piepgras, G. Leinsinger, K. Einhäupl, and C. M. Kirsch

Introduction

Following the publication of the result of the International Cooperative Study on Extra-Intracranial Bypass Surgery, which had failed to show any beneficial effect of this operation in reducing the risk of stroke, the indication for this procedure has been almost entirely abandoned (Bogouslavsky and Regli 1986; EC-IC Bypass Study Group 1985). It has been argued, however, that the indications previously used for bypass surgery, which were mainly based on clinical and angiographic criteria, did not take into consideration the rather complicated pathophysiology of stroke. Using positron emission tomography (PET) which allows the simultaneous measurement of cerebral blood flow (CBF), cerebral blood volume (CBV), and various parameters of brain oxygen metabolism, it is now possible to identify a particular subgroup of patients with cerebrovascular insufficiency, namely those with hemodynamic cerebral ischemia (Gibbs et al. 1984; Powers and Raichle 1985; Powers et al. 1987). According to these studies, hemodynamic cerebral ischemia may occur in patients with cerebrovascular occlusive disease with poor collaterization and is characterized by a low CBF to CBV ratio, reflecting a decreased cerebral perfusion pressure. Instead of using PET, which has only a limited range of application because of its expense and limited availability, the assessment of the cerebral vascular reserve capacity (CVRC) can also be used to identify patients with hemodynamic cerebral ischemia. Here, the physiologic response of an increase in CBF during CO_2 inhalation or following intravenous administration of acetazolamide (Diamox; Lederle, Wolfratshausen, FRG) will be found to be impaired or even absent in patients with hemodynamic compromise of the cerebral circulation (Ringelstein et al. 1988; Vorstrup 1988). Assuming that patients with hemodynamic cerebral ischemia due to cerebrovascular occlusive disease are at higher risk for developing subsequent strokes, it is then reasonable to perform extra-intracranial bypass surgery in this particular subgroup of patients in an attempt to improve the collateral blood flow to the brain. The present prospective study was conducted to evaluate the effect of bypass surgery on CBF and CVRC in patients with proven hemodynamic cerebral ischemia.

Clinical Material and Methods

Patient Population

This series includes 27 patients who underwent extra-intracranial bypass surgery over a 5-year period from 1986 until 1990. There were 24 male and 3 female patients. The mean age of the total group was 57 years, with an age range of 31–75 years. All patients had a history of cerebral ischemia. The majority of 16 cases had previous attacks of transient cerebral ischemia (TIA), and the remaining 11 patients presented with symptoms of prolonged reversible ischemic neurologic deficits (PRIND). Patients with completed stroke were not included.

Diagnostic Studies

For all patients, preoperative evaluation included computerized tomography (CT) of the head, complete cerebral angiography and measurement of CBF which was performed under resting condition and following Diamox injection in order to study the individual CVRC.

For measurement of CBF, the xenon-133 inhalation technique was used with a Tomomatic 64 (Medimatic Inc., Denmark), which utilizes a rotating array of 64 NaI crystals to monitor the cerebral uptake and washout of the isotope from three brain slices simultaneously, which are oriented parallel to the orbital-meatal line and centered 1.5 and 9 cm above it (Stokely et al. 1980). After a 1-min period of Xenon-133 inhalation, counts from the head are collected and an arterial input curve is estimated from a single detector positioned over the right lung. Using a conventional filtered-back projection algorithm, flow values are calculated for each pixel in a 32x32 matrix (Kanno and Lassen 1979). For further analysis of data, a computer program is used to provide flow values according to the presumed vascular territory of the three hemispheric arteries. The flow values given in this study thus primarily represent CBF within the middle cerebral artery territory. All measurements were performed first with the patients under resting conditions, and then repeated after a 30-min waiting period and another 15 min after intravenous administration of 1 g Diamox. Blood pressure and arterial pCO_2 were measured for each study. CVRC was calculated from the difference between the Diamox-activated study and the resting flow study and expressed in ml/100 g per minute. Administration of Diamox was well tolerated, and no serious side effects were noticed after a single dose of the drug. Likewise there were no effects on blood pressure or arterial pCO_2 which could be attributed to Diamox. To interpret CBF and CVRC values, normative data from previous studies in our laboratory were used (Leinsinger et al. 1988).

Follow-up Protocol

All patients with documented hemodynamic cerebrovascular insufficiency were operated on. A standard extra-intracranial bypass procedure was performed using either the frontal or the parietal branch of the superficial temporal artery and connecting it to a cortical branch of the middle cerebral artery close to the Sylvian fissure. During the early postoperative period, bypass patency was evaluated by Doppler sonography.

Before the patients were discharged from the hospital, usually at the end of the 1st postoperative week, measurement of CBF was repeated, as was determination of CVRC after Diamox administration. At around 3 months postoperatively, all patients were readmitted for angiography to document patency of the bypass and the extent of extra-intracranial collateralization. CBF and CVRC studies were also performed at this time and thereafter repeated at yearly intervals. The mean follow-up period for all patients included in this study is 2.5 years.

Results

Preoperative Findings

Preoperative CT revealed normal findings in five patients with no evidence of hypodense areas suggestive of a previous ischemic event. One patient who was operated on early in this series showed an area of infarction related to the right presylvian middle cerebral territory. In 21 patients, distinctive areas of hypodensity were seen located between the vascular territories of the middle cerebral and the anterior or posterior cerebral arteries, thus showing the characteristic finding of border zone ischemia (Bogouslavsky and Regli 1986). Cerebral panangiography showed a unilateral occlusion of the cervical internal carotid artery in 22 patients. Five patients had bilateral occlusion of the internal carotid artery. The degree of collateralization was also evaluated using angiography. In one patient, the hemisphere on the side of occlusion was exclusively supplied over the anterior communicating artery. In 16 patients, two collaterals, namely the anterior and the posterior communicating arteries supplied the hemisphere of occlusion. In the remaining ten patients, in addition to the already mentioned collaterals, there were also collaterals from the external carotid artery system to the intracranial circulation, usually involving the ophthalmic artery.

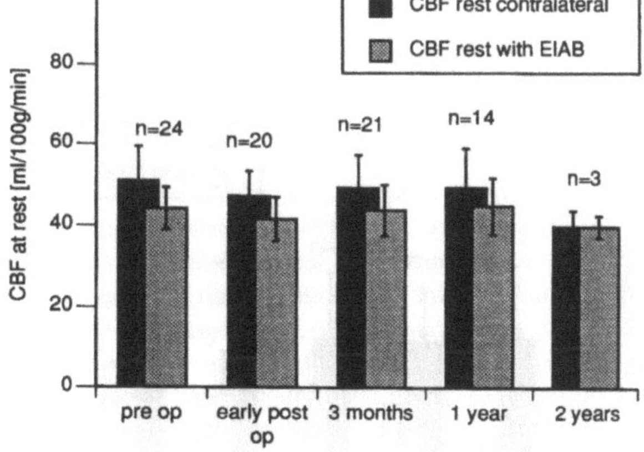

Fig. 1. Mean pre- and postoperative resting CBF values. (*EIAB*, extra-intracranial artery bypass; for details see text.)

Cerebral Blood Flow

Mean values of CBF measured at rest, and before and at various intervals after surgery are shown in Fig. 1. Although preoperative CBF values were found to be lower over the occluded hemisphere, this difference, when compared with the contralateral side, did not reach statistical significance. Postoperativley, these values were found to be essentially unchanged, with only a slight increase found over the operated side. After 2 years, follow-up studies revealed the same resting flow values over both hemispheres. This finding, however, must be attributed to a small decrease in CBF over the contralateral side rather than to an increase over the operated side.

Cerebrovascular Reserve Capacity

In contrast to the changes found in resting CBF values, significant changes were found with regard to CVRC values (Fig. 2). Preoperatively, the mean values of CVRC over the contralateral side were found to be within the normal range, and this did not change considerably over the follow-up period. Also preoperatively, over the side of the carotid occlusion, the reserve capacity was found to be almost exhausted, with a mean value of 2.2 ml/100 g per minute. Although not all patients had such a severe impairment of CVRC, this low value is due to the fact that five patients showed a paradoxical flow decrease (steal phenomenon) when the study was performed after administration of Diamox (Vorstrup et al. 1985). Postoperatively, CVRC over the operated side showed a steady increase, which was found to be significant when compared with preoperative values of CVRC.

Clinical Outcome and Bypass Patency

One patient died suddenly, after an initially uneventful postoperative course, at 10 days after surgery from a massive myocardial infarction. Two patients, developed postoperative strokes. One of them had bilateral carotid artery occlusion and additional atheromatous changes in the vertebrobasilar artery system. A massive infarction of the

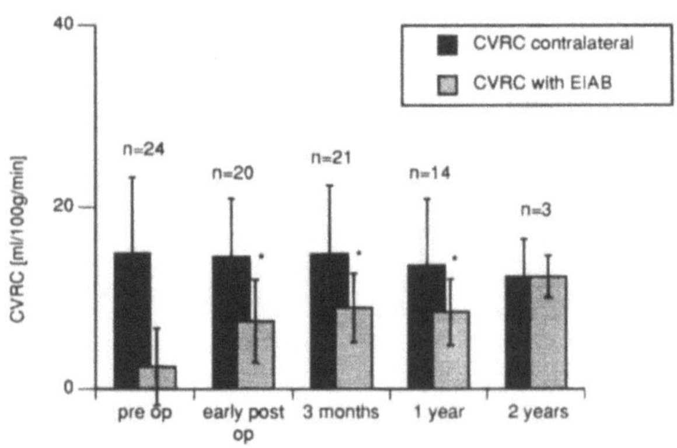

Fig. 2. Mean CVRC values pre- and postoperatively (*EIAB*, extra-intracranial artery bypass; for details see text.)

middle cerebral artery on the operated side was seen on an early postoperative CT scan, and the patient was finally discharged in a severely disabled state. The other patient, a 63-year-old man who had recurrent TIA preoperatively and a carotid occlusion, deteriorated postoperatively with development of a contralateral hemiplegia, which subsequently showed incomplete recovery. The postoperative course was uneventful in the remaining 24 patients. Only one patient reported another TIA during the follow-up period. Postoperative control angiography was performed in 25 patients and demonstrated excellent bypass function with ante- and retrograde filling of the entire middle cerebral artery territory in 15 cases. Eight patients had angiograms showing filling of two branches of the cortical brain circulation, and one patient had only filling of one branch of the middle cerebral artery.

Discussion

In this study we were able to show that extra-intracranial bypass surgery can improve the CVRC in symptomatic patients with proven hemodynamic ischemia. While no effect of the procedure was seen when pre- and postoperative resting flow values were compared, CVRC values significantly increased following surgery. Furthermore, excluding the patient who died from myocardial infarction and those two patients with early postoperative stroke, the clinical course was uneventful, with only one TIA episode reported over a mean follow-up period of 2.5 years in 24 patients. These results seem promising because they lend support to the concept that extra-intracranial bypass surgery may be regarded as the logical treatment for patients with hemodynamic cerebral ischemia due to occlusion of major brain supplying arteries. Before this concept can be more generalized, however, there remain several questions to be answered. First, the natural history of patients with hemodynamic cerebral ischemia has not been thoroughly investigated, particularly with regard to their stroke risk. The few studies which have addressed this question come to the conclusion that these patients do have a higher stroke risk than the larger group of all those patients with previous episodes of cerebral insufficiency (Kleiser et al., this volume) (Rutigliano et al. 1989). Secondly, the question has been raised, whether in patients with an exhausted CVRC inherent adaptative mechanisms of the cerebral circulation could not compensate for this impairment, which then would make any surgical intervention superfluous.

Respective studies have been performed in a small group of patients in our laboratory and have shown that a natural restoration of an impaired CVRC is exceptionally rare, and, therefore, it is highly unlikely to occur in most patients (Piepgras et al., this volume). Finally, there is no definite information available as yet concerning the incidence of hemodynamic cerebral ischemia. From clinical experience it can be concluded, however, that only a small percentage of all patients exhibit this particular impairment of the cerebral circulation. Further assessment of this uncertainty is needed, eventually requiring another controlled study where patients with hemodynamic cerebral ischemia are either operated on or treated medically. We do believe, however, that the results of this study and also of similar observations made by others, all of which are admittedly limited by a small number of operated patients, do justify further interest in extra-intracranial bypass surgery. This is certainly not meant in the sense of a revival of bypass surgery, but rather as an attempt to offer a selected group of patients the best form of treatment which is based on a sound knowledge of the underlying pathophysiology.

References

Bogouslavsky J, Regli F (1986) Borderzone infarctions distal to internal carotid artery occlusion: Prognostic implications. Ann Neurol 20:346–350

EC-IC Bypass Study Group (1985) Failure of extra-intracranial arterial bypass to reduce the risk of ischemic stroke. N Engl J Med 313:1191–1200

Gibbs JM, Leenders KL, Wise RJS, Jones T (1984) Evaluation of cerebral perfusion reserve in patients with carotid artery occlusion. Lancet i:310–314

Kanno L, Lassen NA (1979) Two methods for calculating cerebral blood flow from emission computed tomography of inert gas concentration. J Comput Assist Tomogr 3:71–76

Leinsinger G, Schmiedek P, Kreisig T, Einhäupl K, Bauer W, Moser E (1988) 133-Xe-DSPECT. Bedeutung der zerebrovaskularen Reservekapazität für Diagnostik und Therapie der chronischen zerebralen Ischämie. Nucl Med 27:127–134

Powers WJ, Raichle ME (1985) Positron emission tomography and its application to the study of cerebrovascular disease in man. Stroke 16:361–376

Powers WJ, Press GA, Grubb RL, Gado M, Raichle ME (1987) The effect of hemodynamically significant carotid artery disease on the hemodynamic status of the cerebral circulation. Ann Intern Med 106:27–35

Ringelstein EB, Sievers C, Ecker S, Schneider PA, Otis SM (1988) Noninvasive assessment of CO_2-induced cerebral vascular response in normal individuals and patients with internal carotid artery occlusions. Stroke 19:963–969

Rutigliano MJ, Yonas H, Johnson DW (1989) Natural history of patients with compromised cerebral reserves. J Cereb Blood Flow 9 [Suppl 609]

Strokely EM Sveinsdottier E, Lassen NA, Rommer P (1980) A single photon dynamic computer-assisted tomograph (DCAT) for imaging brain function in multiple cross sections. J Comput Assist Tomogr 4:230–240

Vorstrup S (1988) Tomographic cerebral blood flow measurements in patients with ischemic cerebrovascular disease and evaluation of the vasodilatory capacity by the acetazolamite test. Acta Neurol Scand 77 [Suppl. 114]

Vorstrup S, Lassen L, Henriksen O et al. (1985) CBF before and after extracranial-intracranial bypass surgery in patients with ischemic cerebrovascular disease studied with 133-Xe inhalation tomography. Stroke 16:616–626

Follow-up Studies of Cerebrovascular Reserve Capacity in Patients with Cerebrovascular Disease

A. Piepgras, P. Schmiedek, G. Leinsinger, R. L. Haberl, C. M. Kirsch, and K. M. Einhäupl

Introduction

There has been an increasing number of reports of the assessment of cerebrovascular reserve capacity (CVRC) in patients with cerebrovascular disease since it was first described by Vorstrup et al. in 1984. These reports almost exclusively deal with changes in CVRC after any kind of treatment, mostly revascularizing or recanalizing procedures. However, little is known on the natural history of the CVRC in patients with obstructive cerebrovascular disease, so far. In this series, therefore we studied the spontaneous course of the CVRC in those patients.

Subjects and Methods

In 14 patients symptomatic for various forms of cerebral ischemia, 3 women and 11 men between 25 and 70 years (mean age 49±12 years; median 52), CVRC was calculated using dynamic single photon emission computed tomography (D-SPECT) measurements at 2 different time points. An angiographically or sonographically proven occlusion of one internal carotid artery was found in 9 subjects, a high grade stenosis (>90%) in 3. In one patient we found a high grade stenosis of a middle cerebral artery (MCA) and an additional stenosis of the contralateral carotid artery was found in another. One patient had an occlusion of one vertebral artery and a high grade stenosis of the other one. One patient with a bilateral traumatic carotid dissection had recanalized carotids at follow-up (no. 10). This case was evaluated separately and was not considered in the statistical evaluations.

Mean time interval between initial and follow-up examination was 311±210 days (range 35–700 days). The patient data are summarized in Table 1.

Regional cerebral blood flow (CBF; ml/100 g per minute) was measured by inhalation of ^{133}Xe and D-SPECT, a rapidly rotating detector system with 64 separate sodium iodide crystals (Tomomatic 64; Medimatic, Copenhagen, Denmark) for tomographic recording of axial slices. Spatial resolution within a slice was 17 mm. Quantified CBF was calculated in three solices, 2, 6, and 10 cm above the canthomeatal line. Each slice was divided into regions of interest by a special computer program. Only data from the second slice in an area representing the perfusion territory of the MCA was analyzed. CVRC was calculated as the absolute increase of regional cerebral blood flow (△CBF, ml/100 g per minute) 15 min after stimulation on baseline CBF at rest. This calculation is based on our previously published protocol (Kreisig et al. 1987).

Table 1. Clinical data for 14 patients with occlusive intracranial artery disease

Patient no.	Age	Sex	Clinical symptoms	Vessel status
1	52	f	PRIND	ICA-O l
2	61	m	TIA	ICA-S r (>90%); ICA-S l (60%)
3	57	m	TIA	ICA-O l
4	44	m	PRIND	ICA-O l, S-60% r
5	57	m	CS	VA-O l, VA-S r
6	38	f	TIA	ICA-S l
7	56	n	TIA	MCA-S l
8	25	m	TIA	ICA-O l
9	38	m	TIA	ICA-O l
10	34	m	TIA	ICA-O l; ICA-O r
11	60	m	CS	ICA-O r
12	51	f	PRIND	ICA-S l
13	47	m	PRIND	ICA-O r
14	70	m	PRIND	ICA-O l

ICA, internal carotid artery; MCA, middle cerebral artery; O, occlusion; S, stenosis; TIA, transient ischemic attacks; PRIND, prolonged reversible ischemic neurologic deficit; f, female; m, male; r, right; l, left; CS, completed stroke

Basis for interpretation of $\triangle$CBF results is our nomogram: In 26 healthy normals a linear reciprocal relationship of $\triangle$CBF on CBF at rest ($\triangle CBF = -0.6 x CBF_{rest} + 50$; $r=0.77$) describes the proportionally higher increase of CBF after stimulation in individuals with low CBF at rest and lower increases on high CBF at rest. In each D-SPECT study, we measured blood pressure, pCO_2 and pO_2 at rest and after stimulation from arterial blood gas punctures.

Comparisons between the two measurements of CVRC in each patient were based on individually corrected CVRC, according to our nomogram. For each patient the individual difference to the mean CVRC based on the respective resting CBF was calculated and named corrected CVRC (CVRC-corr.). Differences of follow-up CVRC-corr. and initial CVRC-corr. were calculated according to the formula:

$$\text{Difference} = (-0.6 \text{ x } CBF_{rest(2)} + 50) - (CBF_{stim(2)}) - CBF_{rest(2)}) - (-0.6 \text{ x } CBF_{rest(1)} + 50) - (CBF_{stim(1)} - CBF_{rest(1)})$$

Results

There were no statistically significant changes in CBF at rest ($p=0.4$) or CVRC corrected for CBF at rest (CVRC-corr.: $p=0.2$) between initial examination and follow-up (Fig. 1) ipsi- or contralaterally. Mean CBF at rest at the initial examination was 53.9±8.6 ml/100 g per minute ipsilaterally and 60.8±10.1 ml/100 g per minute contralaterally. The side differences in CBF at rest were statistically significant ($p=0.0002$). Mean CBF at rest at the follow-up examination was 55.8±6.7 ml/100 g per minute versus 61.6±6.8 ml/g per minute. These side differences were statistically significant ($p=0.001$). The side differences in CVRC-corr. were statistically highly signi-

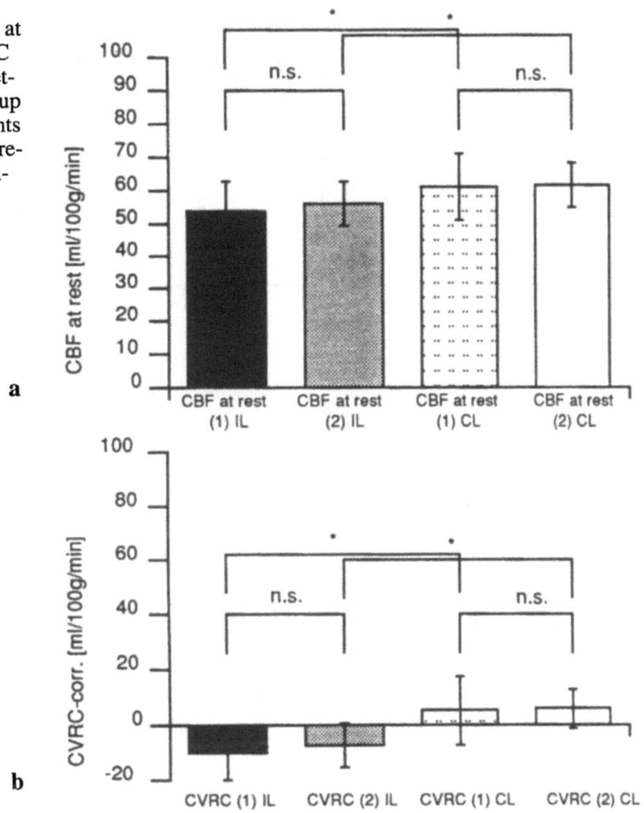

Fig. 1a, b. Changes in CBF at rest (**a**) and corrected CVRC (**b**; ml/100 g per minute) between initial *(1)* and follow-up *(2)* examination in 14 patients suffering from occlusive cerebrovascular disease. *IL*, ipsilateral; *CL*, contralateral

ficant (values at initial examination, with follow-up in brackets, in ml/100 g per minute): −10.5±9.7 (−7.4±8.1) ipsilaterally, and 4.8±12.6; p=0.0009 (5.6±7.1; p=0.0002) contralaterally.

The one case with bilateral carotid dissection (no. 10), presented with TIAs for the right hemisphere. Initial examination showed a "high-normal" CVRC for the left hemisphere combined with a "steal phenomenon" (a decrease in CBF after stimulation) in the right MCA territory. The patient refused surgical intervention by means of an extra-intracranial bypass. Follow-up examination after a symptom-free interval of 3 months revealed spontaneous recanalization on both sides. CVRC on the left side stayed "high-normal" and had improved to normal values on the right side (see Fig. 2).

Figure 2 shows the individual changes for the 14 patients during initial examination and follow-up. In one patient (no. 7) with an MCA stenosis an improvement was noted both ipsi- and contralaterally. Patient no. 10, who had a bilateral, traumatic carotid dissection, had improved in CVRC on one side at follow-up, but not on the other. Control angiography revealed bilateral reperfused carotid arteries.

Because of interindividual differences in the follow-up period a correlation of time interval and CVRC-corr. was calculated but could not be proven. There were no significant changes in pCO_2 at rest and after acetazolamide-induced stimulation of CBF.

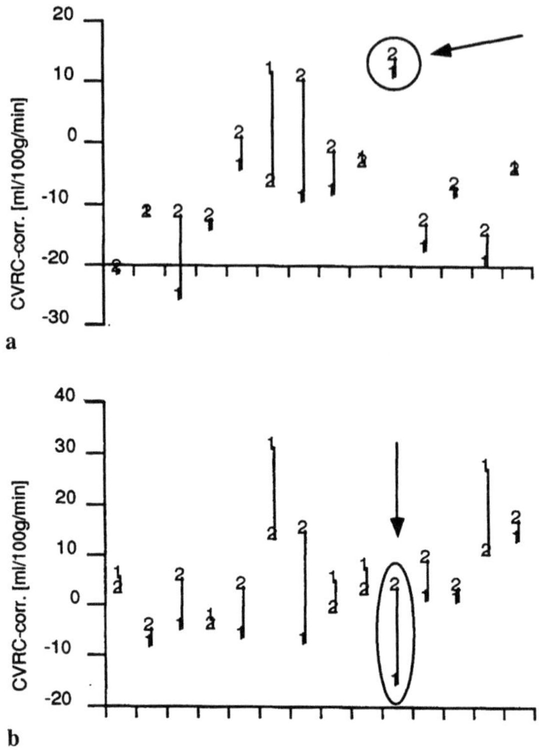

Fig. 2a, b. Individual changes in ipsilateral **(a)** and contralateral **(b)** corrected CVRC (ml/100 g per minute) between initial *(1)* and follow-up *(2)* examination in the same 14 patients suffering from occlusion cerebrovascular disease. *Arrows* depict findings in the patient with bilateral carotid dissection

Discussion

No significant spontaneous improvement of the CVRC could be demonstrated in this group of patients suffering from occlusive cerebrovascular disease. There was s slight improvement in some cases, not related to the severity of the disease. We used D-SPECT to calculate CVRC. The method is based on the Kanno/Lassen algorithm (Kanno and Lassen 1979) and allows calculation of regional CBF from the ^{133}Xe clearance. An emission computer tomograph is used, giving the advantage of three-dimensionality over stationary detectors. With standardized "region-of-interest" software (Büll et al. 1983) accuracy for quantified CBF is high and also provides satisfactory spatial resolution. The combination of D-SPECT with acetazolamide for assessment of CVRC was introduced by Vorstrup et al. in 1984. Our findings of CVRC in patients are interpreted on the basis of a nomogram, reported previously for 26 normal subjects (Vorstrup et al. 1986). Increase in cerebral blood flow (△CBF) shows a linear reciprocal dependency on CBF at rest. In order to compare the CVRC of two different baseline CBF measurements at rest correctly, in this study the difference was calculated between the actual change in CBF after stimulation and the calculated mean normal CVRC, according to the nomogram.

The use of acetazolamide stimulation in combination with ^{133}Xe inhalation for assessment of the CVRC in patients with occlusion of the carotid artery is reported by several groups. In a study including 72 patients with occlusion of the internal carotid artery, symptomatic for TIAs, PRIND or stroke, Derlon et al. (1988) found a normal or slightly decreased CVRC in the contralateral, asymptomatic hemisphere, ipsilateral to the occlusion in 32% of the patients there was a permanently decreased CVRC. In seven cases of carotid dissection, they noted a spontaneous normalization, too. The combination of carotid occlusion and normal CVRC does not necessarily have to do with the collaterals seen in the angiogram.

Our study suggests that the CVRC in patients with occlusive cerebrovascular disease treated medically does not improve significantly statistically speaking. This is in contrast to a recently published series of patients treated surgically with an extra-intracranial bypass (Schmiedek et al. 1988). Thirteen patients symptomatic for cerebral ischemia were operated on. A significant improvement in CVRC during the follow-up examinations was noted.

The predictive value of the CVRC for development of stroke remains to be determined. A prospective study should clarify this issue.

References

Büll U, Moser EA, Kirsch CM, Schmiedek P (1983) [^{133}Xe-DSPECT (Dynamik Single Photon Emission CT). Results of a new noninvasive method for measuring regional cerebral blood flow (rCBF). Comparison with cranial angiography and transmission CT]. Fortschr Geb Röntgenstr. 139:351–358

Derlon JM, Bouvard G, Petit MC, Thenint JP, Viader F, Khoury S, Dupuy B, Houtteville JP (1988) Single photon emission study of hemodynamic reserve in internal carotid occlusion. Value of combined measurement of cerebral blood flow and cerebral blood volume. In: Suzuki J (ed) Advances in surgery for cerebral stroke. Springer, Berlin Heidelberg New York, pp 605–607

Kanno I, Lassen NA (1979) Two methods for calculating regional cerebral blood flow from emission computed tomography of inert gas concentrations. J Comput Assist Tomogr 3:71–76

Kreisig T, Schmiedek P, Leinsinger E, Einhäupl K, Moser E (1987) ^{133}Xe-D-SPECT: Normalwerte von zerebraler Ruhedurchblutung und Reservekapazität. Nucl Med 26:192–197

Schmiedek P, Kreisig T, Moser E, Leinsinger G, Einhäupl K (1988) Investigation of the cerebrovascular reserve capacity tp identify patients with chronic brain ischemia who may benefit from bypass surgery. In: Suzuki J (ed) Advances in surgery for cerebral stroke. Springer, Berlin Heidelberg New York, pp 171–172

Vorstrup S, Engell HC, Lindewald H, Lassen NA (1984) Hemodynamically significant stenosis on the internal carotid artery treated with endarterectomy. J Neurosurg 60:1070–1075

Vorstrup S, Brun B, Lassen NA (1986) Evaluation of the cerebral vasodilatory capacity by the acetazolamide test before EC-IC bypass surgery in patients with occlusion of the internal carotid artery. Stroke 17:1291–1298

Subject Index

AAE (acetazolamide asymmetry enhancement) 233
acetazolamide (Diamox) 65, 67, 71, 88, 91, 95, 113, 116, 146, 164, 171, 186, 232, 257
– activation 88
– asymmetry enhancement (AAE) 233
– challenge 215
– pre- and postacetazolamide CBF studies 216
– stimulated cerebral blood flow by laser, continious measurement 66
– stimulation with 250
– test 71, 174, 232
– vasodilatory challenge 217
acidosis 4, 51
– extracellular 76, 147
activation
– acetazolamide 88
– behavioral 121
– cerebral 19
– cognitive activities 204
– cortical 28
– functional 130, 131, 144
– – deactivation 128
– neuronal 4, 50–52
– physiological 144
– selective 200
– studies 121
adenosine 4, 51, 153
alkaline shift 51
Alzheimer's disease 122
amaurosis fugax 233, 237
aminoisobutyric acid 25
amybarbital 145
anaerobic glycolysis 129
aneurysmal rupture 90
angiographic steal 89
angiography 90
– cerebral 142
angioma
– cerebral 121
– venous 129
angioplasty, endovascular 90
angle-independent double-beam technique 232
aphasia 122
application
– microapplication 3
– perivascular microapplication 50
arachidonic acid 6, 38, 44
arterial
– boundary zones 178
– occlusion, temporary 91
– oxygen content 150
– spasm, chronic 37
– xenon buildup curve 216
arteriolar dilation 147
arteriosclerotic lesions, ulcerative 250
arteriovenous malformation, intracranial 82
artery
– (see also ICA, internal carotid artery) 94, 226, 237
– MCA (middle cerebral artery) 113, 226
– PCA (posterior cerebral artery) 205
artificial CSF 67
asymmetry
– index, hemispheric 95
– side-to-side 72, 108, 172
autocoids 6
– and circulation hormones 3
autoradiography, carbon-14 iodo-antipyrine 176
autoregulation/autoregulatory 7, 37, 44, 86, 124, 154, 172, 175, 178
– capacity 150
– cerebral 5
– of CBF following SAH 221
– disturbances 91
– impaired/impairment 106, 222
– lower limit of 5
– reserve, exhausted 228
– – and incidence of ipsilateral neurological deficits 230
– response 100, 204
– test 173
– – stress test 171
axon-like reflex 52

barbiturates 79, 145
barium chloride 30
basal membrane 12
behavioral activation 121
benzodiazepines 145
bicompartmental model 232

bicuculline 50
blood
- cisternal 222
- content, intravascular 144
blood flow
- capillary 66
- regulation of 28
- values, fast (gray matter) 232
- velocity 158, 200, 237
-- averaged MCA 226
-- changes 204
blood velocity 90, 142
blood volume, cerebral (CBV) 113, 116, 122, 141, 158, 171
blood-brain barrier 6, 8, 25, 184
bradykinin 6, 43
brain
- capillary endothelium 65
- damage, ischaemic 175
- edema/oedema 6, 88, 184
- protection syntheses 65
- tumor 122, 130
- work, intrinsic 145
breakthrough 5
bypass surgery, extracranial-intracranial arterial (ECIC) 91, 97, 116, 164, 171, 173, 257

calcitonin-gene related peptide (CGRP) 6
calcium
- antagonists 46
- concentration 4
canine basilar artery 40
capillary
- blood flow 66
- density 12, 15, 152
- endothelium, brain 65
- network 61
- perfusion 12
- recruitment 16, 64, 111, 152
- reserve capillaries 16
carboanhydrase inhibition 67, 164
carbogene 226
carbon dioxide 150
- stimulation 113
carbon-14 iodo-antipyrine autoradiography 176
carbonic anhydrase 76, 186, 196
carotid
- artery disease 250
-- functional test 250
-- internal (ICA) 94, 226, 237
-- obstructive lesions, hemodynamic assessment of 94
-- stenotic lesions 250
carotid
- dissection, traumatic 263
- endarterectomy 161, 168, 237
-- follow-up after 253
-- prophylactic 232
- flow, ultrasonic common (CCF) 232
- occlusion/occlusive disease 71, 91
CBF (cerebral blood flow) 12, 84, 122, 150, 175, 186, 200
- autoregulation of CBF following SAH 221
- global 221
- imaging, clinical 92
- mapping CBF 216
- regional (see rCBF) 141, 158, 232, 250
- reserve, hemodynamic compromise 217
- studies, pre- and postacetazolamide 216
- values, preoperative and postoperative 232
CBV (cerebral blood volume) 113, 116, 122, 141, 158, 171
- local (CBV) 122
- regional (rCBV) 158
CCF (ultrasonic common carotid flow) 232
- values, preoperative and postoperative 232
cerebral fastigial nucleus (FN) 24
cerebral
- activation 19
- angiography 142
- angiomas 121
- artery
-- (see also ICA, internal carotid artery) 94, 226, 237
-- middle cerebral artery (MCA) 113, 226
-- posterior cerebral artery (PCA) 205
- autoregulation 5
- blood flow (see CBF) 12, 84, 122, 150, 175, 186, 200
-- regional (see rCBF) 141, 158, 232, 250
- blood volume (see CBV) 113, 116, 122, 141, 158, 171
- clearance of xenon^{-133} 221
- flow reserve, stress test of 215
- infarction 90
- ischemia 55, 123, 250
-- delayed (vasospasm) 90, 220
-- hemodynamic 257
- ischemia/low CO_2 reactivity, correlation between 228
- metabolic activity 20
- metabolic rate for oxygen 123
- perfusion 90, 161
-- pressure (CPP) 94, 154, 175
-- reserve 71
- reserve capacity 226
- revascularization 82
- vascular
-- pathophysiology 121
-- reserve capacity (CVRC) 257, 263
-- resistance 76
- vasodilation
-- global 232
-- regional 124
- vasodilatory capacity 171
- vasomotor reactivity (VMR) 158
- vasoreactivity 75
- vasospasm 8, 38, 90

cerebrospinal compliances 196
cerebrovascular
– disease 75, 263
–– chronic 111
– innervation 5
– insufficiency 257
– occlusive disease 257
– premeability 6
– reactivity 113
– reserve 186
–– technique 250
– resistance 3, 50–52
cerebrovasodilation 25–28
cervical sympathetic ganglion 5
CGRP (calcitonin-gene related peptide) 6
chemical factors, local 3
– metabolic 3
cholinergic nerves, parasympathetic 5
cimetidine 6
circulation
– collateral 183
– hormones and autacoids 3
circumventricular organs 25
cisternal blood 222
CLSM (confocal laser scanning microscopy) 61
CO_2
– reactivity
–– absolute 151
–– exhausted-/hemodynamic infarction, correlation between 230
–– local 151
–– low reactivity-/cerebral ischemia, correlation between 228
–– normalized (NCR) 227
–– relative 151
– stimulation 111
– test, transcranial Doppler CO_2 test 226
cognitive activities 204
collateral/collateralization 257
– circulation 183
– efficiency of 226
– potential 90
compensatory flow 173
computed tomography
– dynamic single photon emission (see D-SPECT) 251, 263
– single photon emission (see SPECT) 71, 86, 94, 142, 172, 200, 251
conductance vessels 142
confocal laser scanning microscopy (CLSM) 61
contralateral disease, degree of 243
cortical
– activation 28
– blood flow 85
– projections 123
coupling of flow 4
CPP (cerebral perfusion pressure) 175
cranial window 38, 61
– closed 61, 66
CSF, artificial 67
CT/xenon (Xe/CT) 215
CVRC (cerebral vascular reserve capacity) 257, 263
– spontaneous course of 263

D-SPECT (dynamic single photon emission computed tomography) 251, 263
deactivation, functional 128
decreased
– metabolic demand 100
– perfusion pressure 123
dementia 122
density
– capillary 12, 15, 152
– synaptic 135
dialysis, microdialysis technique 51
Diamox (see acetazolamide)
DID (delayed ischemic deficits) 220
– peak incidence 220
diffusion flow techniques, thermal 79
dissociation in vasoreactive properties 88
diuretics 79
DMRF (dorsal medullary reticular formation) 24
Doppler
– laser Doppler (LD) 66, 116
– sonography, transcranial (TCD) 71, 90, 150, 158, 200, 210
–– CO2 test 226
–– technique 141
dorsal medullary reticular formation (DMRF) 24
double-beam technique, angle-independent 232
dual isotope scanning 147
duplex ultrasound scanning 237
dynorphin 6

ECIC (extracranial-intracranial arterial bypass surgery) 91, 97, 116, 164, 171, 173, 257
EDCF (endothelial-derived constricting factors) 7
edema 86, 101
– allerted 80
– brain 184
EDRF (endothelial-derived relaxing factors) 7, 29, 40, 41
EDTA (ethylenediaminetetraacetic acid) 4
EEG responses 195
efficiency of the collaterals 226
eicosanoids 6
embolism 94
emotional speech 132
end-tidal xenon curve 216
endarterectomy 101, 250
– carotid 161, 169
–– follow-up after 253

endothelial factors 3, 7
endothelial-derived
– constricting factors (EDCF) 7
– relaxing factors (EDRF) 7, 28, 40, 41
endothelium-dependent relaxations and contractions 37, 38
endovascular
– angioplasty 90
– techniques 89
energy metabolism 121
enkephalin 6
epidural pressure transducer 190
epilepsy 122, 128
– temporal lobe 131
epileptiform discharges, focal 122
epileptogenic dysfunction 130
erythrocyte
– flow 63
– – in cerebral capillaries 61
– – intracapillary 61
– labeling 95
– supply rate 63
ethylenediaminetetraacetic acid (EDTA) 4
extracellular
– acidosis 76, 147
– space 4
extracranial-intracranial arterial bypass surgery (ECIC) 91, 101, 116, 164, 171, 173, 257
extraction fractions 17
extraparenchymal vessels 20, 50

fast (gray matter) blood flow values 232
feeding capacity, local 146
fibronectin 12
FITC (fluoresceinisothiocyanate) 12, 13
flow
– acetazolamide-stimulated cerebral blood flow by laser, continuous measurement 66
– augmentation surgery 217
– blood flow
– – capillary 66
– – cerebral (see CBF) 12, 84, 122, 150, 175, 186, 200
– – cortical 85
– – regulation of 28
– – tissue 90
– – velocity 158, 200, 204, 237
– – – changes 204
– compensatory 173
– coupling of 4
– erythrocyte flow 63, 64
– – in cerebral capillaries 61
– – intracapillary 61
– fast (gray matter) blood flow values 232
– low-flow
– – infarction 166, 168
– – ischemia 94
– paradoxal augmentation of 88
– redistribution of 88, 173
– regional cerebral blood flow (see rCBF) 141, 158, 232, 250
– stress test of cerebral flow reserves 215
– techniques, thermal diffusion 79
– volume flow changes 200
flow-to-volume ratio 116
flowmetry 66
fluoresceinisothiocyanate (FITC) 12, 13
fluorescent
– fibronectin antibody 13
– markers, intravascular 15
– microscopic studies 17
– staining 12
– – intravascular 14
fluorochrome 12
FN (cerebellar fastigial nucleus) 24
focal
– epileptiform discharges 122
– ischemia 125
foci, dysfunctional 133
foramen of Monroe 193
free radicals 50, 52
functional
– activation 129, 130, 131, 144
– deactivation 128
– hyperemia 51
– mapping 144
– neuroanatomy 121
– recovery 127
– recruitment 127
– reserve capacity 133
– test, carotid artery 250

GABA (g-aminobutyric acid) 50
ganglion, cervical sympathetic 5
ganglionectomy 52
GEF (glucose extraction fraction) 123
glucose
– hypometabolism 129
– utilization, local 12
glycolysis, anaerobic 129
guanylate cyclase 41

haemorrhagic hypotension 175, 183
head injury 79, 175
hemispheral values 221
hemispheric asymmetry index 95
hemodilution 153
hemodynamic
– assessment of carotid artery obstructive lesions 94
– cerebral ischemia 257
– – prospectiv study 257
– compromise 109, 161
– deficit 102
– derangements 82
– disturbances 85, 86, 91
– failure 250
– infarction/exhausted CO_2 reactivity,

correlation between 230
– information 82
– origin 171
– sequelea 90
– state 91
– stroke 123
– studies 95
hemodynamically uncompensated ischemia 124
hemorrhage 86
– subarachnoid (SAH) 7, 8, 31, 90, 92, 175, 220
hemorrhagic stroke 128
hippocampus 26, 55
histamine 6, 38
HMPAO (99Tcm-hexamethyl-propyleramine oxim) 143
Hunterian ligation 90
hydrogen
– clearance technique 55, 66, 176
– ion activity 4
hypercapnia 65, 67, 113, 121, 153, 226, 237
– to ICA blood flow velocity, response of 238
– stress test 237
hyperdynamic therapy 91
hyperemia 4, 82
– functional 51
hyperemic
– complications 86, 87, 89
– syndromes 101
hypermetabolism 130
hyperperfusion 55, 56
hyperventilation 79, 82, 159, 226
hypometabolism 125
hypoperfusion 55, 85, 91, 124
hypotension 221
– haemorrhagic 175, 183
hypoxia 153

ICA (internal carotid artery) 94, 226, 237
– blood flow velocity to hypercapnia, response of 238
– occlusion 226
– stenosis 237
– unilateral 160
ICP (intracranial pressure) 79, 186
imaging, quantitative 121
immunohistochemical methods 5
impaired autoregulation 222
indicator dilution techniques 17
indomethacin 44, 52, 147
infarction, cerebral 90
– incomplete 186
– low-flow 166, 168
– massive 102
initial slope (IS) 232
– index (ISI) 95, 232
interhemispheric
– assymetries 95
– ratio 95
internal carotid artery (see also ICA) 94, 226, 237
interstitial space 51
intracapillary erythrocyte flow 61
intracellular pH 197
intracranial
– arteriovenous malformation 92
– pressure (ICP) 79, 186
– pressure 191, 193
– vascular malformations 82
intraparenchymal vessels 3, 50
intravascular
– blood content 144
– fluorescent markers 15
– fluorescent staining 14
intrinsic brain work 145
intrinsic neural
– networks 20
– pathways 20
– system 31
IS (initial slope) 232
ischemic
– brain damage 175
– deficit, immediate 222
ischemia 4
– cerebral 55, 123, 250
– chronic regional 121
– delayed cerebral ischemia (vasospasm) 90, 220
– focal 125
– hemodynamic cerebral 257
– hemodynamically uncompensated 124
– low-flow 94
– model 55
ischemic
– attacks, transient (TIAs) 161, 171, 237, 251, 253, 258
– complications 85, 89
– deficits 90
– – delayed (DID) 220
– degeneration, chronic 128
– neurologic deficits, prolonged reversible (PRIND) 258
– ophthalmopathy 161
– stroke 122
ISI (initial slope index) 95, 232
isotope scanning, dual 147

lacunar lesions 230
laser
– Doppler (LD) 66, 116
– scanning microscopy, confocal (CLSM) 61
leptomeningeal collaterals 217
leukotrienes 6, 38
ligation, Hunterian 90
light microscopy 61
locus ceruleus 26
look through 143

low-flow
- infarction 164
- ischemia 94

magnetic resonance imaging (MRI) 85, 196
mannitol 79, 183
mapping
- CBF 215
- functional 144
MCA (middle cerebral artery) 226
mean vascular transit time (MVTT) 123
medulla, rostral ventrolateral (RVL) 25
medullary reticular formation, dorsal (DMRF) 24
mental activity 200
metabolic
- artivity, cerebral 24
- changes, stimulation-induced 133
- delay 145
- demand 37, 113
-- decreased 96
- factors, local chemical 3
- mechanism 19
- recruitment 130
metabolism, hypermetabolism 130
methylene blue 41
microapplication 3
- perivascular 50
microdialysis technique 51
micropuncture technique 3, 50
microscopy
- confocal laser scanning (CLSM) 61
- light microscopy 61
microvascular
- architecture 61
- network 63
microvasculature 28
middle cerebral artery (MCA) 113, 226
- averaged, blood flow velocity 226
misery perfusion 129
- syndrome 124
monitoring
- continuous 79
- pathophysiological 90
Monroe-Kelly doctrine 19
morphometric analysis 56
motor areas, supplementary 127
MRI (magnetic resonance imaging) 85, 196
muscarine receptors 5
MVTT (mean vascular transit time) 123
myogenic mechanisms 7

NCR (normalized CO_2 reactivity) 227
neck bruits, asymptomatic 237
nerves, parasympathetic cholinergic nerves 5
neural (see also neuronal)
- networks 30
-- intrinsic 20
- pathways, intrinsic 20
- system, intrinsic 31
neuritic plaques 133
neuroanatomy, functional 121
neurofibrillary tangles 133
neurogenic
- factors 19
- regulation 20
neurological deficits, ipsilateral 230
neuromodulators, vasoactive 20
neuronal
- activation/activity 4, 50–52, 144
- decay, selective 125
- recruitment 121
neurotransmitters, vasoactive 20
nitric oxide (NO) 43
nitroglycerin 148
norepinephrine 5, 38, 172
normal perfusion pressure breakthrough 86
normalized CO_2 reactivity (NCR) 226

O_2 transport rate 153
occlusion
- bilateral 259
- unilateral 259
occlusive disease, cerebrovascular 257
OEF (oxygen extraction fraction) 122
ophthalmopathy, ischemic 161
opioid peptides 6
orthostatic changes 171
osmolarity, perivascular 4
oxygen
- content, arterial 150
- demand theory 153
- extraction fraction, local (OEF) 122
- metabolism, regional 144
- reactivity 152
- transport capacity 118
oxyhemoglobin 41

paradoxal augmentation of flow 88
parasympathetic cholinergic nerves 5
parenchym
- extraparenchymal arteries 50
- extraperenchymal vessels 20
- intraparenchymal arteries 50
- intraparenchymal vessels 3
parenchymal damage 100
pathophysiological monitoring 90
PCA (posterior cerebral artery) 205
PCO_2 values, steady states of 226
- end-tidal 226
peak frequency (PF), maximum 238
penumbral region/zones 155, 183
peptideric innervation 6
perforating vessels, recruitment of 89
perforator recruitment 87
perfusion
- capillary 12
- cerebral 90, 161

- deficit 123
-- regional 121
- hyperperfusion 55, 56
- hypoperfusion 55, 85, 91, 124
- misery 129
- mode 12
- pressure 5, 50, 111, 158
-- breakthrough, normal 86
-- cerebral (CPP) 94, 154, 175
-- decreased 123
-- regional 173
- reperfusion 55
- research, cerebral (CPR) 94, 111
- reserve 75, 76, 88, 91, 111, 150
-- cerebral 71
- syndrome, misery 124
- territory 71. 72
- tissue 142, 143
perivascular
- microapplication 50
- milieu 3
- osmolarity 4
- plexus 20
- space 28
permeability surface area product 16
PET (positron emission tomography) 82, 84, 121, 171, 200
PF (peak frequency), maximum 238
pH, intracellular 197
pharmacological
- manipulation 144
-- indirect 145
- stimulation 141
physiological
- activation 144
- stimulation 113, 131, 141
PI (pulsatility index) 72
pial arteries, superficial 3
plexus, perivascular 20
positron emission tomography (PET) 82, 94, 121, 171, 200
posterior cerebral artery (PCA) 205
potassium 4
potential, collateral 90
pre- and postacetazolamide CBF studies 216
primary vasodilation 26
PRIND (prolonged reversible ischemic neurologic deficit) 258
prolonged reversible ischemic neurologic deficit (PRIND) 258
prostacyclin 44
prostanoids 6, 50, 52
protective vasoconstriction 88
PTI (pulsatility transmission index) 72
pulsatility
- index (PI) 72
- transmission index (PTI) 72

quantitative imaging 121

radioimmunoassay 42
rCBF (regional cerebral blood flow) 141, 158, 232
rCBV (regional cerebral blood volume) 141
reactivity
- index 238
- loss of 241
recognition
- continuous visual 132
- task, visual 123
recovery, functional 128
recruitment 14, 111
- capillary 12, 111, 152
- functional 127
- metabolic 130
- of perforating vessels 89
redistribution of flow 173
regional
- cerebral blood flow (rCBF) 141, 158, 232, 250
- ischemia, chronic 121
- oxygen metabolism 144
- perfusion deficits 121
reperfusion 55
reserve capacity
- cerebral 226
- functional 133
- regional 121
reserve capillaries 16
resistance vessels 76, 142
reticular formation, dorsal medullary (DMRF) 24
revascularization
- cerebral 82
- procedures 94
- surgical 97
rostral ventrolateral medulla (RVL) 24

SAH (subarachnoid hemorrhage) 175, 220
- autoregulation of CBF following SAH 221
scanning
- confocal laser scanning microscopy (CLSM) 61
- dual isotope scanning 147
- duplex ultrasound scanning 237
secondary vasodilation 24
selective vulnerability 55, 57
self-stimulation 130
sensory stimulation 145
serotonergic innervation 6
serotonin 5
side-to-side asymmetry 72, 109, 172
single photon emission computed tomography (see SPECT)
- dynamic (D-SPECT) 251, 263
slope index, initial 221
SP (substance P) 6, 38
spatial resolution 143

SPECT (single photon emission computed tomography) 71, 86, 94, 142, 172, 200, 251
speech, emotional 133
steal 87
– angiographic 89
– effects 123
– index 86
– phenomenon 86, 87, 218, 253, 260, 265
stenosis, effect of 243
stimulation-induced metabolic changes 133
stress test 221
– autoregulatory 171
– of cerebral flow reserves 215
– hypercapnia 237
stroke
– hemodynamic 123, 128
– ischemic 122
– rate, annual 228
subarachnoid hemorrhage (SAH) 7, 8, 31, 90, 92, 175, 220
substance P (SP) 6, 38
superficial pial arteries 3
superoxide
– dismutase 41
– radicals 52
supplementary motor areas 127
surgical revascularization 101
synaptic density 134
sypathetic innervation 5

TCD (transcranial Doppler ultrasound) 71, 158, 200, 210
– temporal resolution of 210
99Tcm-hexamethyl-propyleramine oxim (HMPAO) 143
tedistribution, tolerance of 89
temporal
– lobe epilepsy 131
– resolution of the TCD method 209
temporary arterial occlusion 91
tests
– acetazolamide test, 71, 174, 232
– autoregulation test 171, 173
– functional test, carotid artery 250
– noninvasive testing of vasomotor reserve 158
– stress test 221
– – autoregulatory stress test 171
– – of cerebral flow reserves 215
– – hypercapnia stress test 237
– transcranial Doppler CO_2 test 226
theophylline 51, 147
therapy, hyperdynamic 91
thermal diffusion 82
– flow techniques 79
thermistors 79
three-dimensional reconstruction 63
thrombocytes 5
thromboembolic lesions 230
thromboxane 58
– receptors 44
– synthetase 44
TIAs (transient ischemic attacks) 161, 171, 237, 251, 253, 258
tissue
– acidosis 164
– blood flow 90
– damage, structural 90
– perfusion 142, 143
transcranial Doppler
– CO_2 test 226
– technique 141
– ultrasound (see TCD) 71, 90, 150, 158, 200, 210
transient ischemic attacks (TIAs) 161, 171, 237, 251, 253, 258
transit time 115
transmitters and innervation, vascular 3
traumatic
– carotid dissection 263
– vasospasm 80
treatment, hyperdynamic therapy 91
trigeminovascular nerves 50, 52
trimetaphan 221
tumors, brain 122, 130

ulcerative arteriosclerotic lesions 250
ultrasonic common carotid flow (CCF) 232
undershoot 201

vascular
– disorders, occlusive 215
– innervation and transmitters 3
– malformations, intracranial 82
– nerves 5
– occlusion 183
– pathophysiology, cerebral 121
– reserve capacity, cerebral (CVRC) 257, 263
– resistance 50
– transit time, mean (MVTT) 123
vasoactive
– intestinal polypeptide (VIP) 29
– neuromodulators 20
– neurotransmitters 20
– substances 19
– transmitters 28
vasoconstriction 150
– protective 88
vasoconstrictive capabilities 164
vasodilating stimuli 158
vasodilation 150, 186
– global, cerebral 232
– primary 26
– regional cerebral 124
– secondary 24
vasodilator
– response 195
– theory 153

vasodilatory
– capacity 150
– – cerebral 171
– – regional 171
– challenge with acetazolamide 217
– substance 40
vasomotor
– reactivity, cerebral (VMR) 158
– reserve, noninvasive testing 158
vasopressin 38
vasoreactive properties, dissociation in 88
vasoreactivity 71, 74, 155
– cerebral 75
– intact 88
vasospasm 31
– cerebral 8, 38, 90
– chronic 8, 40, 41
– delayed cerebral ischemia 90, 220
– traumatic 80
velocity 63
– changes 200
– maximum 201
venous angiomas 128
vessel diameter 155
VIP (vasoactive intestinal polypeptide) 29
visual
– image analysis 123
– recognition, continuous 133
– recognition task 123
– stimulus 208
VMR (cerebral vasomotor reactivity) 158
volume flow changes 200
vulnerability, selective 55, 57

133-XE (see xenon-133)
xenon
– buildup curve, arterial 216
– curve, end-tidal 216
– stable 215
xenon-133 (133-XE) 143
– clearance, intra-arterial 176
– cerebral clearance of 221
– inhalation technique 172, 200, 250, 258, 263
– injection technique 200
– intravenous technique 232
xenon/CT (Xe/CT) 215
xenon/oxygen, medical-grade 215

MIX
Papier aus verantwortungsvollen Quellen
Paper from responsible sources
FSC® C105338

If you have any concerns about our products,
you can contact us on
ProductSafety@springernature.com

In case Publisher is established outside the EU,
the EU authorized representative is:
Springer Nature Customer Service Center GmbH
Europaplatz 3, 69115 Heidelberg, Germany

Printed by Libri Plureos GmbH
in Hamburg, Germany